LEGAL RIGHTS

LEGAL WRITING

LEGAL RIGHTS

The Guide for Deaf and Hard of Hearing People

Fifth Edition

NATIONAL ASSOCIATION OF THE DEAF

Gallaudet University Press
Washington, D.C.

Gallaudet University Press
Washington, D.C. 20002

© 1982, 1984, 1986, 1992, 2000 by Gallaudet University.
All rights reserved. First edition 1982
Fifth edition 2000
Printed in Canada

Library of Congress Cataloging-in-Publication Data

Legal rights : the guide for deaf and hard of hearing people / National
Association of the Deaf.—5th ed.
    p.   cm.
    Rev. ed. of: Legal rights / National Center for Law and Deafness. 4th ed.
1992.
    Includes bibliographical references and index.
    ISBN 1-56368-091-2
    1. Deaf—Legal status, laws, etc.—United States.   2. Hearing impaired—
Legal status, laws, etc.—United States.   I. DuBow, Sy. Legal rights.
II. National Association of the Deaf.
    KF480.5.D4 L44   2000
    346.7301′3—dc21   00-029338

All photographs courtesy of the Gallaudet University Archives.
All attempts have been made to obtain permission from the Maine Medical
Center to reprint "Policy for Effective Communication with and Services for
People who are Deaf and Hard of Hearing," copyright 1999. The publishers
have generously given permission to reprint from the following copyrighted
works. "State-wide Services for People who are Deaf and Hard of Hearing,"
and "Directory of National Organizations of and for Deaf and Hard of Hearing
People," both copyright 1999 by the Laurent Clerc National Deaf Education
Center. "Formal Opinion No. 1995-12," copyright 1995 by the Committee on
Professional and Judicial Ethics of the Association of the Bar of the City of New
York.

♾ The paper used in this publication meets the minimum requirements of
American National Standard for Information Sciences—Permanence of Paper
for Printed Library Materials, ANSI Z39.48-1984.

Authors

**National Association
of the Deaf Law Center**

Marc Charmatz, Director
J.D., Northwestern University

Sarah Geer, Senior Attorney
J.D., University of North
Carolina

*Mary Vargas, Staff Attorney/
Skadden Fellow*
J.D., University of Connecticut

**National Association
of the Deaf Department of
Government Affairs**

Kelby Brick, Staff Attorney
J.D., Temple University

*Karen Peltz Strauss, Staff
Attorney*
J.D., University of Pennsylvania

*To the Executive Directors of the National
Association of the Deaf, for their longstanding
support of the goals of the NAD Law Center
and
In memory of Fred Schreiber, the happy warrior for
deaf people's rights*

Contents

Preface

The deaf community is committed to eradicating discriminatory attitudes and practices and is determined to remove barriers to communication. Federal and state laws are intended to break down these barriers to communication and help deaf and hard of hearing people overcome stereotyped assumptions about their abilities. This new edition of *Legal Rights* is the most comprehensive resource yet written on legal rights and remedies available to people who are deaf and hard of hearing. It also discusses flexible, non-litigious ways to ensure effective communication and better understanding through deaf awareness and information technology.

This edition includes vital information on the Americans with Disabilities Act (ADA), landmark legislation for all individuals with disabilities. It discusses the ADA's mandates regarding employment, government services, public accommodations, and telecommunications in the context of the particular needs of people who are deaf and hard of hearing. The new edition also updates information on Federal Communication Commission rules and three laws—the Television Decoder Circuitry Act, the Hearing Aid Compatibility Act, and the Telecommunications Act of 1996—that govern television and telephone access.

The federal and state laws discussed in *Legal Rights* ensure that all citizens with disabilities have an equal opportunity to access vital community services, find employment, and lead productive lives. Deaf people now have a variety of options, including legal tools, to help them secure this fundamental equity. It is up to all of us to help ensure that the federal and state laws are followed and enforced, so that the words on paper become a reality for all Americans.

MARC CHARMATZ

Acknowledgments

The authors would like to thank the co-authors of prior editions of this book: Sy DuBow, legal director of the National Center for Law and Deafness, or NCLD (1976–1996); Larry Goldberg, associate director of the NCLD (1976–1983); Elaine Gardner, associate legal director of the NCLD (1983–1996); Andrew Penn, NCLD staff attorney (1978–1981); and Sheila Conlon Mentkowski, NCLD staff attorney (1981–1988).

The authors also thank Michelle Buescher, a former law student at the NAD Law Center, for her contributions on employment law and architectural barriers; and Karen Peltz Strauss, co-author, who continued editing her contributions to this book after leaving the NAD to become Deputy Chief of the Consumer Information Bureau at the Federal Communications Commission.

LEGAL RIGHTS

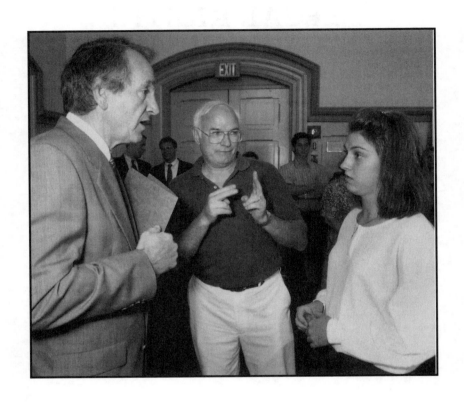

Chapter 1

Communicating with People Who Are Deaf or Hard of Hearing

Almost ten percent of all Americans (more than twenty-eight million people) have some kind of hearing loss.[1] It is difficult to generalize about deaf and hard of hearing people because of the wide range of hearing loss, the variety of communication methods, and the differences in the age of the disability's onset. Hearing loss can be more than a barrier to sound perception, it also can impede communication and understanding.

Deaf and hard of hearing people frequently rely on information they can see—processing information through their eyes, not their ears. Sign language, speech, amplification, and writing are some of their preferred methods of communication. In order to communicate as effectively as possible, many use more than one method. It is important to know, however, that with the use of an auxiliary aid or reasonable accommodation, along with the sensitivity to establish clear lines of communication, they can communicate and participate fully and easily in most settings.

Frequently, deaf and hard of hearing people have not received fair treatment from professional, social, and government service providers, including the courts and police. Some accommodations can make a critical difference in whether they receive necessary services, and whether they can participate satisfactorily in society. The material cost of such accommodations is modest in comparison with the benefit.

As we review the various methods that deaf and hard of hearing people use to communicate, one general rule to bear in mind is that each person has a preferred method, because he or she has spent a lifetime knowing what works most successfully. Whatever method is natural for that person is the approach that should always be used, preferably from the first moment of contact.

SIGN LANGUAGE AND INTERPRETERS

American Sign Language (ASL) is a visible language that is linguistically independent of English. Its signals are handshapes and movements that represent words and concepts. Many deaf and hard of hearing people use ASL rather than English as their primary mode of communication. For many, it is a native language with rich cultural associations.

An interpreter is a skilled professional who can translate the meaning of spoken English words into ASL, and can translate ASL into English. Interpreting written or spoken English into ASL requires a high degree of education. It takes as much time and effort to learn sign language as any other language.

Sometimes, a specialized interpreter must be used. For example, a person who is both deaf and blind may need an interpreter skilled in tactile communication. Some deaf and hard of hearing people do not use sign language but require an "oral" interpreter who silently mouths the speaker's words to them. The oral interpreter is usually a person whom the deaf or hard of hearing person finds easy to speechread and who knows how to substitute synonyms for words that are difficult to speechread. Another instance when a specialized interpreter may be needed is when the deaf or hard of hearing person has rudimentary language skills or does not use conventional ASL. In this situation, another deaf or hard of hearing person may provide interpretation into conventional ASL, which can then be interpreted into English by the regular interpreter.

Qualified interpreters can be found through local and state chapters of the National Association of the Deaf (NAD) or the Registry of Interpreters for the Deaf (RID). Both organizations have their own rigorous certification requirements. Deaf and hard of hearing people may themselves suggest local interpreters. Other sources of interpreters include:

+ local interpreting agencies specifically serving deaf and hard of hearing people,
+ organizations of deaf and hard of hearing people,
+ your state association of the deaf,
+ state commissions or agencies for deaf and hard of hearing people, or
+ school programs for deaf and hard of hearing children.

Professional offices and service agencies should develop their own lists of interpreters whom they know to be reliable and competent. A few states, such as Texas and Missouri, have adopted certification or licensing standards for interpreters.

Regularly using the same interpreter can enhance the quality of communication, since interpreters who are familiar with a speaker's verbal style and customary phrases will be able to interpret more effectively. Interpreters also can provide valuable assistance to service providers by advising them about effective use of an interpreter and about other means of communicating with deaf and hard of hearing people.

While professional certification may be useful in evaluating the skills of an interpreter, the ultimate authority on an interpreter's qualifications should be the deaf or hard of hearing person. An interpreter who is unable to provide effective communication for a particular person is unqualified, despite professional certification.

Relying on amateurs who know some sign language is a frequent error, because the ability to make or read signs or to fingerspell is no substitute for proficient interpreting. An amateur or a beginning signer will not know sign language well enough to

---

Interpreter Guidelines

A professional interpreter should uphold the NAD's or RID's codes of ethics, which carefully define the role of an interpreter. These codes prohibit an interpreter from continuing in any assignment if attempts to communicate are unsuccessful for either party.

When communicating with a deaf person through a sign language interpreter, keep in mind the following guidelines:

+ When addressing a deaf person, look directly at him or her, not the interpreter. Speak to the person as if the interpreter were not present. For example, say, "The meeting will be on Tuesday," rather than, "Tell her that the meeting will be on Tuesday." The interpreter will sign exactly what is said.
+ Some deaf people use their own voice while signing. Others do not, so the interpreter will say in English what the person signs. In both cases, respond by talking to the deaf person, not the interpreter.
+ The interpreter should stand or sit directly beside the speaker so that he or she is easily visible to the deaf person.
+ The interpreter should not be placed in shadows or in front of any source of bright light, such as a window.

---

interpret or to communicate effectively with most deaf and hard of hearing people.

Many inexperienced interpreters do not sign in ASL but use signs borrowed from ASL in an English word order. They may frequently impose a completely incorrect English meaning on a sign, such as using the sign for the adjective "fine," meaning "good," to connote the noun "fine," meaning "penalty." An unqualified interpreter might fingerspell words when he or she does not know a sign; but in ASL, directly translated English idioms are meaningless. For example, a direct translation of the English idiom "have to" would mean "possess" in ASL.

✦ No private conversation should occur with the interpreter or with anyone else in the deaf person's presence. The interpreter must interpret everything that is said in front of the deaf person. Any discussion of the deaf person's language or communication level should take place privately with the interpreter. Ask the deaf person, not the interpreter, if he or she understands what is being said.

✦ Speak naturally and not too fast. Remember that names and some other words must be fingerspelled and that this takes more time than signing. The interpreter will indicate whether it is necessary to slow down. Avoid jargon or other technical words with which the deaf person may be unfamiliar. If possible, meet with the interpreter before the interview to discuss the best way to interpret certain technical concepts into ASL without losing any of the meaning.

✦ Make sure that the interpreter understands the need for complete confidentiality. Do not expect or allow the interpreter to participate in the conversation. The interpreter's only role is to facilitate communication with the deaf person.

COMMUNICATION BARRIERS

Problems with Note Writing

Many deaf and hard of hearing people rely on written notes to communicate with hearing people or to supplement other modes of communication. However, written communications may pose problems and may not alway be effective or appropriate. A written conversation is tedious, cumbersome, and time-consuming. Written messages are frequently condensed. The writer omits much of the information that would otherwise be exchanged, so the deaf or hard of hearing person does not get the same amount of detail that a hearing person would.

A common misconception is that deaf and hard of hearing people compensate for their inability to hear by reading and writing. Deaf and hard of hearing people are just like the general population. Some deaf and hard of hearing people are highly educated. Others are not. Some people are very literate while others are not. Therefore, one should not assume that deaf and hard of hearing people are able to communicate easily or effectively in writing.

Most people learn their native language by hearing it spoken around them from infancy. But a person who is born deaf or hard of hearing or who loses the ability to hear when very young cannot learn English in this way. Therefore, educational strategies have to be different in order to enable such a child to learn fluent English. This is frequently done by emphasizing visual methods such as sign language or oralism. Some of these educational programs succeed, while others fail.

The extensive use of idioms in English also poses significant reading problems for people who are deaf or hard of hearing. For example, the expression "under arrest" in the Miranda warnings (discussed in chapter ten) would be puzzling to many people because "under" in ASL means only "beneath."

Because a person often can not fully convey all the necessary information by writing notes, and because everybody has different levels of literacy, the limitations of note-writing as a communication method should be observed carefully to avoid miscommunication.

Speechreading Comprehension

A common misconception about deaf and hard of hearing people is that they all speechread and do so with good comprehension. Very few people can read lips well enough to understand speech, even under optimum conditions. One survey concluded: "even the best speechreaders in a one-to-one situation were found to understand only twenty-six percent of what was said and many bright deaf and hard of hearing individuals grasp less than five percent."[2]

This low level of comprehension occurs because many English speech sounds are not visible on the mouth or lips. Certain spoken words or sounds create similar lip movements. The ambiguity of speechreading is demonstrated by the fact that the sounds of *T, D, Z, S,* and *N* all look identical on the lips. The words *right, ride,* and *rise* would be indistinguishable to a deaf or hard of hearing person, as would the sentences, "Do you have the time?" and "Do you have a dime?" The meaning of entire sentences can be lost because a key word is missed or misunderstood.

The amount of training and practice a person has in speechreading is important. There are many factors that can hinder one's ability to speechread, such as when:

- ✦ there is more than one speaker (e.g., any group setting or conversation),
- ✦ the speaker is not directly in front of the speechreader,
- ✦ the speaker is in motion or not directly facing the speechreader,
- ✦ the lips are obscured by hands, beards, or mustaches,
- ✦ the speaker does not articulate carefully or has distorted speech,
- ✦ the speaker has a regional or foreign accent,
- ✦ the speaker is using technical or unfamiliar words,
- ✦ the speechreader is not familiar with the grammar or vocabulary of spoken English,
- ✦ the speaker is not well-lighted,
- ✦ the speechreader must look into a glare or light, and
- ✦ the speechreader has poor vision.

Speechreading often supplements other modes of communication, but it is seldom sufficient in itself to ensure effective communication. Do not rely on extensive use of speechreading, unless the deaf or hard of hearing person indicates such a preference. When a deaf or hard of hearing person does not understand a sentence, the speaker should repeat the thought more slowly. If this is not successful, try using different words. The speaker should use gestures freely, for example, pointing to a wristwatch to indicate time.

Environmental Interferences

Environmental factors can interfere when communicating with a deaf or hard of hearing person. The room should be adequately lighted, without glare. Although profoundly deaf people will not be affected by background noises, they will be distracted by a great deal of background movement or changes in lighting. A person who uses a hearing aid or who has residual hearing may be seriously distracted by background noises. One should try to talk in a quiet place, away from the noises of machinery, other conversations, and distractions.

When talking to someone who is deaf or hard of hearing, speak directly to the person without moving around, turning away, or looking down at papers or books. Speak naturally, without shouting or distorting normal mouth movements.

Early hearing loss interferes with language and speech acquisition. Some deaf and hard of hearing people have normal and intelligible speech. Others do not use their voices at all. Many deaf and hard of hearing people who speak exhibit unusual tones, inflections, or modulations. Whether or not a deaf or hard of hearing person uses speech is a matter of individual preference. Difficulty in understanding a deaf or hard of hearing person's voice can often be relieved by listening without interruption for a while until the person's particular voice patterns become familiar.

The phrases "mute" (whether deaf-mute or deaf and mute) and "deaf and dumb" are considered insulting by deaf people and should never be used.

COMMUNICATION DEVICES

Telecommunications

One frustration of hearing loss is the inability to use a conventional telephone. Hearing people rely heavily on the telephone and take it for granted in communicating with businesses, friends, government agencies, and emergency services. With new devices for deaf and hard of hearing people coming into more frequent use, the telephone has become a means rather than a barrier to communication.

A TTY (also called a TDD or telecommunication device for the deaf) is a machine with a typewriter keyboard connected by an acoustic coupler to a regular telephone. Two people with compatible equipment can have a typed conversation over the telephone, enabling deaf people to have the same functional telephone service as other people. The devices are inexpensive and easy to use. Software is now available to permit many personal computers to be used as TTYs.

Each state has a relay service center. The relay service allows hearing people who do not have a TTY to communicate with deaf and hard of hearing people who do have a TTY. The relay centers are staffed with people known as communication agents (CAs) who act as live intermediaries between the hearing person and the deaf or hard of hearing person. One person will call the relay center and give the CA the other person's telephone number. The CA will dial the number and stay on both lines, relaying the entire conversation by typing the hearing person's spoken words and reading the deaf or hard of hearing person's typed words. All calls placed through relay services are completely confidential. The Federal Communications Commission (FCC) prohibits the reporting of any activity of any kind overheard during a relay call.

Some states are now starting to offer video relay services. This functions the same way as a TTY relay service, but allows the deaf or hard of hearing person to communicate visually with the CA through a videophone. This enables the person to communicate verbally by signing or speaking/speechreading instead of typing and reading everything on a TTY.

Some deaf and hard of hearing people who can enunciate for themselves use relay services with a voice carry over (VCO) option. This allows the deaf individual to speak directly to the other person over a regular telephone receiver. The CA will then type the other person's response back to the deaf person, who reads it on his or her TTY.

Many deaf and hard of hearing people are now using alternative telecommunications methods such as e-mail, pagers, and faxes. Other devices can adapt telephones to the individual needs of people who are deaf or hard of hearing. Amplifier switches can be added to telephone receivers. Telephones and other auditory systems—alarms, doorbells, or in-home buzzers—can be connected to a blinking light that alerts a deaf or hard of hearing person to a ringing telephone. Many hearing aids are equipped with inductive coil "telephone switches." These hearing aids use electromagnetic leakage from compatible telephone receivers to transmit the message. If, in a job situation, a person using this kind of hearing aid is assigned to an incompatible telephone, a compatible model can be acquired at reasonable cost.

Computer-Assisted, Real-Time Transcription

Some deaf and hard of hearing people use a system of transcription in which a trained stenographer takes down spoken information. A computer then translates the stenographer's notes almost instantly into English words and displays them on a monitor. The deaf person can then read a simultaneous transcript. This system is known as computer-assisted, real-time transcription (CART), because it is available as the words are spoken. Until this technology was developed, transcripts had to be made from recordings of spoken information and were not available for hours or days. One advantage of a CART system is that the stenographer can also produce a printed transcript of the spoken information.

A CART system is ideal for individuals who have excellent reading skills, and for those who do not know sign language and therefore cannot use a sign language interpreter. Because of the speed of the transcription, it is not appropriate for individuals who are slow readers. Despite advancements in the technology, many disconcerting errors can still appear in a real-time transcription.

CART systems are frequently used in courts, since they were first developed using the skills of court stenographers. CART is increasingly being used in classrooms, lecture halls, and other settings. The success of the transcription depends on the skills of the stenographer and the sophistication of the translation program.

When voice recognition software is perfected, it is likely that automatic computerized transcription systems will be available. For the present, a trained stenographer is needed to reliably recognize and transcribe human speech.

Assistive Listening Systems

Background noise and reverberation make it difficult for individuals who are deaf or hard of hearing—whether or not they wear hearing aids—to distinguish the words and sounds around them. Thus, deaf and hard of hearing people have difficulty participating on equal terms with hearing people in rooms that are not equipped with an assistive listening system. Even the best in sound systems technology, combined with the best in hearing aid technology, cannot solve these problems. Therefore, the 1990 Americans with Disabilities Act included requirements for installing assistive listening devices in places of public accommodation.

The purpose of an assistive listening system is to transmit the sound as directly as possible to the ear. Such systems should not be confused with audio systems (such as public address systems) generally designed to enhance sound quality or simply make sound louder. Rather than enhancing all the sounds in a room, an assistive listening device can bring specific sounds directly to the user's ears. There are three basic wireless technologies available for this purpose: induction loop, FM broadcast, and infrared light. No single technology is best for all applications. All three types of assistive listening systems can be installed in new and old facilities alike, as long as their individual limitations are kept in mind.

Induction Loop Technology

Induction loop technology is based on electromagnetic transmission. It has a unique advantage in that the signal is received directly by the user's hearing aid if the aid is equipped with a telecoil circuit or "T" switch. There is no need for an additional receiver, as is required by all other technologies. For example, by flipping the "T" switch, the user can receive the signal in his or her own hearing aid rather than using headphones. However, if the listener does not have a hearing aid equipped with a telecoil, or has no hearing aid at all, then induction receivers must be used. An induction receiver takes the place of a hearing aid with a "T" switch by bringing the sound directly to the ear, like headphones. There are three types of receivers: a wand-like device, a pocket-sized device with headphones, and a telecoil installed inside a plastic shell that looks like a hearing aid. The first two are most common.

FM Broadcast Technology

FM systems operate at FCC-designated frequencies. Since each system may use its own broadcast frequency, several systems may operate simultaneously at one location without interfering with one another. However, unlike the loop system, the FM system requires a special receiver for each person, whether or not she or he has a hearing aid. Several options for coupling a hearing aid to an FM system are available. The most convenient methods for public places are either a neckloop or a silhouette inductor used with the hearing aid's telecoil circuit.

Infrared Light Technology

From a practical point of view, the infrared receiver system is in many ways similar in operation to the FM system. However, receivers must be in the line of sight of the emitter (transmitter); the signal can only be received inside the covered room. As with FM technology, each person—hearing-aid wearer or not—must use a receiver. The options for coupling the infrared receiver to the hearing aid are the same as for FM systems.

The communication methods and the assistive listening systems described above are methods to cross and thus eliminate many of the communications barriers that separate deaf, hard of hearing, and hearing people from one another.

NOTES

1. John Wheeler, president of Deafness Research Foundation, March 1999, cited by the Northern Virginia Resource Center, "Frequency of Hearing Loss" [online], available: http://www. nvrc.org/Information/statistics-demo.htm.
2. M. Vernon and E. Mindel, *They Grow in Silence: The Deaf Child and His Family* (Silver Spring, Md.: National Association of the Deaf, 1971), p. 96.

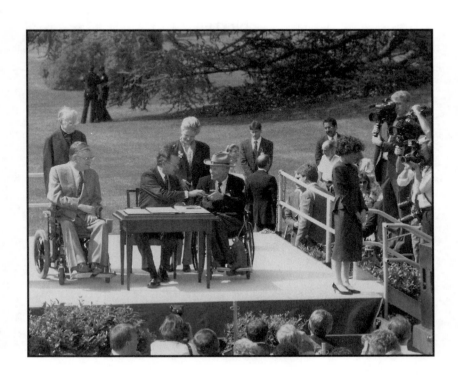

Chapter 2

The Americans with Disabilities Act

The Americans with Disabilities Act (ADA) is landmark civil rights legislation for all citizens with disabilities.[1] The ADA is of tremendous benefit to deaf and hard of hearing people in their efforts to gain equal access to all aspects of society. The ADA requires the removal of communication barriers in many significant places.

Prior to ADA's passage, federal and state laws prohibited discrimination against people with disabilities in some limited areas. For example, Title V of the Rehabilitation Act of 1973 prohibited discrimination in federal programs and federally assisted programs (see chapter three). The Architectural Barriers Act addressed the removal of architectural barriers to access and to communication in federally funded buildings (see chapter nine). The Individuals with Disabilities Education Act (IDEA, originally titled the Education for All Handicapped Children Act) provided important procedural and substantive protections in public school systems (see chapter four). All of these laws established critical principles of equal access, but their impact was blunted by the limited application of the laws.

The ADA took the important principles in these laws and extended them to the broad mainstream of American public life.

The ADA prohibits discrimination in almost every aspect of society. This legislation provides legal protections in employment (Title I), access to state and local government and public transportation (Title II), public accommodations (Title III), and telecommunications (Title IV). Under the ADA, virtually all employers with fifteen or more employees must eliminate discriminatory practices, not just those with federal contracts or receiving federal financial assistance. Private businesses and professionals and nonprofit organizations must make their facilities and services accessible to people with disabilities. Under the ADA, all state and local government activities must be accessible, even if the government entity does not receive federal funds. The statute applies to a wide range of new construction of private buildings and workplaces, so that new construction standards will include accessibility features as a matter of standard practice.

The ADA was adopted with strong bipartisan support by Congress, and was signed by President George Bush to wide acclaim. It has not eliminated all disability-based discrimination. It does, however, provide a powerful tool for alleviating discrimination against people with disabilities.

DEFINITION OF "DISABILITY"

Federal disability laws protect people with many different kinds of physical and mental disabilities. The definition of "disability" adopted by the ADA is very broad. It includes any person who (1) has a physical or mental impairment that substantially limits one or more major life activity, (2) has a record of such an impairment, or (3) is regarded as having such an impairment.[2]

Major life activities are defined as "taking care of oneself," walking, hearing, doing manual tasks, seeing, speaking, breathing, learning, and working. Federal law therefore protects almost anyone with a disabling condition, whether due to a congenital disability, disease, accident, or almost any other reason.

For example, federal law protects deaf, hard of hearing, and blind people; people in wheelchairs; people with cerebral palsy, diabetes, epilepsy, cancer, speech defects, or mental illness; recovering alcoholics and other recovering drug abusers; and people with mental retardation. A person who is not actually disabled, but who is considered disabled in some way, is still protected by the ADA. For example, people who experienced mental illness in the past may encounter employers unwilling to hire them because of their history of illness. Such people are protected even though they are not ill at the present time. The law also protects people who were misdiagnosed or misclassified as disabled.

Defining "Disability" in the Courts

The person must have a disability that "substantially limits" the ability to perform a major life activity. However, a person need not be profoundly or severely deaf to be protected by the ADA. People who are hard of hearing are substantially affected in their ability to hear, and so they are entitled to the protections of the law. The ADA regulation for employment states that the term "substantially limits" generally means that the person is unable to perform a major life activity that the average person in the general population can perform.[3]

In June 1999, the U.S. Supreme Court decided three cases dealing with the definition of an "individual with a disability." The major issue in these cases is whether corrective devices and medication should be considered in determining whether a person is an "individual with a disability."

In *Sutton v. United Airlines,* two airline pilots were not hired as commercial pilots because they were nearsighted. With glasses, their vision can be corrected to 20/20. They said that they were individuals with disabilities because without eyeglasses their vision was 20/100 or less.[4] In *Murphy v. United Parcel Service,* an individual was fired from his job as a mechanic because he had high blood pressure, even though it was controlled with medication.[5] And in *Kirkingburg v. Albertsons,* an individual with vision in only one eye was denied continued employment as a truck driver. Although he had a waiver of the vision standards of the U.S. Department of Transportation, the Supreme Court found he was not disabled because he could still see out of one eye.[6]

These cases affect many individuals who thought they were

entitled to the legal rights afforded by the ADA and the Rehabilitation Act. The U.S. Supreme Court ruled that a person is not considered an individual with a disability if corrective measures (such as glasses or medication) mean that they are not "substantially" impaired in a major life activity.

How does this affect deaf and hard of hearing individuals? We should not overreact to these decisions. The U.S. Supreme Court stressed that determining whether a person is an individual with a disability needs to be done on a case-by-case basis. Deaf and hard of hearing individuals should not be seriously affected by these decisions. Under the ADA and the Rehabilitation Act, a deaf or hard of hearing individual is considered an "individual with a disability" because of a substantial impairment to the major life activity of hearing.

A major concern relates to hearing aids and cochlear implants and to people with mild or moderate hearing loss. Some people have argued that a deaf or hard of hearing individual does not have a disability if he or she wears a hearing aid, but this is an overreaction.

For most individuals, eyeglasses correct vision to 20/20. This is simply not the case with hearing aids and assistive listening devices. Many hearing aid users still have great difficulty understanding speech, especially in noisy work settings. The major legal issue is whether an individual who uses a hearing aid, assistive listening device, or a cochlear implant has a substantial impairment to a major life activity. If that person has a "substantial impairment," then he or she is entitled to the legal protections of the ADA and the Rehabilitation Act. This will be true for most deaf and hard of hearing individuals. Some people have a degree of hearing loss that can be brought within "normal" limits with a hearing aid and assistive listening devices. They will be challenged when demonstrating that they are individuals with disabilities under the federal laws. However, they may still be entitled to the legal protection of the ADA or the Rehabilitation Act if they can show, among other things, that even with hearing aids they have a substantial impairment to a major life activity, for instance, they cannot distinguish all words due to interference or background noise. These future decisions will have to be made on a case-by-case basis.

TITLE I: EMPLOYMENT

Title I of the ADA and regulations adopted by the U.S. Equal Employment Opportunity Commission (EEOC) prohibit an employer from discriminating against a "qualified individual with a disability" in the following areas: (1) job application procedures, (2) hiring, (3) discharge, (4) compensation, (5) advancement, and (6) any other terms, conditions, and privileges of employment.[7]

Employers Covered Under the ADA

Employers with fifteen or more employees (including part-time and seasonal) are covered by Title I. Employment agencies, unions, and joint labor/management committees also are covered by Title I. Exempted from ADA's requirements are the United States government, Indian tribes, and tax-exempt private membership clubs.[8]

Discrimination Prohibited

The ADA and the EEOC regulations make it unlawful for an employer to discriminate on the basis of disability against a qualified individual in the following areas:

- recruitment, advertising, and job application procedures;
- hiring, upgrading, promotion, award of tenure, demotion, transfer, layoff, termination, right of return from layoff, and rehire;
- rates of pay;
- job assignments, job classifications, position descriptions, and seniority lists;
- leaves of absence, sick leave, or any other leave;
- fringe benefits;
- selection and financial support for training;

+ activities sponsored by the employer including social and recreational programs; and
+ any other term, condition, or privilege of employment.[9]

Employers are required to provide reasonable accommodations to people with disabilities during the application process and on the job. A reasonable accommodation is any change or adjustment to an environment that permits a qualified applicant or employee to participate in the job application process, perform the essential functions of a job, or enjoy benefits and privileges of employment.

Some examples of prohibited discrimination against a deaf or hard of hearing person include:

+ being denied a qualified interpreter for a job interview,
+ not being hired or promoted because the employer says communication is required and does not consider an accommodation to be reasonable,
+ receiving a lower rate of pay for doing the same job as hearing workers,
+ not being provided special equipment such as TTYs or visible signaling devices, and
+ being denied an opportunity to participate in training because the employer refuses to pay for a qualified interpreter.

Employer's Defense of "Undue Hardship"

An employer who is asked to make a reasonable accommodation may claim that the requested accommodation would be an "undue hardship," meaning a significant difficulty or expense. In deciding whether an accommodation would be an undue hardship to the business, the following conditions should be considered:

1. the nature and net cost of the accommodation needed, taking into consideration the availability of tax credits and deductions, and/or outside funding;
2. the overall financial resources of the business site providing the accommodation, the number of employees, and the effect on resources;
3. the overall financial resources of the business, including its

size in terms of number of employees and number and type of business sites; and

4. the type of operation of the business and the relationship of the facility to the overall business.

The EEOC analysis to the regulations gives the following example involving a deaf applicant: An independently owned fast-food franchise receives no money from the parent company that gives out the franchises. The franchise refuses to hire a deaf person because it says it would be an undue hardship to provide an interpreter for monthly staff meetings. Since the financial relationship between the local franchise and the parent company is only a franchise fee, only the financial resources of the local franchise would be considered in deciding whether providing the accommodation would be an undue hardship. However, if there is a financial or administrative relationship between the parent company and the local franchise, then the parent company's resources should be considered in determining whether the hardship is undue.

Enforcement Provisions

Employment practices under the ADA are enforced by the EEOC, along with state and local civil rights agencies who work in conjunction with the commission. Individuals with disabilities have the same remedies available to all other minorities under Title VII of the Civil Rights Act of 1964, as amended by the Civil Rights Act of 1991. An employer found in violation of the employment section of the ADA may be ordered to discontinue discriminatory practices, to correct policies and practices, to hire a qualified individual with a disability, or to rehire the person with back pay and provide the person with a reasonable accommodation. Compensatory and punitive damages may be available for intentional discrimination, but damages may not be awarded where the employer demonstrates "good faith efforts" to identify and make reasonable accommodations. Employers who lose a case will be required to pay the disabled person's attorney's fees and costs. (See chapter eight for extended discussion of employment rights under the ADA and other laws.)

TITLE II: STATE AND LOCAL GOVERNMENTS

Title II of the ADA requires all state and local government agencies to make all of their services accessible to individuals with disabilities. It also requires public transportation agencies to be accessible. Title II became effective in 1992. The U.S. Department of Justice adopted regulations implementing and explaining the requirements of Title II.[10]

These requirements are important because they extend protection against discrimination to many agencies that were not covered by Section 504 of the Rehabilitation Act of 1973 because they did not receive any federal funding (see chapter three). For example, many courts and police departments do not receive federal financial assistance. Deaf people could not use Section 504 to complain about discrimination when these law enforcement agencies did not provide interpreter services. Now, they can look to the ADA to require equal access.

The goal of Title II is to make sure that people with disabilities may use all services, programs, and activities of state and local governments. Any person with a disability who meets the essential eligibility requirements for getting services or participating in a government program is protected by the ADA.

Agencies That Must Be Accessible

Title II of the ADA applies to all state and local "public entities," as well as to AMTRAK and commuter transportation agencies. The term is defined broadly to include "everything a state or local entity does." Public agencies include:

- school systems,
- motor vehicle departments,
- police and fire departments,
- parks and recreation programs,
- jails and prisons,
- libraries,
- food stamp offices,
- welfare and social service agencies, and
- public hospitals, clinics, and counseling centers.

limit   Although federal courts are not covered by Title II, state and local courts, as well as city, county, and state legislatures, must comply with the statute. Government activities carried out by private contractors also are covered by the ADA. For example, state park concession activities often are operated by private contractors; shelters and halfway houses may be operated by private non-profit agencies but receive state and local government contracts.

Federal government agencies, however, are not covered by Title II. Federal buildings and federal executive agencies are required to be accessible, but they are covered by the Rehabilitation   *limitation* Act and the Architectural Barriers Act, not by the ADA.

Defining Discrimination under Rehabilitation/Access Statutes

If a person with a disability meets the "essential eligibility requirements" for a government service, the government agency cannot use the disability as a reason to (1) exclude the person from participating in the service, (2) deny the benefits or services, programs or activities of the agency, or (3) subject the person to discrimination. In addition, government agencies must comply with the following guidelines:

1. A government agency cannot exclude or refuse to serve people because of a disability. For example, city recreation programs may not turn away or impose additional requirements on people who are deaf. A counseling or health service may not refuse to accept a deaf client because of difficulty in communication.
2. A government agency must modify policies and practices that are unfair to people with disabilities. For example, an agency that requires a driver's license as the only acceptable means of identification must change its policy because blind individuals or individuals with other disabilities may not be able to get drivers' licenses. If the agency imposes safety requirements that are necessary for the safe operation of the program (such as a requirement to have a valid driver's license), the requirement must be based on actual risk and not on mere speculation, stereotype, or generalizations

about individuals with disabilities. If an agency has a "no pets" policy, it may be required to modify that policy for dogs or other animals that are trained to provide assistance to deaf or blind people.

3. A public park that leases boats or other equipment cannot ask a deaf individual to pay a higher deposit than hearing people or take out additional insurance to rent equipment.

4. A government agency must remove architectural, communication, or transportation barriers. The agency does not have to remove physical barriers in every part of every public building, as long as the programs it offers can be made available to people who cannot use the facility. For example, the agency could serve a person with a disability in an accessible location, or provide an aide, an assistant, or a device that would enable the person with a disability to use the service. Not all pay telephones in public buildings have to be equipped with TTYs, but at least some phones should be usable by deaf people.

5. Most importantly to deaf individuals, a government agency must also provide the "auxiliary aids and services" the person needs in order to communicate.

Auxiliary Aids and Services

Which Auxiliary Aids Should Be Provided?

Government agencies are required to provide deaf people with auxiliary aids so that they may have an equal opportunity to participate in and enjoy the government services, programs, or activities.[11] The appropriate auxiliary aid will depend on the type of activity being accommodated and the needs of the person wanting to take part in that endeavor. For example, a deaf person who uses sign language may need an interpreter to understand a PTA meeting or to talk to a county social worker or police officer. However, an interpreter would be useless for a deaf or hard of hearing person who does not use sign language. In that case, the appropriate accommodation may be a transcription or amplification system.

The Justice Department defines a qualified interpreter as one who can "interpret effectively, accurately, and impartially both receptively and expressively, using any necessary specialized vocabulary.[12] An interpreter who is qualified for one type of interpreting assignment may not have sufficient skills for interpreting in another situation.

What are Auxiliary Aids and Services?

State and local governments must ensure effective communication with individuals with disabilities.[13] In order to make sure that communication for a person who is deaf, blind, or hard of hearing is as effective as communication with others, the public agency must provide appropriate auxiliary aids.

Auxiliary aids include any device or service that is needed to make spoken information accessible for a deaf person, or visual information accessible for a blind person. The regulation specifically lists:

qualified interpreters

assistive listening systems (loop, FM, and infrared systems)

television captioning and decoders

TTYs

video text displays

transcriptions

readers

taped texts

brailled materials

large print materials

However, this list is not inclusive, and new types of auxiliary aids will be required under ADA standards as new technology becomes available. Also, just having the assistive equipment is not enough. An agency must adopt and publicize procedures on available equipment and how to request it.

In determining its needs for an interpreter, a government agency should consider the context in which the communication is taking place, the number of people involved, the importance of the communication, and whether the information being communicated is complex or lengthy. A family member or friend may not be qualified to interpret because of factors such as emotional or personal involvement or considerations of confidentiality.[14]

Although the public agency has the final decision about the type of auxiliary aid that will be provided, the deaf individual is in the best position to evaluate his or her own needs and the effectiveness of the service. The Justice Department rule states that in determining what type of auxiliary aid or service is necessary, the government agency must give "primary consideration" to the requests of the individual with disabilities.[15] The Justice Department's analysis to its ADA rule states:

> The public entity must provide an opportunity for individuals with disabilities to request the auxiliary aids and services of their choice. This expressed choice shall be given primary consideration by the public entity. The public entity shall honor the choice unless it can demonstrate that another effective means of communication exists or that use of the means chosen would not be required under the regulation.[16]

Deaf individuals should notify government agencies if interpreters are not sufficiently skilled or if an auxiliary aid does not give them equal access to a program.

Who Pays for the Interpreters and Other Auxiliary Aids?

The government may not charge a person with a disability any extra fee for providing an interpreter or other auxiliary aid.[17] For example, courts may not include an interpreter fee as "court costs" when a deaf person is involved in a trial and is ordered to pay the "costs" of the trial.[18] The ADA does not require an agency to provide an auxiliary aid if it would result in an undue burden or if it would fundamentally alter the nature of the services the agency provides. Interpreters would seldom be considered an undue burden on an agency since the cost is compared to the overall budget of the state or local government.

Even if a particular auxiliary aid is considered to be too expensive or burdensome, the agency must then offer another auxiliary aid, if available, that does not cause a fundamental alteration or undue burden on the agency.

What TTY Services are Required?

Government agencies that communicate by telephone must have TTYs or equally effective telecommunication systems in order to communicate with deaf people.[19] Title IV of the ADA established a nationwide relay system that may be adequate to give TTY users access to many government services. But public agencies must still provide TTYs for outgoing and incoming TTY calls, if the relay service will not give consumers equal access to services offered by telephone.

Telephone emergency services must provide direct access for deaf and hard of hearing individuals.[20] Local governments that provide 911-type services must make sure that a TTY user can call directly, without going through a relay system or a separate telephone number. Emergency-service operators must be trained to recognize and respond to TTY calls.

When a public agency offers use of a telephone as part of its services, it must also be able to offer TTYs and hearing aid-compatible telephones. For example, patients in hospitals or other residential facilities are entitled to equal access to telephones. Agencies that provide pay telephones for public use must make sure that some of their telephones are equipped with a TTY. New and renovated public buildings must meet a high standard of accessibility, including requirements for visual flashing alarms, TTY equipment, and intercom accessibility.

When a relay system does not adequately give access to a telephone service, the government office should have its own TTY for incoming calls. For example, offices with frequent contacts with the public or with clients who use TTYs should have on-site TTYs to provide for direct communication between the government agency and the individual.

Filing a Complaint

A person who believes that he or she is a victim of discrimination by a state or local government may file a lawsuit or administrative complaint under the ADA. The remedies, such as damages and injunctive relief, are the same as those provided under Section 504 of the Rehabilitation Act of 1973 (see chapter three).

Administrative complaints may be filed with any agency that provides financial assistance to the program, with the U.S. Department of Justice, or with the federal agency with enforcement authority over that subject area. Complaints should be made in writing, and signed by the complainant or an authorized representative. The complaint must contain the complainant's name and address and a description of the discrimination by the public entity. For more information, or to file a complaint, contact:

Disability Rights Section
Civil Rights Division
U.S. Department of Justice
P.O. Box 66738
Washington, DC 20035-6738

TITLE III: PUBLIC ACCOMMODATION

The most dramatic expansion of disability rights is the application of Title III of the ADA to give equal access to "places of public accommodation." For the first time, thousands of private businesses, professionals, and nonprofit organizations must remove communication and physical barriers for people with disabilities. For deaf and hard of hearing people, Title III and its regulations will be of tremendous help in removing communication barriers.[21] The title states that:

No individual shall be discriminated against on the basis of disability in the full and equal enjoyment of the goods, services, facilities, privileges, advantages, or accommodations of any place of public accommodation by any person who owns, leases (or leases to), or operates a place of public accommodation.[22]

Title III covers a wide range of commercial and non-profit places such as hotels, theaters, restaurants, doctors' offices, lawyers' offices, retail stores, banks, museums, parks, libraries, daycare centers, and private schools. A "place of public accommodation" is a facility operated by a private entity, whose operations affect commerce, and that falls within at least one of the following categories:

1. an inn, hotel, motel, or other place of lodging (except for an establishment in a building that has not more than five rooms for rent and is the residence of the proprietor);
2. a restaurant, bar, or other establishment serving food or drink;
3. a movie theater, theater, concert hall, stadium, or other place of exhibition or entertainment;
4. an auditorium, convention center, lecture hall, or other place of public gathering;
5. a bakery, grocery store, clothing store, hardware store, shopping center, or other sales or rental establishment;
6. a laundromat, dry cleaner, bank, barber shop, beauty shop, travel service, shoe repair service, funeral parlor, gas station, office of an accountant or lawyer, pharmacy, insurance office, professional office of a health care provider, hospital, or other service establishment;
7. a terminal, depot, or other station used for public transportation;
8. a museum, library, gallery, or other place of public display or collection;
9. a park, zoo, amusement park, or other place of recreation;
10. a nursery, elementary, secondary, undergraduate, or postgraduate private school, or other place of education;
11. a day care center, senior citizen center, homeless shelter, food bank, adoption agency, or other social service establishment; and
12. a gymnasium, health spa, bowling alley, golf course, or other place of exercise or recreation.[23]

The examples given in each category help illustrate and define the category, but they are not the only entities that are covered. For example, even though the "sales or rental establishment" category does not list jewelry stores, all stores including jewelry stores are covered. Even though the "service establishment" category does not list photo finishing shops or housecleaning services, all service and professional service agencies are included. Even though the "education" category does not list driving schools or computer training specialists, all such educational activities are covered.

It does not matter whether an entity has one employee or one thousand employees. If it fits within the definition of one of the twelve categories, it is covered by Title III of the ADA. However, not all "public" activities are covered by Title III. For example, television broadcasters offer services to the general public, but they do not fit within any of the twelve categories. Furthermore, Title III of the ADA does not cover private clubs, religious organizations, or places of worship.

Auxiliary Aids

A public accommodation must provide an "auxiliary aid or service" where necessary. The Department of Justice regulations to implement Title III provide a comprehensive list of auxiliary aids and services required by the ADA, including qualified interpreters.[24]

Other examples of auxiliary aids listed in the regulations are note takers, transcription services, written materials, telephone handset amplifiers, assistive listening devices, assistive listening systems, telephones compatible with hearing aids, closed-caption decoders, open and closed captioning, telecommunication devices for deaf people (TTYs), videotext displays. The list is not intended to be exhaustive. The Justice Department noted that new devices will become available as technology advances, and they will be considered "auxilary aids and services."

The costs of compliance with the auxiliary aids requirements may not be financed by charging a fee to a deaf person. However, if a public accommodation loans out special equipment to a customer (such as a decoder or an assistive listening device), it is permitted to charge a reasonable, refundable deposit to assure that the equipment will be returned. However, such deposits would be permissible only if the business also demands a deposit for the loan of equipment to people without disabilities.

Defense to the Requirements

The ADA does not require a public accommodation to provide any auxiliary aid that would result in an "undue burden" or in a fundamental alteration in the nature of the goods and services provided by a public accommodation. An undue burden is defined as a "significant" difficulty or expense to the public accommodation. However, the public accommodation is not relieved from the duty to furnish an alternative auxiliary aid, if available, that would not result in an undue burden.

The Justice Department strongly encourages public accommodations to consult with an individual before providing him or her with a particular auxiliary aid or service. The department's analysis to the regulation points out that an interpreter may be necessary to ensure effective communication. According to the analysis, there is a wide range of communication situations, including areas such as health, legal matters, and finances, that would be sufficiently lengthy or complex to require an interpreter for effective communication.

TTY Requirements

Title III also requires public accommodations to provide TTYs upon request when such facilities offer a customer, client, patient, or participant the opportunity to make outgoing telephone calls on more than an incidental convenience basis. Where entry to a place of public accommodation requires use of a security entrance telephone, a TTY or other effective means of communication must be provided for use by a deaf person. Hotels should also provide a TTY at the front desk in order to take calls from guests who use TTYs in their rooms.

Decoders and Captioning

Hospitals that provide televisions for patient use and places of lodging that provide televisions in five or more guest rooms must provide a means for decoding captions upon request. While movie theaters are not required to present open-captioned films, other public accommodations that impart verbal information through soundtracks on films, videotapes, or slide shows are required to make such information accessible through such means as captioning.

Conferences and Performances

Education and training organizations, trade associations, or performing artists that lease space for a conference or performance at a hotel, auditorium, convention center, or stadium must comply with the ADA. The analysis to the Justice Department regulation states that the renter should be responsible for providing auxiliary aids and services for the participants in its conference or performance. The determination of who actually provides auxiliary aids (the landlord or the renters) can be decided during the lease negotiations. For example, if a theater rents space to a performing artist, the question of who provides for a requested interpreter will be decided by their contract. Both the landlord and tenant are subject to the requirements of the ADA.

Use of Service Animals

The Title III regulation also provides broad protections for the use of service animals.[25] Public accommodations have to modify their policies and practices to allow the use of service animals. Service animals are broadly defined to include any dog or other animal that is trained to provide assistance to a person with a disability. The ADA does not require service animals to be professionally trained or certified by state agencies.

Examinations and Courses

The ADA requires private organizations that offer examinations or courses for licensing, certification, or credentials to provide appropriate auxiliary aids such as interpreters.[26] This applies to high school or college education and to professional and trade training. The private organization would not be required to provide an auxiliary aid if it could show the provision of the auxiliary aid would fundamentally alter the skills or knowledge the examination intends to test. Examinations must be used that best reflect an individual's aptitude or achievement level rather than reflecting the person's impaired sensory, manual, or speaking skills. The only exception is where those skills are what the examination seeks to measure.

Existing vs. New Facilities

The ADA requires the removal of structural communication barriers from existing facilities.[27] This can be accomplished by installing flashing alarm systems, permanent signage, pay TTYs, assistive listening systems, and adequate sound buffers.

For newly constructed buildings, the U.S. Architectural and Transportation Barriers Compliance Board (Access Board) has developed ADA Accessibility Guidelines (ADAAG).[28] According to these guidelines, all new construction and building alterations must be accessible to disabled people. The requirements for TTYs, public telephones, assistive listening systems, and visual alarms are as follows:

1. One TTY must be provided inside any building that has four or more public pay telephones, including both interior and exterior phones. In addition, one TTY must be provided whenever there is an interior public pay phone in a stadium or arena; a convention center; a hotel with a convention center; a covered shopping mall; or a hospital emergency, recovery, or waiting room.
2. One accessible public pay phone must be provided for each level of a public accommodation. If a level has two or more banks of phones, there must be one accessible phone for each bank.
3. Fixed-seating assembly areas that accommodate fifty or more people or that have audio-amplification systems must have a permanently installed assistive listening system.
4. Hotels must make eight percent of the first one hundred

rooms and approximately four percent of the remaining rooms accessible to deaf and hard of hearing people. These rooms must contain visual alarms, notification devices, volume-control telephones, and an accessible electrical outlet for a TTY. Half of these rooms must also be accessible to people with physical disabilities.

Enforcement

Individuals with disabilities can bring lawsuits for court orders to stop discrimination, but they cannot collect money damages. If the individuals win their court case, they can recover attorney's fees and costs. Individuals with disabilities can also file complaints with the U.S. attorney general, who has the power to initiate lawsuits in cases of public importance or where a "pattern or practice" of discrimination is alleged. In such cases, the attorney general may seek money damages and civil penalties. In many cases, the Justice Department will refer a case for mediation rather than investigating.

TITLE IV: TELECOMMUNICATIONS

Title IV of the ADA requires telephone companies to provide both local and long distance telecommunications relay services across the nation. (See chapter 12 for a complete discussion of telecommunication issues.) These relay services enable people who use TTYs to have telephone conversations with people who use conventional voice telephones any time, any place, and for any reason whatsoever.

Title IV of the ADA also requires all television public service announcements that are produced or funded by the federal government to include closed captioning. Occasionally, federal agencies develop television announcements about AIDS, aging, drug use, and other general health and consumer issues. In the future, the vital information in these and other federally assisted announcements will finally reach individuals who rely on closed captions to receive the verbal content of television.

NOTES

1. PL 101-336, 42 U.S. Code 12101 *et seq.*
2. 42 U.S.C. 12102(2). See also 29 U.S.C. 706(8)(A) (Rehabilitation Act); 42 U.S.Code 3602(h) (Fair Housing Act Amendments Act of 1988); 49 U.S.C. 1374(c)(2) (Air Carrier Access Act).
3. 29 C.F.R. §1630.2(j)(1).
4. *Sutton v. United Airlines,* 119 S.Ct. 2139 (1999).
5. *Murphy v. United Parcel Service,* 119 S.Ct. 2133 (1999).
6. *Kirkingburg v. Albertsons,* 119 S.Ct. 2162 (1999).
7. 29 C.F.R. §1630.
8. 29 C.F.R. §1630.2.
9. 29 C.F.R. §1630.4.
10. 28 C.F.R. Part 35.
11. 28 C.F.R. §35.160(b).
12. 28 C.F.R. §35.104.
13. 28 C.F.R. §35.160.
14. *56 Fed. Reg.* 35,701 (July 26, 1991).
15. 28 C.F.R. §35.160(b).
16. *56 Fed. Reg.* 35,711–35,712 (July 26, 1991).
17. 28 C.F.R. §35.130(f).
18. The analysis to the Justice Department ADA regulation states that "the costs of interpreter services may not be assessed as an element of court costs. The [Justice] Department has already recognized that imposition of the cost of courtroom interpreter services is impermissible under section 504 . . . Accordingly, recouping the costs of interpreter services by assessing them as part of court costs would also be prohibited." *56 Fed. Reg.* 35,706 (July 26, 1991).
19. 28 C.F.R. §35.161.
20. 28 C.F.R. §35.162.
21. 28 C.F.R. Part 36.
22. 42 U.S.C. 12182(a).
23. 28 C.F.R. §36.104.
24. 28 C.F.R. §36.303.
25. 28 C.F.R. §36.302.
26. 28 C.F.R. §36.309.
27. 28 C.F.R. §36.304.
28. 28 C.F.R. §36.401.

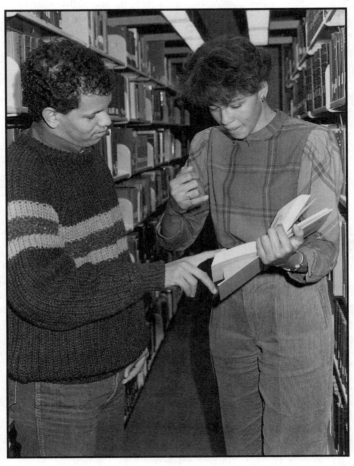

Chapter 3

The Rehabilitation Act of 1973

Historically, people with disabilities have been unemployed and underemployed. In 1920, Congress passed the first federal laws to help disabled people get job training and find employment.[1] But these laws were clearly inadequate; even highly qualified people with disabilities could not find good jobs because of widespread discrimination by private employers and by federal, state, and local governments. Congress addressed the problem by enacting the Rehabilitation Act of 1973.

Title V of the Rehabilitation Act has been hailed as a "bill of rights" for people with disabilities. The purpose of Title V is to make sure that programs receiving federal money can be used by all disabled people, so that the federal government will no longer be implicated in discriminatory activities. This chapter will look at the implementation, regulation, and application of Section 504, which prohibits discrimination in federally-supported programs.

SECTION 504

As amended in 1978, Section 504 of the Rehabilitation Act reads:

The five major sections of Title V prohibit discrimination and require accessibility in employment, education, health, welfare, and social services.

Section 501 applies to federal government employment practices.[2] It requires each executive department and agency to adopt an affirmative action plan for the hiring, placement, and advancement of qualified people with disabilities. (For more information, see chapter eight.)

Section 502 created the Architectural and Transportation Barriers Compliance Board, or Access Board.[3] The Access Board's primary functions are to ensure compliance with the Architectural Barriers Act (a 1968 federal law prohibiting architectural barriers in federally funded buildings) and to eliminate barriers from public buildings. (For more information, see chapter nine.)

Section 503 requires affirmative action in the hiring, placement, and promotion of qualified people with disabilities by employers who have contracts or subcontracts with the federal government of more than $2,500 a year.[4] Contractors with fifty or more employees or contracts for more than $50,000 are also required to have written affirmative action plans. (See chapter eight.)

Section 504 prohibits discrimination against qualified people with disabilities in any federally-supported program or activity.[5] Recipients of federal financial assistance include most public and some private institutions, from schools and nursing homes to museums and airports.

Section 508 requires federal agencies to procure and use electronic and information technology that is accessible to individuals with disabilities.[6] Examples of this technology are: hardware and software for computers, telecommunications equipment, Internet-based information and applications, and multimedia applications. The Architectural and Transportation Compliance Board has the responsibility of establishing accessibility standards under Section 508. Each federal agency must use these standards to develop its own policies for procuring and using electronic and information technology.

No otherwise qualified individual with a disability in the United States . . . shall, solely by reason of his or her disability, be excluded from the participation in, be denied the benefits of, or be subjected to discrimination under any program or activity receiving Federal financial assistance or under any program or activity conducted by any Executive Agency or by the United States Postal Service.

The statute is implemented by detailed regulations that every federal agency giving financial assistance must promulgate, spelling out the Section 504 obligations of its recipients.[7] In 1977 the U.S. Department of Health, Education, and Welfare (HEW)* became the first agency to publish its regulation and detailed analysis.[8] The department also issued a set of standards for other agencies to use in developing their own Section 504 rules. A 1980 Executive Order gave the Justice Department primary authority to monitor the agencies' regulations.[9]

Who Must Obey Section 504?

The federal government assists many programs and activities around the country. The HHS regulation defines "federal financial assistance" as any grant, loan, contract, or any other arrangement by which the department provides assistance in the form of funds or services of federal personnel or property.[10] Procurement contracts are specifically excluded. As a result, private manufacturers of items purchased by the government do not have to obey Section 504. However, they are subject to Section 503, which prohibits employment discrimination. Organizations that have both procurement contracts and that receive federal financial assistance have to obey both Sections 503 and 504 of the law.

Section 504 applies to an organization whether it receives federal assistance directly or indirectly, for example, through a state

*HEW was divided into two cabinet-level departments—the Department of Education and the Department of Health and Human Services (HHS) effective May 4, 1980. Hereafter, references to HEW will be restricted to actions taken before that date. Unless noted otherwise, HEW policies remain in effect at HHS and the Department of Education.

The Evolution of Section 508

The U.S. Congress originally enacted Section 508 in 1986. At that time, all federal agencies were directed to make their electronic equipment accessible in compliance with guidelines developed by the General Services Administration. Although a few federal agencies did comply with these mandates, most agencies ignored the directives of Section 508 during the decade that followed.

As the need for access to electronic and information technology grew in the 1990's, consumers with disabilities became frustrated with the failure of the federal government to comply with Section 508. In the mid-1990's, consumers went back to the U.S. Congress, and asked for a new version of Section 508 that contained some teeth—i.e., enforcement mechanisms. In 1998, consumers were successful, and a new version of Section 508 was enacted in the Workforce Investment Act of 1998.[11]

The "new" Section 508 contains strict requirements for federal agencies to obtain and use electronic and information technology that is accessible to (1) federal employees with disabilities and (2) individuals with disabilities outside the federal government who need government information. Under this law, access to and use of information and data must be comparable to access and use available to federal

or local government. A "recipient" is defined as any institution that receives federal assistance or that indirectly benefits from such assistance.

Certain types of significant federal involvement are not considered to be assistance in the form of funds or services. For example, the federal government awards broadcast licenses to radio and television broadcasters, but these licenses are neither federal assistance nor federally conducted programs.[12] Commercial airlines benefit from the federal air traffic control system furnished employees and members of the public who are not disabled, unless doing so would impose an undue burden on the agency. If providing access would result in an undue burden, a federal agency must (1) provide documentation on why access would result in such a burden, and (2) provide the information that was requested through an alternative means of access. Consumers will be able to bring a complaint against agencies that do not comply with these requirements.

Section 508 is expected to have a significant impact on the ability of deaf and hard of hearing individuals. In addition to requiring access to technologies themselves, the new law will require mainstream technologies to work with adaptive technologies. For example, if a particular piece of equipment connects to phone lines, the law requires that TTYs be able to connect to the device in question. The new law will also require all materials presented in an audio format to have either open or closed captioning. Finally, a piece of technology that transports information will be required to transmit the information in a manner that does not eliminate access. For example, if a particular software program contains captions, the technology used to transmit that program may not eliminate those captions.

by the government, but the U.S. Supreme Court has held that operation of the federal system is not federal financial assistance to the airlines themselves.[13]

Because the definition of federal financial assistance is so broad, many private and public institutions must obey Section 504. The types of institutions usually receiving some form of federal financial assistance include elementary and secondary schools, colleges and universities, hospitals, nursing homes, vocational rehabilitation agencies, public welfare offices, state and local governments, police and fire departments, correction and probation departments, libraries, museums, theater programs, parks, recreational facilities, mass transit systems, airports and harbors, subsidized housing programs, legal services programs, and most parts of the judicial system.

Sometimes it is difficult to determine whether and from what agency an institution gets federal financial assistance. If the institution is public, citizens usually can examine its financial records and reports to see if it receives federal assistance. Many federal agencies keep public lists of the programs and activities they fund. If the agency does not have such a list, or if the particular institution is not listed, a request can be filed under the Freedom of Information Act (FOIA) with each federal agency thought to be the funding source.[14]

The FOIA request should identify the possible recipient, state that the information is being sought under the Freedom of Information Act, and ask if the particular institution receives federal financial assistance and, if so, for what purpose. It is important to identify the institution fully and correctly and to give the name and address of any parent organization(s) to which it belongs. For example, a local branch library may not be listed as a direct recipient of federal assistance. Instead, the state, regional, or county association may be the formal recipient. The federal agency is supposed to respond to a FOIA request within ten days.

A complaint against an institution for violation of Section 504 can be filed with a federal agency even if it is not clear whether that institution gets financial assistance from that agency. If the agency does not financially support that institution, the agency will simply refuse to accept the complaint.

If an institution receives any federal financial assistance for one part of its activities, then it must obey Section 504 in all of its activities which benefit from the financial assistance—even if those other activities do not receive any direct aid. Section 504 was again amended in 1987 to clarify that the law applies to all of the operations of an agency, department, college, hospital, or other organization that receives any federal financial assistance.[15]

Section 504 applies to federal executive agencies and recipients of federal financial assistance. Because the original 1973 law did not apply to federal agencies, most of the Section 504 regulations apply only to recipients of assistance from the agency and not to the agency itself. Since the adoption of the 1978 amendments, however, the agencies themselves must obey Section 504, whether or not they have adopted specific regulations that apply to their own activities.[16]

Defining a "Qualified" Person with a Disability

Section 504 does not guarantee access to jobs or services merely because a person has a disability. To be protected by Section 504, a person with a disability must also be qualified for the job or service in question. The 504 regulations define a "qualified person with a disability" as:

+ With respect to employment, a person with a disability who, with reasonable accommodation, can perform the essential functions of the job in question.
+ With respect to public preschool, elementary, secondary, or adult education, a person with a disability (i) of an age during which other students are provided such services, (ii) of any age during which it is mandatory under state law to provide such services, or (iii) to whom a state is required to provide a free appropriate public education under the Individuals with Disabilities Education Act (IDEA).
+ With respect to postsecondary and vocational education services, a person with a disability who meets the academic and technical standards requisite to admission or participation in the recipient's education program or activity; and
+ With respect to other services, a person with a disability who meets the essential eligibility requirements for the receipt of such services.[17]

A person must fall under the applicable definition in order to be protected by the nondiscrimination provisions of Section 504.

GENERAL NONDISCRIMINATION PROVISIONS

The Section 504 regulations list general categories of discriminatory behavior that are prohibited. They also establish broad policy guidelines to determine whether a particular discriminatory act is prohibited by Section 504.

Equal Opportunity

The most significant principle of Section 504 is that no recipient or federal agency may deny a qualified person an opportunity to participate in or benefit from its programs or services.[18] A federally-funded program cannot refuse to serve a person with a disability merely because of that disability. A deaf person cannot be denied admission to a mental health counseling program merely because he or she is deaf. If a counseling program is available only to people who live in a certain county, however, and the deaf person does not live in that county, he or she can be denied admission to the program for that nondiscriminatory reason.

A person with a disability must be given an opportunity to participate in or benefit from a program in a manner that is equal to and as effective as the opportunity provided to other people.[19] To be equally effective, a program does not have to produce the identical result or level of achievement for disabled and nondisabled participants; the requirement is only that people with disabilities must be provided an equal opportunity to obtain the same result, to gain the same benefit, or to reach the same level of achievement as other people.[20] For example, the administrator of an adult education program might tell a deaf person simply to read the written materials for a class, rather than attending lectures and discussions. This would be unfair. Because the lectures and discussions help to explain and amplify the written material, the deaf person would not have an equal opportunity to benefit from the class.

Different or Special Treatment

Sometimes people with disabilities need different treatment in order to give them genuine equal opportunity. In the area of race or sex discrimination, equal opportunity usually means treating people in exactly the same way. But a person with a disability may need some special assistance or accommodation in order to get benefits or services equivalent to those of other people. Failure to provide that accommodation would constitute discrimination. As explained in the analysis accompanying the original Section 504 regulation:

> Different or special treatment of handicapped persons because of their handicaps, may be necessary in a number of contexts in order to assure equal opportunity. Thus, for example, it is meaningless to "admit" a handicapped person in a wheelchair to a program if the program is offered only on the third floor of a walk-up building. Nor is one providing equal educational opportunity to a deaf child by admitting him or her to a classroom but providing no means for the child to understand the teacher or receive instruction.[21]

At the same time, Section 504 also prohibits unnecessary special or different treatment if it would tend to stigmatize people with disabilities or set them apart from other people. Different or separate aids, benefits, or services are prohibited unless the separation is necessary to provide services that are as effective as those provided to others.[22] A legal services organization, for example, may designate a special office to serve clients who have disabilities, if the office is physically accessible and has lawyers trained in disability law. But it would be unfair to require all clients with disabilities, regardless of their legal problems, to use only that special office.

Communication Barriers

The general nondiscrimination provisions in the Section 504 regulation apply to the communication barriers faced by deaf people as well as to physical barriers to people in wheelchairs. A deaf woman may be able to walk up a flight of stairs to a job counseling center without difficulty. But if she cannot understand the intake worker's explanations about filling out the forms, she will not be able to do it correctly. She will not know what services are available or how to get them. A deaf man may be able to walk into a hospital or mental health center, but if he cannot communicate with the doctor or counselor he does not have meaningful, equivalent access to the program and its facilities.

The HHS analysis of the regulation gives an example of a welfare office that uses telephones to communicate with clients. Clients can call the office for information or to reach caseworkers. Staff can call clients to schedule appointments. But this office must also provide another method to communicate with its deaf clients. The best alternative might be a TTY-equipped telephone. Another example is a museum exhibit that includes monitors with videotaped interviews or explanations. The exhibit's tape must be captioned to enable deaf or hard of hearing people to have the same information.

Communication problems are specifically addressed in the Justice Department's Section 504 regulations. These rules require recipients to ensure that communications are effectively conveyed to people with impaired vision or hearing.[23] The regulation requires recipients to provide appropriate auxiliary aids in order to give deaf people equal access to programs and services.[24]

When the Justice Department implemented the ADA, it clarified Section 504's definition of auxiliary aids and services. The ADA regulation clearly lists amplifiers, assistive listening devices and systems, hearing aid compatible telephones, television decoders, captioning, TTYs, videotext displays, or "other effective methods of making aurally delivered materials available to individuals with hearing impairments." The Justice Department also defined a qualified interpreter as one who is able to interpret effectively, accurately, and impartially, using any necessary specialized vocabulary.[25]

Interpreters should be available for any meeting, conference, class, or other group activity held by an agency that receives federal financial assistance. Section 504 requires interpreters for cultural events, city government meetings, adult education classes, park programs, or any other event that deaf people may wish to attend. Publicity for meetings should announce the availability of special services and interpreters and should describe the procedures for requesting them.

The needs of deaf people are specifically addressed by one HHS regulation that requires funding recipients to ensure that people with impaired vision or hearing can obtain information about the various services that are accessible to them.[26] For example, incoming telephone lines for inquiries must be TTY-equipped and be identified as such in the phone directory, letterhead, and anywhere else that the recipient's telephone number is given. Televised public service announcements should be signed or captioned. If programs or services are announced by radio, a recipient might ensure that deaf people receive the same information by direct mail or by announcements inserted in local newsletters or newspapers distributed by associations of people who are deaf or hard of hearing.

Program Accessibility

The regulation requires that programs be operated so that people with disabilities can use them easily and have equal opportunity to benefit from them.[27] For people in wheelchairs, "program accessibility" means removing architectural and physical barriers. For deaf people, it means removing communication barriers. Deaf people cannot fully utilize programs and facilities that they do not have equal access to or in which they are unable to communicate effectively. Programs and facilities must be usable. This requirement of the Rehabilitation Act suggests much more than physical accessibility to a site or building. In effect, the act requires that people with disabilities have functionally equivalent services and programs. As a policy concept, program accessibility should be invoked aggressively to help deaf people overcome their isolation and exclusion from many programs and services.

The government regulation lists methods to make programs accessible.[28] While the list does not provide much guidance for making specific programs accessible to deaf people, the phrase "re-design of equipment" encompasses modifications to telephones and auditory alarm systems; captions for films and videotapes; and stage, podium, and audiovisual system designs that include facilities and lighting for interpreters. The phrase "assignment of aides" can be interpreted to mean the provision of appropriate interpreters, note takers, transcribers, or other aides needed by deaf people. Because the list of methods in the regulation is not inclusive, deaf people should feel free to request any other accommodation that would make a program or activity accessible.

ENFORCEMENT OF SECTION 504

A person who believes that a recipient of federal financial assistance has discriminated against him or her on the basis of the disability has several alternative procedures for seeking redress.

Administrative Enforcement

There is no central enforcement mechanism for Section 504. Although the Justice Department has overall supervision, every agency that provides federal financial assistance is required to adopt its own regulations and enforcement procedures. Each agency must make its recipients sign assurances of compliance with Section 504 and use the same enforcement procedures as those established to enforce Title VI of the Civil Rights Act of 1964. Within this framework, the procedures used by the various agencies can differ substantially. However, most of the agencies have adopted procedures that are modeled on those originally developed by HEW and now used by the Department of HHS and the Department of Education.

Self-Evaluation

All recipients must conduct a self-evaluation of their Section 504 compliance, assisted by interested people, including people with disabilities or organizations representing them.[29] Recipients must complete their self-evaluations, modify any policies or practices that were not in compliance with Section 504, and take appropriate remedial steps to eliminate the effects of any discrimination that resulted from past policies and practices. If a recipient has not yet conducted a self-evaluation or made appropriate modifications, a person bringing a complaint can use this fact to focus attention on discriminatory practices. If a recipient refuses to conduct a self-evaluation, any interested person can file a complaint asking the appropriate federal agency to compel compliance.

Internal Grievance Procedure

The Department of Education and the HHS require recipients with fifteen or more employees to adopt grievance procedures for complaints alleging discrimination under Section 504. Such recipients must also designate at least one person to coordinate Section 504 compliance. The grievance procedure must incorporate appropriate due process standards and provide for "prompt and equitable" resolution of complaints.[30] Complaint procedures need not be established for applicants seeking employment or admission to postsecondary institutions.

A grievance procedure can be a useful, inexpensive mechanism to resolve simple complaints, especially those stemming from ignorance or misunderstandings about disabilities and Section 504 obligations. Correspondence, memoranda, and other documents generated in grievance proceedings can be used later as evidence of the recipient's discriminatory attitudes or policies. Because the grievance procedure is set up and operated by the recipient itself, though, it will usually be ineffective to resolve major or contested complaints.

Complaint to the Federal Agency

A person who believes that a recipient of federal financial assistance has violated Section 504 can file a complaint with the federal agency that provided the financial assistance. Complaints against recipients of funding from The Department of Education and HHS should be filed with that agency's regional Office for Civil Rights.

Filing Complaints

Complaints must be filed within 180 days of the alleged discriminatory act. For example, if a deaf person went to a hospital on February 1 and did not get an interpreter, the person must send a complaint to HHS by August 1. If he or she waits longer than that, the department will not be required to do anything about the complaint. However, the time for filing can be extended at the discretion of the department. Many discriminatory acts are continuous; they represent a general policy or course of conduct. When this is the case, the 180-day limit is not a problem. The complainant can try to use the program or service again—reapply for benefits or employment, or renew the request for auxiliary aids—so there will be no question that the discriminatory act took place within the time limits.

The complaint can be a simple letter that merely notifies the federal agency of an alleged discriminatory act. However, it will have more impact if it sets out all of the important facts of the discrimination and fully identifies the parts of the Section 504 regulation that have been violated. The complaint should include the following information:

- the name, address, and telephone number of the person lodging the complaint ("complainant"), and any special instructions for telephoning a deaf complainant;
- the name, address, and telephone number of complainant's attorney or other representative, if any;
- a statement that the complainant is a "qualified person with a disability" under Section 504;
- the name, address, and telephone number of the program or facility that discriminated and a statement that this program receives financial assistance from the federal agency;
- a complete description of the discriminatory acts, in chronological order. The complaint should be as specific as possible about the dates, places, names, and titles of the people involved, and should explain why the conduct was discriminatory and how the complainant was qualified for the job, benefit, service, or program.

+ a description of any attempts to complain about the discrimination and the organization's response;
+ any other information or documents that help explain the discrimination and describe what happened;
+ a list of witnesses, including names, addresses, titles, and telephone numbers;
+ if possible, an analysis of the parts of the Section 504 regulation that have been violated.

Any relevant documents should be photocopied and attached to the complaint. Do not send original documents. Any attached documents should be numbered and clearly identified by number in the text of the complaint.

Agency Investigation

The federal agency will then investigate to determine whether there has been a violation of Section 504. Agency investigators should interview the complainant, representatives of the program, and other relevant witnesses. Although the complainant is not a formal "party" to the investigation, and has no role in the investigation or in the resolution reached by the agency, the complainant should attempt to be actively involved in the investigation. Make sure that the federal investigator has contacted important witnesses and is familiar with the issues. This is particularly important in complaints involving deafness; few investigators are knowledgeable about deafness and the types of auxiliary aids or reasonable accommodations that may be necessary to overcome communication barriers. The investigator may need to meet with experts or other people who can provide relevant information.

If the federal agency finds that a recipient has violated Section 504, it will notify the complainant and the recipient in writing. It will then try to negotiate with the recipient to provide the appropriate relief. The agency can require the recipient to take necessary remedial action to overcome effects of the discrimination. The agency can also require a remedial action plan that shows what steps the recipient will take within a specific time period to come into compliance. Such a plan requires the recipient to document its efforts. If the recipient fails to take the required corrective steps, or if negotiations do not result in a satisfactory resolution, the federal agency will then institute enforcement proceedings to terminate the recipient's federal financial assistance.

Judicial Enforcement

A person has the right to bypass Section 504 agency complaint procedures by bringing a lawsuit in federal court. Investigations by federal agencies can take a long time; by the time they are finished, it may be too late to help the person with a disability. A lawsuit in federal court might provide a quicker, more effective remedy, as well as monetary damages; attorney's fees and other court costs can be awarded. For example, a deaf woman who was about to have a baby found out that her hospital would not allow an interpreter in the delivery room. She could not wait for a federal agency to investigate her complaint, so she filed a lawsuit in federal court and got immediate help. Federal injunctions have also been upheld in cases involving college students needing classroom interpreters on short notice.

Each of these methods to enforce Section 504 should be reviewed carefully to determine which will be most effective in a particular case.

NOTES

1. The earliest laws regarding people who are deaf include PL 236–66 and the Smith-Fess Act of 1920.
2. 29 U.S. Code §791.
3. 29 U.S.C. §792.
4. 29 U.S.C. §793.
5. 29 U.S.C. §794.
6. PL 105-220, Title IV, §408(b), codified at 29 U.S.C. §794(d).
7. Executive Order No. 11,914 (1976), printed in 41 *Fed. Reg.* 17,871 (April 28, 1976).
8. 45 C.F.R. Part 84.
9. Executive Order No. 12,250 (1980), printed in 45 *Fed. Reg.* 72,995 (1980); 28 C.F.R. Part 41.
10. 45 C.F.R. §84.3(h).
11. PL 105-220, Title IV, §508(b), codified at 29 U.S.C. §794(d).
12. 47 C.F.R. §1.1830(b)(6).

13. *United States Department of Transportation v. Paralyzed Veterans of America*, 477 U.S. 597 (1986).
14. 5 U.S.C. §552.
15. Civil Rights Restoration Act of 1987, P.L. 100–259, 29 U.S.C. §794(b).
16. See regulations of the U.S. Department of Justice, which apply to its own "federally conducted" programs, 28 C.F.R. §39.
17. 45 C.F.R. §84.3(k); 34 C.F.R. §104.4(k).
18. 45 C.F.R. §84.4(b)(1)(i).
19. 45 C.F.R. §84.4(b)(1)(ii and iii).
20. 45 C.F.R. §84.4(b)(2).
21. 42 Fed. Reg. 22,676 (1977).
22. 45 C.F.R. §84.4(b)(3).
23. 28 C.F.R. §42.503(e).
24. 28 C.F.R. §35.104.
25. 28 C.F.R. §35.104.
26. 45 C.F.R. §84.22(f).
27. 45 C.F.R. §84.22.
28. Ibid.
29. 28 C.F.R. §41.5(b)(2).
30. 28 C.F.R. §41.5(a).

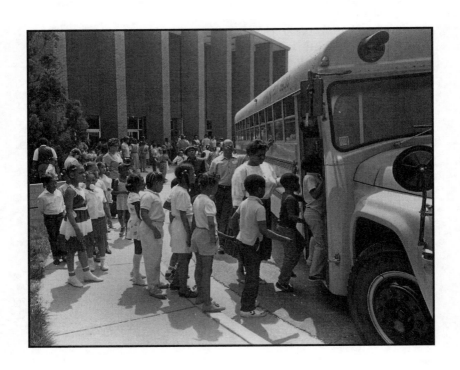

Chapter **4**

Public School Education

In these days, it is doubtful that any child may reasonably be expected to succeed in life if he is denied the opportunity of an education. Such an opportunity, where the state has undertaken to provide it, is a right which must be made available to all on equal terms.

BROWN V. BOARD OF EDUCATION[1]

Education is one of the essential civil rights issues for deaf children and their families. The *Brown v. Board of Education* case was decided in 1954, but many children with disabilities are still denied their right to equal educational opportunity. In 1975 Congress found that more than half of this nation's eight million children with disabilities were not receiving appropriate educational services, and one million were excluded from the public school system entirely.[2] Since then, Congress has taken action to guarantee children the right to qualified teachers, accessible classrooms, and appropriate materials and programs. But parents still have a responsibility to advocate to ensure that their children receive the services they need.

THE INDIVIDUALS WITH DISABILITIES EDUCATION ACT

The Individuals with Disabilities Education Act (IDEA) provides the states with money for special education and imposes procedural and substantive requirements on how that special education should be provided.[3]

The original law (known as the Education for All Handicapped Children Act, or PL 94-142) was passed in 1975, and implemented in 1977. This statute was amended in 1990 and renamed the Individuals with Disabilities Education Act (IDEA). Amendments passed in 1997 attempted to improve educational opportunities for children with disabilities and to give families and other community-based entities a greater role in the decision-making process. In March 1999 the Department of Education issued regulations reflecting the 1997 amendments. The law and its regulations are intended to fulfill four major purposes:

1. to ensure that all children with disabilities have access to a free appropriate public education that emphasizes special education and related services designed to meet their unique needs and prepare them for employment and independent living;
2. to ensure that the rights of children with disabilities and their parents are protected;
3. to assist States, localities, educational service agencies, and Federal agencies to pay for the education of all children with disabilities;
4. to assess and ensure the effectiveness of efforts to educate children with disabilities.[4]

In addition to these federal laws, most states have adopted their own laws or regulations to go along with IDEA requirements. These state laws usually give children with disabilities similar educational rights and establish procedures for getting special education services that meet IDEA standards. In a few states, such as Massachusetts, students are entitled to a higher standard of services than under IDEA.[5]

Defining Children Who are Deaf or Hard of Hearing

The law covers children aged three through twenty-one who need special education and related services because of their disabilities.[6] Infants and toddlers up to age three are also included in IDEA, but under a separate system, discussed below. The law includes children who are deaf or hard of hearing, and other children with disabilities.[7]

Merely having a disability is not enough to qualify for services under IDEA. The disability must affect the child's educational performance, so that the child needs at least some accommodation as a result of the disability. If a child is successfully attending a regular school program without any accommodations or modifications as a result of a disability, then the child is not considered a "child with a disability" for purposes of IDEA.

Appropriate Education and Placement

The heart of the law is the guaranteed right of every child to a free, appropriate public education. Under IDEA and Section 504,

---

Under IDEA

+ "Deafness" means a hearing disability that is so severe that the child is impaired in processing linguistic information through hearing, with or without amplification, and that adversely affects a child's educational performance.
+ "Deaf-blindness" means concomitant hearing and visual impairments, the combination of which causes such severe communication and other developmental and educational needs that they cannot be accommodated in special education programs designed solely for deafness or children with blindness.
+ "Hearing impairment" means a permanent or fluctuating impairment that adversely affects a child's educational performance, but that is not included under the definition of deafness in this section.[8]

every child with a disability has a right to (1) specially designed instruction meeting his or her unique needs and (2) related services that are necessary to help the child benefit from the special program. Moreover, this education must take place in the least restrictive environment. IDEA requires states to ensure that, to the maximum extent possible, children with disabilities are educated with children who are not disabled. Special classes and separate school placements are appropriate only when the disability is of such a nature or severity that placement in regular classes with the use of supplementary aids and services will not meet that child's educational needs. The integration of disabled and nondisabled children in school classrooms is often called "mainstreaming" or "inclusion."

Problems with Total Inclusion

Although mainstreaming can reduce stigma and isolation for many children with disabilities, it is not always appropriate for children who are deaf or hard of hearing. In 1988, the Commission on Education of the Deaf (COED) report warned that mainstreaming has been more detrimental than beneficial for many deaf children.[9] Without substantial support systems and services, placement in a mainstream classroom often constitutes a more socially and educationally restrictive environment for a deaf child than a setting in which the students and teachers have a shared language.

The individual child's specific needs must govern any decision about his or her program. Education consists of more than listening to a teacher. Education involves small group discussions, formal and informal interactions with peers and teachers, physical and recreational education, extracurricular activities and social aspects of learning. There is no one type of placement that is appropriate for all deaf or hard of hearing children. Parents need to be fully involved in determining the placement that will allow the child to achieve the full range of educational goals, and determining the full range of support services that will make that placement successful.

A continuum of alternative placements must be available to meet the needs of children with disabilities. Such placements include mainstream classes, special classes, special schools, residential schools, and combinations of different types of programs. The placement decision is made by a group of people including the parents and representatives of the school district. If this group decides that placement in a special school or residential program is necessary for the child, the program, including travel, tuition, room, and board, must be at no cost to the parents of the child.

THE INDIVIDUALIZED EDUCATIONAL PROGRAM

A school system and the child's parents must devise an appropriate Individualized Education Program (IEP) for each child with a disability. The IEP is a written report that identifies and assesses the child's disability, establishes long- and short-term learning goals, and states which services the school must provide to help the child achieve these goals.[10] Special education and related services are then provided in accordance with the terms of the IEP.

A school violates IDEA if it draws up an IEP and merely presents it to parents for their consent. Parents should work with school officials to develop the plan. The meetings where this work is done should also include the child's current teacher, a representative of the school system who is qualified to provide or supervise the special services, the child (where appropriate), and other people at the discretion of the parents or the school. Parents may ask professional and legal experts to attend the meeting.[11] If the parents are deaf or hard of hearing, the law specifically requires the school system to provide an interpreter or other accommodation so they can participate fully in the meeting. Before the IEP meeting, the parents should exercise their right to review their child's school records to make sure that the information is accurate and complete.[12]

IDEA says that parents must be involved in the identification, evaluation, and placement decisions involving children with disabilities. No child should be placed in a special education program, or have their placement changed, without parental consent. The law requires parents to be fully informed about placement and educational decisions affecting their child.[13]

Contents of the IEP

The IEP must include:

+ a statement of the child's present levels of educational performance;
+ a statement of measurable annual goals, including benchmarks or short-term objectives;
+ a statement of the special education and related services and supplementary aids and services to be provided to the child, or on behalf of the child, and a statement of the program modifications or supports for school personnel that will be provided for the child;
+ an explanation of the extent, if any, to which the children will not participate with nondisabled children in the regular class and in [other] activities;
+ a statement of any individual modifications in the administration of state or district-wide assessment of student achievement that are needed in order for the child to participate in the assessment;
+ the projected dates for the beginning of the services modifications described and the anticipated frequency, location, and duration of those services and modifications; and
+ a statement of how the child's progress toward annual goals will be measured and how the child's parents will be informed of the progress being made.[14]

It is especially important to identify specialized equipment and services early enough so that the school system will have these services in place at the beginning of a school year. IEPs must be reviewed at least once a year, and they should be written in the spring or early summer so they can be implemented when school starts in the fall.

The goals and objectives that are written into the IEP are not limited to academic performance. The goals should relate to social, psychomotor, communication, and emotional needs as well as to conventional academic curriculum goals. The IEP must consider the child's strengths and the results of his or her evaluations before determining the appropriate placement and services. Evaluations and tests used to assess a child must not be discriminatory on a racial or cultural basis and must be performed in the child's native language or other mode of communication.[15]

The IEP is the mechanism parents use to make certain that their child receives an appropriate education. The school is legally required to provide the services that are written into the IEP. Parents should be certain that it includes every special service that the child needs. They should not sign an IEP that does not specify the services they believe the child needs in order to benefit from a special education. Parents who disagree with the proposed service plan should not sign the IEP; they instead should initiate due process procedures (discussed later in this chapter).

Parents should ask for and keep a copy of their child's IEP so they can remember what was agreed upon and hold the school to its promises. If they later have to go to court to obtain the services, the IEP will be the primary item of evidence.

Special Factors

In developing an IEP for a deaf or hard of hearing child, the IEP team must consider the communication needs of the child, including his or her academic level, language and communication needs, and opportunities for direct communication with peers and professional personnel in the child's language and communication mode.[16] These vital aspects of IDEA must be considered to ensure that the deaf or hard of hearing child receives an appropriate education. This may mean that the child needs to be in an environment or classroom that allows the child to speak directly with classmates, teachers, and other personnel in the child's native language (such as sign language or oral communication). To speak directly means to communicate without any third party involvement (i.e., interpreters). If the child is in an environment where direct communication with everyone is not available, an alternative placement may be more appropriate.

Appropriate Language Medium

Controversy over language methods has raged in deaf education programs for years. The original debate was between the efficacy of oral versus sign language. Any consideration of educational methods using manual components is complicated by the existence of sign language variants and by the number of different possible systems for using manual language with children in a learning setting. "Sign language" is a continuum of language systems that can be differentiated by the types of visual components used (signs, fingerspelling, body movement, and facial expression) and by the degree to which a particular system parallels formal English syntax and vocabulary.

American Sign Language (ASL) is linguistically distinct from English and has its own formal syntax, rules of grammar, and idioms. However, a number of other systems used in schools are closely related to English. Some of these are pidgin signed English systems that use signs in a rough approximation of English word order. Other systems have been devised to make English "visible" by providing word-by-word translation of English through signs and fingerspelling, with additional signs to represent word endings and other grammatical forms. Cued Speech is another method that has been introduced in some school systems. Cued Speech is not a language but a system of specific handshapes placed at specific locations around the head; the combination of handshapes and locations represent English sounds. The child speechreads while simultaneously reading the manual cues. Another approach to education is the bilingual approach, which emphasizes both American Sign Language and English and expects the child to become fluent in both languages. (In a bilingual environment, speech is not used simultaneously with ASL.) Finally, some programs for deaf children are purely oral and emphasize the use of residual hearing and speechreading.

In determining the proper educational program and writing the IEP, the critical first step is to identify the language medium appropriate for that child. What is best varies from child to child, depending on his or her native language, the amount and type of residual hearing (if any), the level of the child's communication skills, his or her exposure to manual communication methods, age of onset of deafness, the primary language used by the child's family, and other conditions. What is found to be appropriate should be spelled out in the IEP. If interpreters or teachers will be using sign language, the IEP should also identify the minimum skill level or competency they should have. In a few states, such as Texas, efforts have been made to identify levels of sign language or interpreter competency using state tests.[17] Such criteria should be included in an IEP whenever possible, to assure that teachers and interpreters working with a child will be able to communicate effectively.

Selecting the proper communication medium is important because it makes instruction possible and meaningful. All educators of deaf children are concerned with maximizing the child's use and understanding of the English language. A related but more immediate goal is to make what happens in the classroom accessible to that child. With some children, this might mean providing only a hearing aid; other children will require both an aid and a sign language interpreter; and still others will need a special teacher, a modified curriculum, and a range of support services. The IEP should spell out the individual child's communication requirements.

Assistive Technology and Related Services

The IEP must be worded to ensure the deaf child access to related services and communication technology in the classroom. IDEA specifically mentions speech-language and audiology services, psychological and counseling services, physical and occupational therapy, recreation, early identification, orientation and mobility services, school health services, social work services, and parent counseling and training.[18]

However, this list is not comprehensive and therefore other services can and should be included in the IEP. Typical related services for deaf and hard of hearing children include amplifiers (e.g., hearing aids and/or assistive listening systems), computer-aided, real-time transcription (CART) services, software and computer hardware, and interpreters. Some deaf children benefit from having supplementary hearing devices that range from conventional hearing aids to specialized auditory training devices and amplification equipment. In addition to these services and technologies, a child may need special services to increase his or her use of residual hearing. These services should be specified in the IEP and provided as part of the child's program.

For example, control of background noise may be essential if a child is to receive the full benefit of a hearing aid. If so, this need should be identified so the school can take appropriate steps to improve acoustics in the rooms the child will be using. The Access Board is currently working with private industry to develop standards on classroom acoustics. In a November 1999 *Federal Register* notice, the Access Board announced that it will work with a group headed by the American National Standards Institute (ANSI) and the Acoustical Society of America to develop a standard. According to the Access Board, recent research has shown that "high levels of background noise in classrooms, much of it from heating and cooling systems, significantly compromise speech intelligibility for many young children in classrooms."[19]

Improved lighting also may be necessary to ensure that information presented visually is clear and understandable. Speech therapy, auditory training, and media support services (such as captioned TV and films) are other services that a deaf child might need; if so, these services should be written into the IEP. Related services also include audiology services, interpreters, counseling for parents and the child, and parental training to help parents acquire the necessary skills that will allow them to support the implementation of the child's IEP. The school may have to provide sign language education and training for parents and families to ensure that the child continues language development and educational progress at home.

The school must ensure that the child's hearing aids and other assistive technology devices are functioning properly and are available at no cost if the IEP determines that those devices are necessary. If the IEP also determines that the use of those devices are required in a child's home or in other settings in order for the child to continue to receive access to an appropriate education, the school must allow the child or the parents to take those devices outside the school environment.[20]

Qualified Professional

Childhood deafness is a low-incidence disability. Most school systems have relatively few deaf children in each age group, a factor that increases the difficulty of providing properly trained teachers and highly specialized, related services to ensure an appropriate education in mainstream classes.

A position paper of the International Association of Parents of the Deaf (now the American Society for Deaf Children) noted:

> Currently, many local and public schools lack qualified diagnostic staff for making the placement, lack supportive services, lack trained personnel, lack necessary amplification equipment and a desirable visual environment, lack an understanding of total communication which may be essential for communication with students, and in many cases, lack financial resources required for the education of deaf children and lack commitment.[21]

Although this statement was made in 1976, these problems still exist. School systems are required by law to evaluate children for hearing loss, to create special programs to prevent hearing loss, and to provide counseling and guidance to students, parents, and teachers on issues related to hearing loss. They are responsible for determining a child's need for amplification, for selecting and fitting an appropriate aid, and for evaluating the effectiveness of the amplification. These responsibilities can overwhelm teachers and administrators who lack special training. Opportunities for such training must be made available to school staff so they may become more knowledgeable about deafness and other disabilities, the range of possible solutions and accommodations, and how they may best meet their responsibilities under the law. It may be appropriate for a school system to require in-service training, special certification, and fluency in sign language for teachers who will be working with deaf students.

Personnel providing special education or related services must meet the state educational agency's recognized certification, licensing, registration, or other comparable requirements. This could mean the requirement of certified educators of deaf and hard of hearing children, certified sign language interpreters and licensed audiologists.

SUPREME COURT DECISIONS

In June 1982, the U.S. Supreme Court decided its first case involving IDEA. The case was *Board of Education of the Hendrick Hudson Central School District v. Rowley.* Lower courts had ruled that Amy Rowley, a mainstreamed elementary school student, required a sign language interpreter to make classroom instruction fully accessible. The Supreme Court affirmed the right of all children with disabilities to receive personalized instruction and the support services they need to benefit from their educational program. In Rowley's particular case, however, the Court found that Rowley did not need an interpreter because she was doing well in school without one. The Court said that Rowley was receiving sufficient other support services (i.e., a phonic ear listening device and a personal tutor) to enable her to benefit from her education.[22]

The Court's decision does not mean that other deaf children will be unable to get interpreter services. It merely means children must show that they cannot benefit from their education without such a service. Rowley's speechreading skills, residual hearing, and high intelligence made her a special case.

A majority of the Court found that Congress did not intend to give children with disabilities a right to "strict equality of opportunity or services" because that would require impossible measurements and comparisons. But IDEA does require access to a free, appropriate public education that is "meaningful." The

Court held that a state ". . . satisfies this requirement by providing personalized instruction with sufficient supportive services to permit the child to benefit educationally from that instruction."[23]

The Court upheld the major purposes of IDEA as outlined previously in this chapter. The IEP and the due process hearing for parents were not changed. They remain at the heart of the law and continue to give parents the opportunity to prove that their child needs a particular service or program.

Other Supreme Court decisions support a child's right to related services necessary for "meaningful access" to education. In *Irving Independent School District v. Tatro*, the Court held that a school district must provide a child who has spina bifida with catheterization so that she could remain at school during the day.[24] In 1999, the Court ruled that a school system must provide extensive nursing services to medically fragile students, so that they can attend school in regular settings.[25] This decision sends a clear signal that a school system may not refuse to provide services based on the cost or the "burden" of providing related services.

INFANTS AND TODDLERS

Education begins at birth, and for parents of deaf and hard of hearing children, this period is of special importance because it is the time of optimal language learning. Although the responsibilities of school systems under IDEA do not begin until a child reaches age three, the federal government does provide money to states for the provision of programs and services to children with special needs from birth to age three. Each state participating in this program must offer a comprehensive statewide interagency system for providing "early intervention services" for toddlers and infants with disabilities and their families. Eligible children are those experiencing developmental delays in cognitive, physical, communication, social or emotional development, or those who have a physical or mental condition that has a high probability of developmental delays.[26]

Although in some states the services for infants and toddlers are managed through the state department of education, in other states they are provided through the state health or social service agency. The tool for identifying services for a child younger than age three is an Individualized Family Service Plan (IFSP). Like the IEP, an IFSP must be developed at least once a year. It should cover:

+ any necessary family training, counseling, special instruction, speech-language and audiology services;
+ occupational therapy, physical therapy, psychological services;
+ diagnostic medical services, health services, social work, vision services, and assistive technology devices and services; and
+ transportation, day care and related costs that are necessary for the child's family to take advantage of these services.

Each IFSP must include:

+ a statement of the child's present levels of development;
+ a statement of the family's resources, priorities and concerns as they relate to the child's development;
+ a statement of major outcomes expected for the child and the family, and how and when they should be achieved;
+ a statement of which early intervention services are to be provided;
+ a statement of the setting in which the services will be provided, and a justification for any services that will not be provided in a "natural environment";
+ a statement of when services will begin and how long they will continue; and
+ the name of the case manager responsible for carrying out the provisions of the IFSP and the steps to be taken to help the child transition to a preschool program.

The team that develops the IFSP must include the child's parents; other family members or an advocate whose participation is requested by the parent; the service coordinator; a person directly involved in conducting the evaluation of the child; and any appropriate service providers. Interpreters must be provided for deaf parents.

PROCEDURAL SAFEGUARDS

IDEA provides procedural safeguards by which parents can be assured of both their own participation in the decision-making process and an appropriate education for their child.[27] A school system must give written notice to parents when it wishes to initiate or change the identification, evaluation, or placement of a child with a disability. The notice must describe procedural protections, the action that the school system proposes or refuses to take, and its reasons. The notice must also describe any options the school system considered and explain why those options were rejected, and describe each evaluation procedure, test, record, report, or other relevant factor the school system used as a basis for the proposed change.

The notice must be written in language understandable to the general public and provided in the parents' native language(s) or any other form of communication used by the parents. If the native language is not a written language, the school system has to translate the notice and ensure that the parents understand it. For example, a qualified sign language interpreter must translate and explain the notice to deaf parents who communicate in sign language.

If the parents do not accept the school system's evaluation and proposed placement or if they are not confident that the school system has the resources to provide an appropriate education, they can request a due process hearing. They simply notify the school officials that they are dissatisfied, state their reasons, and ask for a hearing. The hearing and a final decision must be completed within forty-five days of the request. The due process hearing is intended to be an informal dispute-resolution process during which both the parents and the school can present their grievances to a neutral hearing officer. As a practical matter, both parents and school systems are often represented by attorneys. A neutral hearing officer is appointed according to procedures established by the state. Public agencies must keep a list of hearing officers and their qualifications.

Preparation for the Hearing

There are several steps to be taken in preparation for the hearing. One essential step is to find experts in education who can testify in support of the parents' position that the placement is inappropriate. The expert should visit the proposed and current placements before the hearing in order to testify whether the proposed placement can meet the specific needs of that individual child. The parents themselves should visit the proposed placement and see how the IEP could be implemented with the school's resources.

The parents also should examine all school records relevant to their child's placement. Under IDEA, the school system must comply with any reasonable request by the parents to inspect and receive an explanation of their child's records before any hearing. If the parents believe that information in the file is incorrect, they can request amendment of the record. If the parents disagree with the educational evaluation of their child, they have the right to an independent evaluation; the school system is required to take this evaluation into account in deciding the child's placement. Well before the hearing date, the parents should request a list of witnesses who will be testifying for the school.

The key issue at the hearing is whether the proposed placement or service is appropriate to meet the individual needs of the child. At the hearing, the parents can have a lawyer and can call witnesses who are experts in educating children with disabilities. They also have the right to present evidence and to confront and cross-examine any of the witnesses.

Parents can obtain a written or electronic verbatim record of the hearing, which is important in an appeal. The hearing officer must provide written findings of fact explaining his or her decision. Until a decision is rendered, the child must remain in the present educational placement unless the school and the parents agree otherwise. If, however, the complaint involves application for initial admission to public school, the child must be placed in the public school program until completion of all proceedings.

Decisions and Appeals

The hearing officer has the authority to determine the appropriate placement for the child and is not restricted to merely accepting or rejecting the school's program. The hearing officer can order services that are necessary to provide a free, appropriate education for the child. The decision of the hearing officer is final and must be obeyed by the school system, unless it is appealed to the state department of education or the courts.

If an appeal is made to the state education agency, the agency must conduct an impartial review of the decision. The official who conducts the review must:

+ examine the entire hearing record,
+ ensure that the procedures at the hearing were consistent with the due process requirements of the law,
+ seek additional evidence if necessary,
+ afford the parties an opportunity for oral or written argument or both,
+ make an independent decision on completion of the review, and
+ give a copy of written findings and the decision to the parties.

The parents may file a civil lawsuit in state or federal court to challenge the decision of the state agency.

GENERAL ACCESSIBILITY ISSUES: SECTION 504 AND THE ADA

Both public and private schools are subject to the civil rights mandates of the ADA and, if they receive any federal funding, to Section 504 of the Rehabilitation Act. Therefore, schools have the duty to be accessible to people with disabilities.

The ADA and Section 504 apply to all programs and activities offered by a private school or a public school system, including school board meetings, extracurricular programs, teacher conferences, recreational activities, social and cultural activities, adult education, summer school or hobby classes, and children's education programs. Title II of the ADA applies to public school systems. Title III of the ADA applies to all types of private schools and educational programs, for children and adults. Section 504 of the Rehabilitation Act of 1973 applies to school systems and educational agencies (public and private) that receive federal financial assistance, including the federally subsidized school lunch program.

In the Department of Education's Section 504 regulation, public elementary and secondary schools are required to provide a "free, appropriate public education" to qualified children with disabilities, regardless of the nature of their disability.[28] This means that any children with disabilities must be able to participate in a curriculum designed to meet their unique needs, at no cost. If the school system refuses to provide an appropriate education, the Department of Education can cut off federal funds.

Although IDEA governs the provision of most special educational services, Section 504 and the ADA provide additional protection, especially in the context of private schools, architectural accessibility, extracurricular activities, summer programs, adult education, and services for parents, school personnel, and other adults.

The ADA regulations specifically address a school's obligation to remove communication barriers for deaf individuals by providing "appropriate auxiliary aids and services" so that deaf people can participate in the program.[29] The appropriate auxiliary aid depends on the context of the communication and the needs of the individuals. For example, in a school auditorium or a school board meeting, some deaf people may need a sign language interpreter to follow and participate in the proceedings. Other people may need a computer-assisted, real-time transcript (CART) system or an assistive listening device in order to understand and participate in the same activity. If the school has videotapes or films, or if it broadcasts on cable television, captioning is the most appropriate way to give access to deaf viewers. The primary concern is whether or not the auxiliary aid or service is effective and gives the person an opportunity to participate effectively.

Schools must be accessible to parents and the general public as well as to students. The Department of Justice states that school systems must provide auxiliary aids to provide accessibility to parents and other adults with disabilities:

> Some commenters asked for clarification about the responsibilities of public school systems under Section 504 and the ADA with respect to programs, services and activities that are not covered by the Individuals with Disabilities Education Act (IDEA), including, for example, programs open to parents or to the public, graduation ceremonies, parent-teacher organization meetings, plays, and other events open to the public, and adult education classes. Public school systems must comply with the ADA in all of their services, programs, or activities, including those that are open to parents or to the public. For instance, public school systems must provide program accessibility to parents and guardians with disabilities to these programs, activities, or services, and appropriate auxiliary aids and services whenever necessary to ensure effective communication, as long as the provision of the auxiliary aid results neither in an undue burden or in a fundamental alteration of the program.[30]

A federal court has ruled that school systems must provide interpreters when deaf parents meet with teachers or attend school programs such as orientation programs.[31] The Department of Education's Office for Civil Rights has held that Parent Teacher Association (PTA) programs and activities are covered by the ADA because the school district provides significant indirect assistance to the PTA.[32]

In order to ensure that deaf individuals are alerted to a fire or other emergency, school systems should install visual (flashing) fire alarms in areas used by deaf students. Examples of additional accommodations include amplification systems that are compatible with hearing aids and entry systems that do not depend on ability to use an intercom or respond to a buzzer or other auditory device. A TTY may also be necessary, so that the school and parent can communicate directly about illnesses, schedules, discipline of a child and other problems.

Any time a school building is altered or constructed, the building must meet the minimum standards in the ADA accessibility guidelines (ADAAG) or the Uniform Federal Accessibility Standards. The Access Board is proposing changes to the current ADAAG. These architectural accessibility standards may require a school to make structural changes to provide equal access to everyone.

NOTES

1. 375 U.S. 438 at 493 (1954).
2. 20 U.S.C. §1401.
3. 20 U.S.C. §1401 et seq.
4. 34 C.F.R. §300.1.
5. Mass. Gen. L. ch. 71B §2 (1999).
6. 34 C.F.R. §300.7.
7. IDEA also includes children with mental retardation, speech or language impairments, serious emotional disturbance, orthopedic impairments, autism, traumatic brain injury, other health impairments, and specific learning disabilities (20 U.S.C. §1401).
8. 34 C.F.R. §300.7.
9. Commission on Education of the Deaf, Toward Equality: Education of the Deaf. A Report to the President and the Congress of the United States (Washington, D.C., 1988), 30–34.
10. 34 C.F.R. §300.347.
11. 34 C.F.R. §300.344.
12. 34 C.F.R. §300.345.
13. Ibid.
14. 34 C.F.R. §300.347.
15. 34 C.F.R. §300.346.
16. 34 C.F.R. §346(a)(2)(iv).
17. Texas Hum. Res. §81.007 (1997).
18. 34 C.F.R. §300.24.
19. *64 Fed. Reg.* 60,753 (November 9, 1999).
20. 34 C.F.R. §300.308.
21. International Association of Parents of the Deaf, October 1976 position statement.
22. *Board of Education of the Hendrick Hudson Central School District v. Rowley,* 102 S.Ct. 3034 (U.S. 1982).
23. Ibid.
24. *Irving Independent School District v. Tatro,* 104 S.Ct. 3371 (U.S. 1984).
25. *Cedar Rapids Community Sch. Dist. v. Garret F.,* 119 S.Ct. 992 (U.S. 1999).

26. 34 C.F.R. Part 303.
27. 34 C.F.R. §300.500–.517.
28. 34 C.F.R. §104.33.
29. 28 C.F.R. §35.104; 28 C.F.R. §36.303.
30. *56 Fed. Reg.* 35,696 (July 26, 1991); see analysis to ADA's Title II regulations.
31. *Rothschild v. Grottenthaler,* 907 F 2d. 886 (2d. Cir. 1990).
32. Irvine Unified School District, 19 IDELR 883 (OCR 1993).

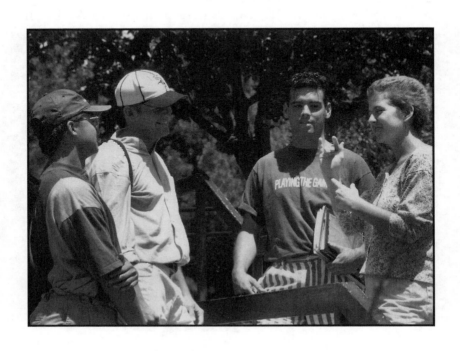

Chapter 5

Postsecondary Education

$\iff$

Since 1973, Section 504 of the Rehabilitation Act has helped make postsecondary education accessible to people with disabilities.[1] Basically, Section 504 requires institutions that receive federal money, including vocational and commercial schools, to not discriminate against students with disabilities in recruitment, admissions, and programs. The Americans with Disabilities Act (ADA) has expanded this requirement to many other schools and universities, both public and private.[2] The ADA now requires that all postsecondary education institutions be accessible, regardless of whether or not they receive federal financial assistance. To accommodate a person with a disability, a college or university is not obligated to substantially change the requirements of its academic program; it must, however, afford equal opportunity for the person to benefit from the program, without segregation from the other students or limits on participation. Auxiliary aids are mandated by the ADA and Section 504, and methods of evaluation are required to measure the student's actual achievement and not his or her ability to take tests.

RECRUITMENT AND ADMISSIONS

Educational institutions may neither refuse to admit applicants because of their disabilities nor subject them to any form of discrimination in admission or recruitment procedures.[3] If the college or university requires pre-admission interviews, a deaf applicant must be interviewed too, with interpreters provided. If there are tours or orientation meetings, the deaf applicant must be able to participate with an interpreter present. If a college sends promotional information or makes recruitment visits to area high schools, then it must do the same for area deaf schools. The institution cannot place a limit or quota on the number or proportion of students with disabilities who may be admitted.

In addition, colleges and universities are generally prohibited from making pre-admission inquiries about disabilities, except in two rare situations: (a) when the school is taking remedial action to overcome the effects of past discrimination, or (b) when it is taking voluntary action to overcome the effects of conditions in the past that limited the participation of persons with disabilities.[4] In either of these circumstances, the school must clearly state that the information sought is intended for use only in connection with remedial or voluntary action.

Educational institutions must ensure that admissions tests are selected and administered so that the test results accurately reflect the applicant's actual aptitude or achievement level and not the effects of his or her hearing loss.[5] For example, oral instructions should be translated into sign language or put into writing. Oral examinations should be conducted with a qualified sign language interpreter or other appropriate aid. If a test is designed to measure some area other than English language skills, then the test should be modified for a deaf applicant who does not have standard English skills. The college might allow the student to take more time or to take a test that is less reliant on English competence.

SUPREME COURT CASE

The issue of preadmission inquiries about disabilities was decided in 1979 by the United States Supreme Court. In its first ruling on the merits of a case brought under Section 504—in *Southeastern Community College v. Davis*—the Court held that a nursing school could require "reasonable physical qualifications for admission to a clinical training program" and reject a student whose disability would require substantial modifications of the program.[6]

The issue in *Davis* was whether Section 504 forbids professional schools from imposing physical qualifications for admission to their clinical training programs. In its decision, the Court also sought to clarify the meaning of "qualified individual with a disability" in postsecondary education and the extent of affirmative relief required by Section 504.

Frances Davis, a licensed practical nurse who was hard of hearing, sought to enroll in a nursing school program to become a registered nurse. Despite evidence that she could perform well in this program, Southeastern Community College rejected Ms. Davis's application due to her hearing disability.

A federal district court in North Carolina upheld the college's decision, noting that in settings such as an operating room, intensive care unit, or postnatal care unit, wearing a surgical mask would prevent Ms. Davis from speechreading to understand what was happening. The court concluded that Ms. Davis's "handicap actually prevents her from safely performing in both her training program and her proposed profession."[7]

The United States Court of Appeals for the Fourth Circuit reversed the decision.[8] In light of the HEW Section 504 regulation (issued after the district court's decision), the appeals court ruled that the college had to reconsider Ms. Davis's application without regard to her hearing disability. The appeals court concluded that the district court erred in considering the nature of Ms. Davis's hearing to determine whether she was "otherwise qualified" for the program rather than limiting its inquiry to her "academic and technical qualifications," which is the requirement of the 504 regulation. Because the college said that it was not prepared to modify its nursing program to accommodate Ms. Davis's hearing disability, the appeals court sent the case back to the district court for it to consider what modifications required by the HEW regulation might accommodate Ms. Davis.

The U.S. Supreme Court agreed to review the case and found

unanimously that the college had not violated Section 504. The Court held that:

> Nothing in the language or history of §504 reflects the intention to limit the freedom of an educational institution to require reasonable physical qualifications for admission to a clinical training program. Nor has there been any showing in this case that any action short of a substantial change in Southeastern's program would render unreasonable the qualifications it imposed.[9]

Writing for the Supreme Court, Justice Lewis Powell found that Section 504 does not compel schools to disregard an applicant's disabilities "or to make *substantial* modifications in their programs to allow disabled persons to participate" [emphasis added].[10] Instead, the Court interpreted Section 504 to mean that mere possession of a disability is not a permissible ground for assuming an inability to function in a particular context.[11]

The Supreme Court also found that under Section 504, an "otherwise handicapped person" is "one who is able to meet all of a program's requirements in spite of his handicap."[12] Ms. Davis was considered unable to meet those requirements since "the ability to understand speech without reliance on lipreading is necessary for patient safety during the clinical phase of the program."[13] The Court stated that on the basis of meager evidence contained in the trial record, it was unlikely that Ms. Davis could successfully participate in the clinical program with any of the accommodations the regulation requires. The Court concluded that either close individual supervision or changing the curriculum to limit her participation to academic classes exceeded the "modification" required by the regulation.

The Supreme Court noted, however, that continuing some requirements may wrongly exclude qualified people with disabilities from participating in programs: "Thus situations may arise where a refusal to modify an existing program might become unreasonable and discriminatory. Identification of these instances where a refusal to accommodate the needs of a disabled person amounts to discrimination against the handicapped continues to be an important responsibility of HEW."[14]

Section 504 Upheld

A significant step forward was the U.S. Supreme Court's 1985 opinion in *Alexander v. Choate.*[15] This case makes clear that Section 504 is not a hollow promise, but a major civil rights statute with teeth.

In *Choate,* the Supreme Court decided that Section 504 requires recipients of federal funding to make reasonable accommodation "to assure meaningful access" to their programs. Support for its view was found in the section's regulations requiring reasonable accommodation in employment, buildings, colleges, and universities.

Significantly, the Court also ruled that federal recipients may be guilty of discrimination when their actions have a discriminatory effect, even if there is no proof they actually intended to discriminate. Justice Thurgood Marshall, writing for the Supreme Court, stated that Congress often saw discrimination against people with disabilities as a result of "thoughtlessness and indifference."[16] The Court pointed out that it would be difficult, if not impossible, to stop discrimination if people with disabilities had to prove that someone actually intended to discriminate against them.

TREATMENT OF STUDENTS

Students with disabilities at colleges and universities must be treated equally with nondisabled students.[17] Programs must be conducted in an integrated setting. Separate facilities for students with disabilities are not permitted.[18] Postsecondary institutions must also ensure that other programs in which students with disabilities participate do not discriminate.[19] Examples of other programs are internships, clinical placement programs, student teaching assignments, or course work at other schools in a consortium. The recipient institution may not continue its relationships with any program that in any way discriminates against students with disabilities.

Colleges and universities must make adjustments to academic requirements that discriminate against a student with a disability.[20] For example, a deaf student should be allowed to substitute a music history or art appreciation course for a required course in music appreciation. Some schools waive foreign language requirements for deaf students or allow them to substitute sign language courses. The individual capabilities and needs of each student must be considered and academic adjustments made as appropriate. Since the *Davis* decision, however, a college is not required to make substantial modifications in its program in order to accommodate students with disabilities. Nor is a college required to change those academic requirements that the college can prove are essential either to the program of instruction or for a particular degree.[21]

Case Study

The issues addressed in *Davis* dealing with the qualifications of a deaf student to participate in a postsecondary education program are best illustrated in one of the first ADA cases to go to jury trial.

Nadelle Grantham was a deaf student who communicated via speechreading, sign language, and speaking, and she used a sign language interpreter for her academic classes. Her career goal was to teach English to deaf children in a public school setting. Her plan was to receive a degree in elementary education from Southeastern Louisiana University (SLU) in Hammond, Louisiana, and then acquire an "add-on" certification for teaching deaf children.

In 1990, Ms. Grantham began taking pre-education courses at SLU. On her application to SLU, Ms. Grantham stated that she intended to major in elementary education. The Louisiana Division of Rehabilitation Services listed Ms. Grantham's career goal as "Teacher of the Deaf (specifically, teaching English to deaf students)," and her major as elementary education. That agency provided sign language interpreter services and note takers while Ms. Grantham was enrolled at SLU.

After being accepted into the SLU Teacher Education Program, Ms. Grantham wrote to the department chairperson, asking to substitute another class for a music class. SLU denied the request. Subsequently, the dean of the College of Education advised Ms. Grantham that she was expelled from the teacher education program based on "concerns about (your) profound hearing impairment . . . concerns about (your) ability to perform the essential functions of a lower elementary teacher in a regular, multi-disciplinary classroom setting," and "concerns over the health and safety of students under (your) supervision in the pre-teaching experience."

Ms. Grantham filed a lawsuit under Title II of the ADA. She was represented by the NAD Law Center and the Advocacy Center for the Elderly and Disabled in New Orleans, Louisiana. Ms. Grantham also took classes at another university which were equivalent to the SLU lower elementary education courses.

At the time of the trial, nine witnesses testified for Ms. Grantham, including experts from Gallaudet University and Lamar University, who testified that Ms. Grantham was qualified for the elementary education program based on her academic performance, as well as the following facts:

+ the few accommodations she required were not difficult or burdensome;
+ SLU would not have to lower its academic standards or substantially modify its elementary education program; and
+ she could perform student teaching in an elementary classroom safely and competently.

The defendants in the case relied on *Davis*. A jury found that the defendants violated the ADA by expelling Ms. Grantham from the lower education program because of her deafness. The jury awarded Ms. Grantham $181,000 in damages.[22] The United States Court of Appeals for the Fifth Circuit affirmed the jury verdict.[23]

The case demonstrates that professional educators may not rely on stereotypical assumptions that are not truly indicative of a deaf individual's ability to participate in a college program.

AUXILIARY AIDS

As a recipient of federal funds, a postsecondary institution has an obligation under Section 504 to be accessible to students with disabilities. As part of this obligation, the Department of Education has determined that colleges and universities must provide necessary auxiliary aids and services, including interpreter services for deaf students.[24] The department's analysis to the Section 504 regulation notes:

> Under §104.44(d), a recipient must ensure that no handicapped student is subject to discrimination in the recipient's program because of the absence of necessary auxiliary educational aids. Colleges and universities expressed concern about the costs of compliance with this provision. The Department emphasizes that recipients can usually meet this obligation by assisting students in using existing resources for auxiliary aids, such as state vocational rehabilitation agencies and private charitable organizations. Indeed, the Department anticipates that the bulk of auxiliary aids will be paid for by private agencies, not by colleges and universities.[25]

Many deaf students are eligible for vocational rehabilitation assistance, which should include interpreter services. However, when the student is not a vocational rehabilitation client, or when funding for interpreters is not forthcoming from vocational rehabilitation, the institution may be responsible for this expense.

The second federal statute which creates the obligation to provide auxiliary aids for colleges and universities is Title II of the ADA (public universities) and Title III of the ADA (private universities).[26] State, community, and private colleges and universities must provide auxiliary aids and services to ensure effective communication with deaf and hard of hearing people.[27] The ADA also requires the removal of structural communication barriers that are in existing facilities.[28]

A comprehensive list of auxiliary aids and services is set forth in the Justice Department's ADA rule, discussed in chapter 2.[29]

For many sign language users, the only effective way to achieve effective communication is through the use of qualified interpreters.[30] In addition to an interpreter, the student will need a competent note taker, because it is impossible to simultaneously watch an interpreter and take notes.

For deaf and hard of hearing people who do not use sign language, a college or university can provide a computer-assisted, real-time transcript (CART) system. A trained stenographer types everything spoken during a class into a computer, which simultaneously converts the stenographer's notes to a written English transcript on a computer screen. In some situations, this system is preferable to a sign language interpreter because it gives the student the exact language of the course. For people who do not use sign language, the CART system may be the best way to ensure effective communication.

COURT DECISIONS

As described in the cases that follow, several courts have decided that a student's college or vocational rehabilitation (VR) agency must cover interpreting expenses. One appellate court found that it is a VR agency's legal duty to pay for interpreters based on Title I of the Rehabilitation Act.[31] A second appellate court held that when a student is a VR client, the state VR agency has primary responsibility under Section 504 to pay for interpreter services for the student's classes.[32]

The first of these two appellate court cases involved Ruth Ann Schornstein, a deaf VR client. Shornstein attended Kean College in New Jersey. Her plan was to earn a college degree in social work/psychology. The New Jersey Division of Vocational Rehabilitation Services accepted Ms. Schornstein as an eligible VR client and developed an individual rehabilitation plan to meet her vocational goal. Although the state agency provided tuition and books, interpreter services were denied. All groups involved agreed she needed an interpreter to participate effectively in her classes.

The National Association of the Deaf Legal Defense Fund (now the NAD Law Center) filed a lawsuit against both the state agency and Kean College. The federal court held that the state agency's policy denying interpreter services to every deaf college student violates Title I of the Rehabilitation Act. Title I requires state VR agencies to provide certain rehabilitation services, including interpreters, to VR clients. The federal court ruled that the state agency policy "completely contradicts the Act's requirements which ensure individualization of programs for handicapped individuals." The district court opinion was affirmed by an appellate court.

The state agency argued that it could decide what services to provide. The court was not persuaded. It found that the Rehabilitation Act specifically requires VR agencies to (1) serve individuals with severe disabilities, including deaf people, first; and (2) provide those services listed in the Rehabilitation Act that are necessary to assist people with disabilities to achieve his or her vocational goal.

Because the state agency accepted Ms. Schornstein as a client and also agreed that she required interpreter services to meet her vocational goals, the court concluded that the agency was legally obligated to provide those services. Since the court decided the case solely on the basis of Title I, it did not find it necessary to rule on the obligation to provide interpreters under either Section 504 or the U.S. Constitution.

In the second case, a deaf student majoring in mechanical engineering at the Illinois Institute of Technology in Chicago needed an interpreter in order to understand and participate in his classes. Although he was an eligible VR client receiving tuition, room and board, and books from the Illinois Department of Rehabilitation Services, the VR agency refused to provide him with interpreters. The college also refused to provide interpreter services.

An Illinois federal court stated that when a student is a VR client, the state VR agency has primary responsibility under Section 504 to pay for interpreter services for the student's classes. The court said that if the student is not a VR client and no other sources are available, then the college has the ultimate responsibility to pay for interpreter services. The Illinois VR agency tried unsuccessfully to persuade the court that it was prohibited from providing interpreters to the student under Title I, if other "similar benefit" programs or community resources were available to pay for these services. The VR agency claimed that the college had a legal obligation under Section 504 to provide interpreters to deaf students; as a "similar benefit" program or community resource, the college should have to pay for those interpreters. The court found that only other rehabilitation services were intended by Congress to be "similar benefit" programs. A federal appeals court affirmed the district court decision.

Other courts have also held colleges and universities responsible for providing their students with interpreting services.[33] In a case the Justice Department brought against the University of Alabama, the U.S. Court of Appeals for the Eleventh Circuit held that the university must provide qualified interpreters for deaf students, even if the students do not have financial need and even if the students are in part-time or other special non-credit categories.[34] The court held that Congress intended colleges and universities to provide free auxiliary aids for students because without this assistance, a deaf student is denied meaningful access to an opportunity to learn.

In *Camenisch v. University of Texas,* the U.S. Court of Appeals for the Fifth Circuit upheld a district court's preliminary injunction requiring the University of Texas to provide an interpreter to a deaf student.[35] The court also ruled that people with disabilities have a right to sue in federal court to enforce their Section 504 rights. Furthermore, said the court, a person with a disability does not have to exhaust administrative remedies before bringing a lawsuit.

The university appealed to the Supreme Court. After accepting the case, the Court refused to decide the Section 504 issues raised by the university.[36] Instead, it sent the case back to the district court to decide whether the university or Camenisch had to pay for the interpreter. The Court held that the university had only appealed a preliminary injunction order and had not waited for a trial on the merits. The Court found the case moot, because the terms of the preliminary injunction had been fulfilled with Camenisch having been provided an interpreter and having already graduated.

Despite these holdings, the allocation of responsibility between state institutions and vocational rehabilitation agencies has been affected by the 1998 amendments to Title I of the Rehabilitation Act, which may transfer responsibility for providing certain services to public colleges.[37] The amendments do not affect the responsibility of vocational rehabilitation agencies for students attending private institutions. As of the time this book went to print, no court had analyzed the impact of these changes for deaf students.

NOTES

1. 29 U.S. Code §794.
2. 42 U.S.C. §12131; 42 U.S.C. §12181.
3. 28 C.F.R. §36.301; 34 C.F.R. §104.42.
4. 34 C.F.R. §104.42(c).
5. 28 C.F.R. §36.309; 34 C.F.R. §104.35.
6. 442 U.S. 397 (1979).
7. 424 F. Supp. 1341, 1345 (E.D.N.C. 1976).
8. 574 F.2d 1158 (4th Cir. 1978).
9. 442 U.S. at 414.
10. 442 U.S. at 405.
11. 442 U.S. at 405.
12. 442 U.S. at 406.
13. 442 U.S. at 307.
14. 442 U.S. at 412–413.
15. *Alexander v. Choate,* 469 U.S. 287 (1985).
16. 469 U.S. 295 (1985).
17. 28 C.F.R. §§36.201, 36.202; 34 C.F.R. §104.43.
18. 28 C.F.R. §36.203; 34 C.F.R. §104.43(c), (d).
19. 34 C.F.R. §104.43(b).
20. 34 C.F.R. §104.44(a).
21. 42 *Fed. Reg.* 22,692 (May 4, 1977).
22. *Grantham v. Moffett et al.,* Civ. A. No.93–4007 (E.D. La. May 23, 1995).
23. *Grantham v. Moffett et al.,* 101 F.3d 698 (5th Cir. 1996).
24. 34 C.F.R. §104.44(d).
25. 45 *Fed. Reg.* 30,954 (Friday, May 9, 1980).
26. 42 U.S.C. §12131; 42 U.S.C. §12181.
27. 28 C.F.R. §§35.160, 36.303.
28. 28 C.F.R. §§35.150, 36.304.

29. See 28 C.F.R. §303(b)(1).
30. 28 C.F.R. §36.104.
31. *Schornstein v. The New Jersey Division of Vocational Rehabilitation Services*, 519 F. Supp. 773 (D.N.J., 1982, affirmed 688 F.2d 824 (3d Cir. 1982).
32. *Jones v. Illinois Department of Rehabilitation Services*, 504 F. Supp. 1244 (N.D. Ill. 1981), affirmed, 689 F.2d 724 (7th Cir. 1982).
33. *Crawford v. University of North Carolina*, 440 F. Supp. 1047 (M.D.N.C. 1977); *Barnes v. Converse College*, 436 F. Supp. 635 (District of South Carolina 1977).
34. *United States v. Board of Trustees for the University of Alabama*, 908 F.2d 740 (11th Cir. 1990).
35. 616 F.2d 127 (5th Cir. 1980).
36. *University of Texas v. Camenisch*, 451 U.S. 390 (1981).
37. PL 105–220, §101(8)(C).

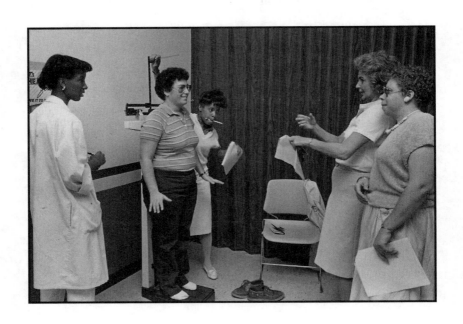

Chapter 6

Health Care and
Social Services

Federal law ensures meaningful access to the complicated web of public and private health care and social services available in most communities. Many agencies receive significant federal assistance and must therefore comply with Section 504 of the Rehabilitation Act of 1973. In addition to Section 504 obligations, public and private health care providers must also comply with the Americans with Disabilities Act of 1990 (ADA). Together, these federal laws require public and private agencies to provide auxiliary aids and services to people with disabilities. Providers are not allowed to discriminate against people with disabilities. Federal law requires them to ensure that their deaf clients, customers, and patients receive effective communication.

This does not mean that deaf people find it easy to get the services to which they are entitled. They are sometimes turned away from a program simply because no one on the staff can communicate with them or understand what they need. Deaf people often get little or no service in situations where hearing people receive good service. A hearing person may get answers to questions about food stamp eligibility, for example, or advice on how to complete an application or information on the details of a program. But the deaf person may be handed a standard written

form with cursory explanations of office and program procedures. He or she may misunderstand the forms and lose benefits
as a consequence.

The sections that follow describe the federal laws that govern
how health care facilities treat patients who are deaf and hard of
hearing. Other considerations include court rulings and state civil
rights and disability laws.

FEDERAL DISABILITY RIGHTS LAWS

Federal disability rights laws include Section 504 of the Rehabilitation Act, the ADA, Justice Department guidelines, and standards set by individual agencies. In each of the following
situations, health care providers violated federal law:

+ The private doctor who refuses to provide an interpreter[1]
+ The federally-funded agency that turns away or discourages
  deaf people, because of communication barriers[2]
+ An agency that provides information or services by telephone but does not have a TTY or refuses to use a TTY
  relay service.[3]

Section 504 of the Rehabilitation Act of 1973

Section 504 of the Rehabilitation Act of 1973 (discussed in chapter three) requires any program with fifteen or more employees
that receives federal financial assistance to be accessible to people
with disabilities. A hospital or doctor's office that takes Medicare
payments receives federal financial assistance; a social service
agency that receives federal grant money is receiving federal financial assistance; health care or social services agencies operated
by state and local government agencies usually receive federal financial assistance.

An agency covered by Section 504 must provide appropriate
"auxiliary aids" to people with impaired sensory, manual, or
speaking skills, when these aids are necessary to afford such people an equal opportunity to benefit from the service in question.[4]

Auxiliary aids are specifically defined to include interpreters, braille, taped material, and other aids.[5] Smaller agencies may also be required to provide auxiliary aids when doing so would not impair the agency's ability to provide its normal benefits or services.[6] Interpreters can be hired for a reasonable hourly fee for occasional deaf clients. TTYs can be acquired for a one-time investment of a few hundred dollars. These expenses are not unduly burdensome for most agencies.

Section 504 applies to many public and nonprofit agencies. For example, food stamp offices must provide an interpreter to assist in explaining the application procedure, eligibility criteria, and available benefits to deaf applicants. Social security offices must also provide auxiliary aids and services, including qualified interpreters. In addition, such offices are required to have a TTY so that deaf people can telephone for information, schedule appointments, or consult with caseworkers. Agencies can also make and receive calls through the relay service (see chapter one).

While such an agency is not required to have an interpreter on staff at all times, deaf people should be able to request an interpreter if needed and to schedule an appointment when an interpreter is available. This appointment procedure is a reasonable method of providing equivalent services, even if applications are ordinarily handled on a first-come, first-served basis. The agency should also post a notice clearly explaining that interpreters are available and how to arrange an interpreted appointment.

Unfortunately, some deaf patients never even receive the opportunity to request auxiliary aids and services. In one case, a deaf woman who was pregnant went to a gynecologist's office with her mother. When the doctor walked into the examining room and discovered that the woman was deaf, he refused to treat her and said that because she was deaf, she must go to a center for high-risk pregnancies. The woman filed suit against the doctor, who received federal financial assistance in the form of Medicaid payments. The court awarded the woman $10,000, finding that the doctor had discriminated against the woman ' violation of the Rehabilitation Act.[7]

The Americans with Disabilities Act of 1990

Under the ADA (discussed in chapter two), deaf people have the right to equal access and participation in health care and social services. They also have the right to effective communication with their health care providers and social service agencies.[8] The ADA prohibits discrimination by public and private agencies, regardless of the agency's size and whether or not it receives federal financial assistance. In this way, the ADA is much broader than Section 504. The ADA obligates hospitals, physicians, social service agencies and public and private health care providers, among others, to provide auxiliary aids and services to individuals with disabilities.[9]

Title II of the ADA prohibits discrimination by state and local governments. This means that public agencies, such as welfare offices and state hospitals, must allow deaf people equal access to their services and programs. For example, the local welfare office must provide interpreters to deaf clients when needed for effective communication. Title II also protects deaf and hard of hearing prisoners seeking health care or social services from discrimination.[10] State and local prisons violate the law if they discourage or prevent deaf prisoners from participating in group therapy or counseling programs because of their disability. When a deaf prisoner needs an interpreter for effective communication, Title II of the ADA directs that a qualified interpreter must be provided.

Private health care providers, such as private hospitals, doctors, and mental health counselors are governed by Title III of the ADA. Under Title III, private health care providers must provide auxiliary aids and services so that people with disabilities can benefit from their services.[11] For deaf and hard of hearing people, this means that their doctors, mental health counselors, training programs, and nursing homes may not discriminate. In fact, any place of public accommodation must provide necessary auxiliary aids and services.

One key element of the ADA is that places of public accommodation may not charge the deaf person for the cost of these auxiliary aids and services.

> A public accommodation may not impose a surcharge on a particular individual with a disability or any group of individuals with disabilities . . . to cover the costs of measures, such as the provision of auxiliary aids . . . that are required to provide that individual . . . with the nondiscriminatory treatment required by the Act . . . [12]

Despite the clarity of the ADA's mandate, deaf people continue to be billed and surcharged for the cost of auxiliary aids in violation of law. Some providers attempt to circumvent the bill for auxiliary aids by asking a family member or friend to interpret for the deaf person. However, the Justice Department specifically cautions against this practice.

> In certain circumstances, notwithstanding that the family member or friend is able to interpret or is a certified interpreter, the family member or friend may not be qualified to render the necessary interpretation because of factors such as emotional or personal involvement or considerations of confidentiality that may adversely affect the ability to interpret "effectively, accurately, and impartially."[13]

Generally, a doctor who has a deaf patient's family interpret for the deaf patient has not provided effective communication. There may be necessary information that the family member fails to communicate in a misguided effort to shield the deaf patient. There may be questions the deaf person will not ask in the presence of a family member or friend. The family member or friend may be too emotionally upset by the situation to interpret correctly. Finally, the family member or friend will seldom meet the interpreter qualification requirements of the law. Therefore, friends or family members should not interpret unless the deaf person specifically requests they do so, and only if the person is competent to provide the service.

Some health care providers covered by the ADA argue that it is too costly to pay for auxiliary aids and services. For example, a doctor might argue that it would be an undue burden to pay for an interpreter. A public accommodation such as a doctor's office may deny an auxiliary aid only if it can demonstrate that providing the auxiliary aid would fundamentally alter the nature of the service or would constitute an undue burden or expense.[14] Whether or not a particular auxiliary aid constitutes an "undue burden" is difficult to decide. It depends on a variety of factors, including the nature and cost of the auxiliary aid or service and the overall financial and other resources of the business. The undue burden standard is intended to be applied on a case-by-case basis. Undue burden is not measured by the amount of income the business is receiving from a deaf client, patient, or customer. Instead, undue burden is measured by the financial impact on the whole entity.

Therefore, it is possible for a business to be responsible for providing auxiliary aids even if it does not make a sale or receive income from a deaf patient or customer, if the cost of the auxiliary aid would not be an undue burden on its overall operation. Even if a public accommodation is able to demonstrate that there is a fundamental alteration or an undue burden, it must be prepared to provide an alternative auxiliary aid if one exists.[15] For example, a doctor who refuses to provide interpreting services will have the obligation to show that effective communication can be achieved by other means.

The cost of auxiliary aids is slight when compared to the overall budget of most health care providers. Effective communication is vital for deaf consumers, but it also benefits health care providers who may be liable for malpractice when a medicine is prescribed or a treatment given without knowing the deaf person's medical history or without obtaining informed consent. It pays for health care providers to communicate effectively with their patients. Under the Revenue Reconciliation Act of 1990, some providers may even be eligible for tax credits for expenses incurred in the course of accommodating patients with disabilities.[16]

AGENCY RESPONSIBILITIES

Deaf people should be aware that many service agencies attempt to evade their legal responsibilities. Small agencies may try to claim that providing auxiliary aids is beyond their financial means. They may seek a waiver of the requirement that they provide aids on the basis of their small size and budget. But some auxiliary aids are critical and most are not excessive in cost. Deaf clients are entitled by law to receive such auxiliary aids free of charge. Under Section 504 of the Rehabilitation Act, the cost is the responsibility of the agency receiving and making use of the federal money. Under the ADA, the cost is the responsibility of the health care provider.

Agency Rules and State Laws

In addition to the requirements of Section 504 and the ADA, most agencies have specific rules that prohibit discrimination against people with disabilities in services they support.[17] Some states have adopted laws that prohibit discrimination against disabled people by government and private social service agencies. Others have laws specifically requiring certain services for deaf people. For example, in New York, the New York Hospital Codes, Rules, and Regulations requires hospitals to produce a sign language interpreter within ten minutes of a deaf patient's arrival in the emergency room.[18]

Most states have civil rights laws prohibiting discrimination by facilities open to the public. Traditionally, these laws have dealt only with racial or religious discrimination; more recently, many of them have been amended to also prohibit discrimination based on disability. In addition to commercial enterprises—such as restaurants, hotels, and stores—these laws apply to service agencies that are open to the public.[19]

Additionally, the American Medical Association (AMA) has revised its policy regarding interpreters for patients who are deaf or hard of hearing. The AMA's Office of the General Counsel, Division of Health Law can provide guidance concerning physician's responsibilities regarding provision of interpreters, and the association offers several resources to help physicians understand their responsibilities under the ADA.[20]

The American Medical Association's
Position on Interpreters

Although the American Medical Association (AMA) initially encouraged health care providers to use deaf patients' relatives as interpreters, it has since revised its guidelines. The AMA currently advises providers to be more proactive in taking their patients' preferences into account when determining how best to facilitate communication. However, the association's policy statement still states "The prohibition against discrimination on the basis of disability includes an obligation to make reasonable accommodations to meet the needs of patients with disabilities. This has been interpreted by some as creating a requirement that physicians provide and pay for the cost of hearing interpreters for their patients who are hearing disabled. While there will be instances where a physician must provide a hearing interpreter, there is no hard and fast requirement for the provision of such services."

The physician's responsibility to make aurally delivered materials accessible to deaf patients may be met "through multiple means, including qualified interpreters, note taking, written materials, and telecommunications devices for deaf persons." The following excerpts from the AMA's policy statement are interesting in that they recognize that the patient's preferred method for communication should be given primary consideration, yet leave the final determination to the physician.

The first step is to determine, in consultation with the patient, the appropriate auxiliary aid or service. In some instances, such as when a conversation is particularly important relative to the care and services being provided, or is particularly complex, effective communication may only be ensured through the use of a qualified interpreter. No special accreditation is needed to meet ADA standards, and qualified interpreters may include: family members or friends, as long as they are effective, accurate, impartial (especially in personal or confidential situations), and an acceptable choice to the patient; personnel from the practice or facility; or interpreters from interpreter services.

The ADA does not mandate the use of interpreters in every instance. The health care professional can choose alternatives to interpreters as long as the result is effective communication. Alternatives to interpreters should be discussed with hearing impaired patients, especially those not aware that such alternatives are permissible under the Act. Acceptable alternatives may include: note taking; written materials; or, if viable, lip-reading. A health care professional or facility is not required to provide an interpreter when:

+ it would present an **undue burden**. An undue burden is a significant expense or difficulty to the operation of the facility. Factors courts use to determine whether providing an interpreter would present an undue burden include the practice or facility's operating income and eligibility for tax credits, and whether it has sources of outside funding or a parent company. Courts also consider the frequency of visits that would require the services of an interpreter. However, the single factor of the cost of an interpreter exceeding the cost of a medical consultation generally has not been found by the courts to be an undue burden.

or,

+ it would **fundamentally alter** the nature of the services normally provided. For example, in sensitive situations, utilizing a family member as an interpreter, or an interpreter not affiliated with the practice or facility, may be inappropriate . . .

Although the health care professional makes the final decision regarding use of an interpreter or other alternative, the patient's choice should be given primary consideration. Also, the reasonableness of a determination *not* to provide an accommodation may be challenged in court in an enforcement action. If there is a disagreement between the health care professional and the patient over the need for a qualified interpreter, the effectiveness of each viable option should be discussed. . . .

Courts have found an ADA violation where the health care professional decides not to use an interpreter and there is evidence that the method used did not result in effective communication.

The health care professional or facility responsible for the care must pay for the cost of an interpreter. Health care professionals or facilities cannot impose a surcharge on an individual with a disability directly or indirectly to offset the cost of the interpreter. The cost of the interpreter should be treated as part of overhead expenses for accounting and tax purposes.[20]

HOSPITAL COMMUNICATION BARRIERS

Before the passage of Section 504 and the ADA, deaf and hard of hearing people had virtually no right to effective communication in hospitals. When deaf people entered a hospital, they had to take what was offered them, sometimes settling for ineffective or even life-threatening health care because they did not understand what was being said. Complicated medical terms were used with the hope that the deaf patient would understand them. Drugs were prescribed without any explanation of how to take them. Sometimes deaf people took these drugs with other medicines, not knowing the possible reactions. Hospital admissions procedures were rarely explained. If they wanted assistance from the nursing staff, they could not use the intercom. If a pregnant woman went into the labor room, she could not bring an interpreter with her; she could not understand what her doctor wanted her to do, because the doctor's surgical mask made speechreading impossible. Under current federal law, these kinds of discrimination are no longer tolerated.

It is not possible to have equal access to services without communication. Communication is, perhaps, the most important ingredient of health care. Without communication, the patient cannot explain the symptoms of his or her illness to the medical staff. Without communication, the patient cannot comprehend the routines of treatment or preventive medicine. If all medical patients were treated like this, the general population would be outraged. Yet deaf people face these circumstances daily.

Compounding the Stress

A person in a medical situation may be apprehensive, nervous, confused, and in pain. When these feelings are compounded by the stress of trying to understand what a health provider is saying, the experience can be traumatic.

In the past, many hospitals have relied on the exchange of written notes, speechreading, or other less-than-satisfactory means to communicate with deaf patients. Yet for a person with limited English skills, written English can be ineffective, frustrating, and dangerous. Written communication also tends to be a summary of a discussion rather than effective communication with all the nuances and contextual clues that are so important in medical situations. Understanding is further hampered by unfamiliar medical terms and the need for fast, efficient communication during a medical emergency.

Some hospitals have attempted to get by with a staff member who has some knowledge of sign language, instead of bringing in a skilled interpreter from outside the hospital. This might be acceptable if the staff member is qualified, but this is rarely the case. More often the staff member's limited understanding of sign language creates serious misunderstandings, leading to ineffective treatment and even misdiagnosis.

Communication that is "effective" and aids that are "appropriate"—two terms used in federal regulations—are best determined by the deaf patient. According to the Department of Health and Human Services (HHS), deaf patients' assessments of their own communication needs must be given great deference.[21] Hospital personnel often assume that they are better able than deaf patients to decide how to communicate. For example, hospital staff might insist that because they can understand the deaf person, the patient can therefore understand them. Hospitals might assume that communication by pen and paper is adequate and that the decision to use an interpreter is up to the doctor. A hospital may claim to have an interpreter on its staff, yet the staff member has only studied sign language for one semester and can not read most signs.

Planning for Deaf and Hard of Hearing Patients

Federal law requires health care providers to offer a full range of communication options (auxiliary aids) so that deaf and hard of hearing persons receive effective health care services. For more than twenty years, the government has required providers to prepare in advance for the reality that deaf and hard of hearing patients will at some time need to use their services. In order to be prepared so that these patients can receive the access required by law, the government asks providers to select a range of communication options through consultation with deaf persons and organizations advocating for the rights of deaf persons. The options which must be provided, at no cost to the deaf patient, include:

+ formal arrangements with interpreters who can accurately and fluently express and receive in sign language;
+ supplemental hearing devices such as amplified telephones, TTYs, televisions equipped with captioning equipment and loop systems for meetings;
+ written communication;
+ staff training in basic sign language; and expressions related to emergency treatment.[22]

These guidelines mean that each health care provider must make its staff aware of local interpreters' names, addresses, phone numbers, and hours of availability. In addition, health care providers must have TTYs so that deaf patients can make appointments, notify providers that they will be needing auxiliary aids, and communicate with family and friends to the same extent as hearing patients.

Yet preparing a range of communication methods in anticipation of the arrival of deaf patients is meaningless if the local deaf community is not aware of these options. Health care providers also have a responsibility to make sure that deaf people seeking treatment are given advance notice of the various communication options. Advance planning makes it possible for deaf patients to access the auxiliary aids that will enable them to communicate with providers.

In most circumstances, deaf people are in the best position to judge what is needed so that they have equal access to health care. The government has repeatedly stressed that when choosing methods for effective communication, patients' judgments must be considered to be of utmost importance. HHS, for example, has repeatedly stated that patients' assessments of their communication needs must be given great deference:

> In most circumstances, we believe that the hearing impaired person is in the best position to determine what means of communication is necessary to insure an equal opportunity to benefit from health care services. Therefore, the patient's judgment regarding what means of communication is necessary to insure effective communication must be accorded great weight . . . The presumption favoring the hearing impaired patient's self assessed need is not overcome merely by a showing that the hearing impaired patient suffered no harm. Rather the recipient [of federal financial assistance] must demonstrate that the hearing impaired patient actually understood what was being communicated through the alternative communication option.[23]

Deaf patients have nothing to gain by requesting an inappropriate auxiliary aid. The risks for both the patient and the provider are too serious. Even in those rare circumstances when an emergency facility is unable to immediately provide a specific type of communication, providers are still obligated to provide the most effective communication in view of the limits of time in the emergency situation.

Advance Preparation for Emergency Care

The emergency health care regulations are especially important. Hospitals are required to establish a special emergency health care procedure for effective communication with deaf people in emergency rooms. The hospitals should be able to locate qualified sign language interpreters on very short notice. They should also have TTY-equipped telephones so that deaf people can alert the hospital that a deaf patient is coming in and will need an interpreter or other special services. The TTY equipment also will permit a hospitalized deaf person to make calls to family or medical personnel when in the emergency room. Emergency room staff can be trained to use and recognize basic sign language necessary for emergency care. They should be trained to quickly recognize that a person is deaf and should know how to find appropriate auxiliary aids.

Hospital Compliance

Services must be equivalent for both hearing and deaf patients. There are many ways a hospital or health center may accommodate deaf patients. For example, a hospital that ordinarily allows only one person to accompany a woman through natural childbirth may have to alter its delivery room rules to allow both the husband and an interpreter to be present during the delivery. A hospital that prohibits admission of deaf people to its psychiatric unit unless they speechread will have to change its policy to comply with Section 504 and the ADA.

Patients in a hospital room have many devices to make the hospital stay easier. Yet many of these devices are useless for deaf patients without modification. For example, if a deaf patient presses the intercom button, the nurse at the station will answer—but they cannot communicate. The deaf patient assumes the nurse knows that he or she is deaf, not realizing that the nurse may be unaware that he or she is deaf. After repeated attempts to contact each other, the nurse and the deaf patient may become exasperated with one other. This typical problem can be prevented by "flagging" deaf patients' charts and intercom buttons so that all pertinent hospital personnel know to respond in person to an intercom summons. Deaf patients should also have TTYs and televisions equipped with decoders for captions.

Hospitals must also provide ongoing staff training to sensitize personnel to other special needs of deaf and hard of hearing people: adequate, glare-free lighting; control of background noise for all hearing-aid wearers; modifications to auditory fire alarm systems; and changes in oral evaluation procedures. Freedom of movement, especially for hands and arms, is crucial in allowing a deaf patient to sign and/or gesture.

Health care facilities should take special steps to make sure that deaf people know about services the hospital normally offers and about any special services to which they may be entitled because of their disabilities. For example, many hospitals provide new patients with an orientation to the hospital, its personnel, and its services. All such information should be available in writing at a level of English that most people can understand. It should include an easy-to-read notice about the availability of sign language interpreters, portable TTYs, and other special services. If a facility gives information by telephone, it should ensure that deaf people can get the same information using a TTY-equipped telephone.

Some deaf people do not know about hospitals' legal obligations. They may not know how to request an interpreter. It is the hospital's responsibility to provide this information. Hospitals also should have easy-to-read notices posted in the emergency room, outpatient clinic, and all admitting areas to inform deaf people of how they can obtain interpreter services or other assistance.

Hospitals often ask patients to sign a written consent to treatment or legal waivers of rights before they will treat them. Federal law requires hospitals to take any necessary steps so that deaf people understand these rights. A deaf patient should ask the hospital to have the consent papers explained in sign language. The consent and waiver papers also should be written in language that the deaf patient can understand.

There are many ways an agency, health center, or hospital can make its services available and useful to deaf people. In 1997 the National Association of the Deaf (NAD) Law Center and a private law firm filed an ADA and Section 504 complaint on behalf of a deaf woman in Maine who was denied interpreter services in a hospital. The Justice Department also filed suit against the hospital. The law firm developed a model policy for making hospitals accessible for deaf patients and their families (see appendix).[24] The purpose of the policy was to provide deaf and hard of hearing people with an equal opportunity to receive and benefit from hospital services, and to facilitate accurate, effective, timely, and dignified communication between hospital personnel and people who are deaf or hard of hearing.

The policy describes a model system where deaf patients receive qualified interpreters; TTYs; captioned televisions; assistive listening devices; trained note takers; computer-assisted, real-time transcription (CART) services; telephone flashers to indicate incoming calls; and other aids and services. Other important elements of the policy include signs explaining the rights of deaf patients, training for hospital staff, and initial patient surveys that would notify hospital staff that a patient is deaf or hard of hearing.

Other hospitals are discovering that not complying with federal civil rights laws can be very costly. One New Jersey hospital recently agreed to pay $700,000 to four deaf residents for failure to provide interpreters, closed captioning, and telecommunication devices over a ten-year period.[25] In Connecticut, deaf and hard of hearing people, along with the Connecticut Association of the Deaf, sued ten acute care hospitals for failing to provide effective communication. The lawsuit settled for approximately $350,000, along with an agreement to remove barriers that prevent effective communication in hospitals.[26] As a result, Connecticut will have a comprehensive, on-call system for obtaining interpreters that will be the first cooperative, hospital-sponsored system in the country. In New York, a jury awarded $250,000 to a deaf woman who was denied interpreter services in the hospital.[27]

Guidelines for Hospitals

The following NAD guidelines help hospital administrators develop procedures for serving the needs of their deaf patients and comply with federal regulations

1. A central office should be designated to supervise services to deaf patients. This office should establish a system to obtain qualified sign language and oral interpreters on short notice twenty-four hours a day.
2. The unit to which a deaf patient is admitted should immediately notify the designated office when a deaf patient is admitted.
3. An interpreter, if available within the hospital, should be sent to the patient immediately to consult with the patient as to the appropriate method of communication, which may include:

   a. use of a qualified sign language and/or oral interpreter
   b. speechreading
   c. handwritten notes
   d. supplemental hearing devices
   e. any combination of the above

   The interpreter should give the patient notice of the right to a qualified sign language and/or oral interpreter to be provided by the hospital without charge to the patient. If no interpreter is available within the hospital, the patient should be given written notice of these rights.

4. The interpreter assists in communication between the patient and the staff to ensure that the deaf patient is receiving equal services and equal opportunity to participate in and benefit from hospital services. These situations include but are not limited to:

    a. obtaining the patient's medical history
    b. obtaining informed consent or permission for treatment
    c. diagnosis of the ailment or injury
    d. explanations of medical procedures to be used
    e. treatment or surgery if the patient is conscious, or to determine if the patient is conscious;
    f. those times the patient is in intensive care or in the recovery room after surgery
    g. emergency situations that arise
    h. explanations of the medications prescribed, how and when they are to be taken, and possible side effects
    i. assisting at the request of the doctor or other hospital staff
    j. discharge of the patient

5. Friends or relatives of a deaf patient should not be used as interpreters unless the deaf patient specifically requests that they interpret. Deaf patients, their friends, and their families should be told that a professional interpreter will be engaged where needed for effective communication.
6. The deaf patient should be informed that another interpreter will be obtained if the patient is unable to communicate with a particular interpreter.
7. Any written notices of rights or services and written consent forms should be written at no higher than a fifth-grade reading level. An interpreter should be provided if the deaf patient is unable to understand such written notices.
8. A TTY should be obtained and used for making appointments, giving out information, and assisting in emergency situations. Portable TTYs should be available on request for deaf inpatients. Telephone amplifiers should be provided for patients who are hard of hearing. All telephones should be hearing aid compatible.
9. Alternative methods to auditory intercom systems, paging systems, and alarm systems should be provided for all deaf patients.
10. Ongoing efforts should be made by the hospital to sensitize staff to the various special needs of deaf patients.
11. Contact with local deaf people, organizations for and of

the deaf, and the community agencies serving deaf people should be maintained for assistance in drawing up a list of qualified interpreters and in developing a program of hospital services that is responsive to the needs of deaf patients.

Direct Care Staff

Hospital staff can do many things to enable communication with a deaf patient and to make the patient more comfortable with the hospital environment, thereby providing better service. Common sense and basic information about deafness will help hospital staff provide good health care.

The deaf patient is the best resource regarding the preferred mode of communication and should be consulted about this and about any problems that arise. The isolation of deaf people can be overcome to a great extent by explaining what is happening and answering any questions the patient might have.

The importance of using a qualified interpreter to ensure effective communication cannot be overemphasized. However, there may be many routine situations—such as bringing dinner or taking temperatures—where an interpreter is not necessary. The following guidelines on working with deaf patients will help compensate for the absence of an interpreter in those circumstances where an interpreter is not needed for effective communication. These guidelines, if implemented, will also improve the quality of care provided.

A. Make added efforts to communicate in such a way that the patient understands what is happening.
   1. Allow more time for every communication, not rushing through what is said. To make sure the patient understands, some thoughts should be repeated using different phrases.
   2. Lip movements should not be exaggerated. Speak at a normal rate of speed and separate words.
   3. Patients' arms should not be restricted; they should be free to write and sign.

    4. Make cards or posters of usual questions and responses that can be pointed to quickly.

    5. Keep paper and pen handy, but be sensitive to the patient's level of English language fluency and writing skills.

B. Be sensitive to the visual environment of deaf patients by adjusting lighting and using visual rather than auditory cues and reassurances.

    1. Use charts, pictures, and/or three-dimensional models when explaining information and procedures to deaf patients.

    2. Do not remove a deaf patient's glasses or leave a deaf patient in total darkness.

    3. Remove any bright lights in front of the deaf person when communicating; glare makes it difficult to read signs or lips.

    4. Face the patient when speaking, without covering your face or mouth.

    5. Keep facial expressions pleasant and unworried so as not to alarm the patient.

C. Alert all staff to the presence and needs of the deaf patient and be sensitive to those needs.

    1. "Flag" the intercom button so that workers will know the patient is deaf and requires a personal visit rather than a response over the intercom.

    2. "Flag" the patient's charts, room, and bed to alert staff to use appropriate means of communication.

D. Inform hospital personnel of the special needs of people with hearing aids.

    1. Allow the patient to wear his or her hearing aid.

    2. Don't shout at the patient.

    3. Be sure that the patient has fully understood what is said.

MENTAL HEALTH ISSUES

Very few deaf or hard of hearing individuals have access to mental health services provided by qualified therapists who are knowledgeable about deafness and are able to communicate effectively with deaf individuals.[28] Progressive programs exist in some states and the District of Columbia, but there are few mental health facilities functioning specifically for deaf patients.[29] Also, few regular facilities are even modestly staffed and equipped to help deaf patients, despite the relative ease and modest expense of these services.

The primary problem is the lack of mental health professionals who have experience working with deaf people. Even with an interpreter present, the mental health professional must be empathetic to deaf people and their culture if therapy is to be effective. There is a gross shortage of psychologists, therapists, clinical social workers, and other mental health professionals who are able to provide counseling and psychotherapy services in sign language.[30]

The most extreme result of lack of communication is interpreting the patient's deafness and speech as psychopathology or mental retardation. Such misdiagnoses result in improper placement, misguided treatment and case management, unjustified exclusion of the patient from hospital programs and activities, and inappropriate aftercare. The result is the patient's isolation, bewilderment, and even rage, all of which run counter to the purposes of the facility and its staff.

Surveys of psychiatric hospitals and institutions for people who are mentally retarded frequently reveal that a disproportionate number of patients are deaf. Dr. McCay Vernon, a psychologist noted for his work with deaf people, observes, "It has been established that IQ is essentially normally distributed in the deaf population. Obviously gross error had been made in the fundamental but relatively easy-to-make diagnosis of mental retardation."[31]

Misdiagnosis can result in a deaf patient being inappropriately assigned and confined to an institution for many years before the mistake is discovered. There are numerous accounts of inappropriate institutionalization. Vernon, for example, reported the case of a patient who spent thirty-five years at Idaho's state school and hospital for the mentally retarded when deafness was the patient's primary disability. Similar cases have been reported in the District of Columbia and in North Carolina.[32]

Increased attention to the needs of deaf and hard of hearing patients has resulted in vastly improved knowledge of effective mental health services. Research, training, and clinical service models are now available. The NAD has developed a model plan known as *Standards of Care for the Delivery of Mental Health Services to Deaf and Hard of Hearing People.*[33] The standards identify guidelines for resources, criteria, and methods of administration and financing for statewide systems of mental health service delivery. The standards also identify the specialized demands for appropriate mental health services in diagnosis, treatment modalities, treatment personnel, treatment settings, access to care, and organization and financing of services. Using the legal tools described below and the professional standards being developed by knowledgeable clinicians, deaf people can have access to public and private mental health services.

Mental Health Programs for Deaf People

Treatment methods and modalities for deaf patients require special interventions, communication methods, and equipment. Few mental health professionals have experience treating deaf patients. As a result, deaf patients often do not receive appropriate care in mental health facilities.[34] Deaf and deaf-blind patients are sometimes the target of abuse or hostility in mental health institutions. Unable to summon help or to identify attackers, they and their food and property are easy targets for more aggressive patients. Even in well-managed facilities where these abuses are rare, deaf people may find the very process of institutionalization brutal to the psyche. Deaf-blind patients may be particularly isolated, frustrated, and unable to understand what is happening.

Responding to these problems, some hospitals and mental health administrations have begun to develop specific programs for deaf people. Such programs are usually characterized by an intake system that permits deaf patients to be consolidated in one unit. The unit is staffed with mental health professionals who know sign language and have knowledge of the cultural and psychosocial implications of deafness and the common dynamics within families with deaf members. Sign language interpreters are provided for staff members who do not have sign language skills. The units are equipped with TTYs and captioned television, and necessary assistive listening devices. Patients in the deaf unit are taught sign language, which is used in all individual and group therapy sessions. Often these units incorporate a treatment philosophy that recognizes the impact of deafness and communication in personality development and mental health. Some units provide education, consultation, diagnostic, and evaluation services to other community mental health programs. They may provide outreach or consultation services to other mental health facilities and outpatient clinics.[35]

Some states fund deaf units through their departments of mental health; other states channel such funding to departments of vocational rehabilitation. Some deaf units have a mix of federal and state grants to pursue their work. Because such grants are temporary, though, new ones must be sought constantly.

When no leadership exists in a state mental health system or vocational rehabilitation department, or when the legislature is indifferent, alternate methods for improving treatment of deaf patients with mental illness must be found. Courts are increasingly recognizing that mental patients have legal rights, so legal action may serve to improve mental health services for deaf patients.

Legal Action for Mental Health Services

Because of the difficulty in bringing individual suits and the limitation of the remedy only to the patient who brought the suit, class action lawsuits have been more effective means of achieving institutional change. A class action suit is filed by a patient who claims to represent all people similarly situated. Because the remedy resulting from the action applies to all such people, some class action litigation has resulted in the definition and articulation of rights of mental patients, minimum standards for care and treatment, and responsibilities and liabilities of the treating staff.

A famous class action suit, *Wyatt v. Stickney,* later called *Wyatt v. Aderholt,* resulted in the recognition and establishment of a mental patient's constitutional right to be treated and not merely held in custodial care.[36] The court issued a far-reaching and effective decision, ruling specifically that patients involuntarily committed through noncriminal procedures to a state mental hospital have a constitutional right to receive such individual treatment as will give them an opportunity to improve or cure their mental condition. The court decreed minimal constitutional standards for adequate treatment, including an individual treatment plan that provides a statement of the least restrictive treatment conditions necessary to achieve the purposes of commitment. The decision recognized a deaf patient's rights to a humane psychological and physical environment, privacy, dignity, and freedom from isolation. The court also established a human rights committee to investigate violations of patients' rights and to oversee implementation of the plan. It also ordered a minimum number of treatment personnel per 250 patients and other changes to ensure more humane living conditions.

Under the *Wyatt* decision, an individualized treatment plan for a deaf person could potentially include programs such as a specialized deaf unit with qualified clinicians knowledgeable about deafness and sign language. By including training and therapy in sign language, the program would allow the patient to participate fully in therapy and to interact with staff and other deaf patients, who themselves would know or be learning sign language. The emphasis on communication skills would be a central aspect of therapy and rehabilitation, allowing the patient the opportunity for social adjustment and eventual integration into society.

State Statutes

State law is often an effective basis for suit. From the point of view of increasing the number and quality of good laws and achieving effective levels of resource allocation, work with the state legislatures is absolutely necessary. Good laws have as far-reaching an impact as legal victories. Concerned people and organizations—mental health professionals, state mental health and vocational rehabilitation administrators, legislators, jurists, and disabled advocates and activists—ought to be natural allies in the effort to produce solutions that are effective, sensible, and not merely cosmetic. The NAD *Standards of Care* can be used as a model state service plan for comprehensive and specialized services.[37] Experts in the mental health needs of deaf individuals have made suggestions for development of appropriate, effective mental health services for deaf patients.[38]

Several states have set the pace. Illinois, North Carolina, and South Carolina have established strong mental health/deaf service program networks. Oklahoma has a law establishing a comprehensive mental health care program for deaf people, including inpatient and outpatient mental health services and counseling to family members of deaf patients.[39] The law requires cooperation with other state health programs and agencies. The professional staff of this statewide program are required to have experience in working with the mental health problems of deaf individuals and their families.

The Oklahoma statute is a good model for a legislative program that directly addresses the needs of the deaf community. Deaf people should be able to receive the entire range of housing and treatment environments: emergency treatment, long- and short-term residential treatment, community mental health centers, nursing homes, personal care homes, foster homes, and halfway houses.

Federal Laws

As discussed at length above, two federal laws have significant impact on the provision of health care services, including mental health care. Both the ADA and Section 504 of the Rehabilitation Act require mental health practitioners to provide effective communication for deaf individuals.

Section 504

Section 504 of the 1973 Rehabilitation Act requires mental health facilities and agencies receiving funding from HHS to provide effective benefits or services in a manner that does not limit the participation of qualified people with disabilities in the program. A mental health agency or facility with fifteen or more employees must provide appropriate auxiliary aids to people with impaired sensory, manual, or speaking skills, where necessary to afford such people an equal opportunity to benefit from the service in question.

Mental health service providers thus bear the responsibility of providing interpreters and specialized personnel to deaf patients. Facilities that refuse to provide them risk a private lawsuit or having HHS cut off their federal funds. Several successful lawsuits have been brought against hospitals, universities, and social service agencies requiring them to provide interpreter services.[40]

The Office for Civil Rights (OCR) of HHS has investigated complaints against several mental health facilities for failure to provide appropriate services. As a result of a complaint brought by the North Carolina Association of the Deaf, a comprehensive, long-range plan has been developed and is being implemented by the North Carolina Department of Human Services.[41]

In a complaint brought by the NAD against the Ohio Department of Mental Health, OCR found that sixteen psychiatric hospitals did not have appropriate policies for serving deaf patients. OCR found that deaf patients not assigned to the existing deaf unit were maintained in a state of social isolation and sensory deprivation. Treatment team members routinely attempted to communicate with deaf patients by exchanging notes. Even when arrangements were made for securing qualified interpreters, the treatment team staff generally did not possess training on the psychosocial issues pertaining to deaf people who are mentally ill. In the course of the investigation, the agency implemented procedures for securing qualified interpreters, established TTY services, and trained staff about deafness and the use of auxiliary aids.

The agency was ordered to establish comprehensive service planning on a statewide basis, with adequate availability of specialized deaf units staffed by mental health professionals with sign language competency and training in the psycho-social issues of deafness.[42] Section 504 generally prohibits hospitals or other agencies from establishing different or separate facilities for people with disabilities. In the context of mental health services for deaf individuals, however, OCR found that the treatment needs of deaf individuals justify separate units staffed by professionals with appropriate communication skills and expertise.

> It is the opinion of Deaf Unit staff, corroborated by research conducted by experts in the field, that such units are the only way most deaf patients can receive an equal opportunity to participate in and benefit from services. This is due to lack of understanding by most people in the field of mental health of the unique communication and psychosocial problems of the deaf and misinterpretation of their use of gestures and nonstandard written English.[43]

Americans with Disabilities Act

The ADA has also been an effective tool for securing specialized mental health services for deaf individuals. Unlike Section 504, which applies only to recipients of federal financial assistance, the ADA applies to all mental health professionals, regardless of the size of the office or sources of funding. Under the ADA, psychologists, psychiatrists, psychiatric social workers, and other therapists have a duty to ensure access to mental health services by providing auxiliary aids and services.

The requirement to provide auxiliary aids does not apply if the mental health provider can demonstrate that providing an auxiliary aid would be an undue financial or administrative burden, or a fundamental alteration of the mental health service. In one case, a federal court ruled that a community mental health center must provide mental health counselors who have sign language skills and knowledge of the psychosocial implications of deafness and the mental health needs of the deaf community, so that deaf clients can receive equal and direct access to competent counseling services without going through an interpreter.[44]

The Maine Medical Center's Model Policy

One of the most comprehensive court judgments was handed down in the Maine Medical Center case discussed earlier. The

Successful Lawsuits

Deaf individuals have achieved victories in several important lawsuits. A deaf woman committed to a Maryland mental hospital received no treatment for more than twenty years. In *Doe v. Wilzack,* brought on her behalf by the NAD's Legal Defense Fund, she won individual relief and the state of Maryland agreed to establish an inpatient treatment unit for her and other deaf inpatients in state facilities.[45]

In a similar case in Minnesota, brought by the Legal Advocacy Project for Hearing Impaired People, the state agreed to establish comprehensive treatment programs for deaf mental health patients. A detailed settlement agreement addresses services for the four plaintiffs as well as staffing, program services, and obligation to secure funding in state facilities for the state's other deaf patients.[46]

In a third case, a deaf child won $1.5 million dollars when he proved that it was medical malpractice to diagnose him as mentally retarded when he was a normal, bright, deaf child.[47]

case was brought by a deaf patient who sought emergency psychiatric services. The hospital was unable to treat her because it failed to provide an interpreter. The patient was left without treatment, isolated and alone. Another federal district court in Maine had previously approved a consent decree that established detailed standards for the care and treatment of mentally retarded people who are placed in community settings.[48] Maine recognized that, regardless of their age and degree of retardation or other disability, people released from institutions into the community have the right to receive "habilitation." Habilitation specifically includes the right to an individualized plan of care, education, and training and to services including physical therapy, psychotherapy, speech therapy, and medical and dental attention.

The Maine Medical Center consent decree was the first one

that obligated a state to consider specifically what was required in order for deaf people to benefit from state services. These requirements included the following: (1) hearing-impaired outpatients who could not acquire speech would be taught sign language, (2) the state would provide sign language training to staff and others working with deaf citizens, (3) screening for hearing ability would be conducted with each patient, (4) treatment and further evaluation would be provided by qualified speech and hearing professionals, and (5) hearing aids, when needed, would be provided and maintained in good working order. The court appointed a master to monitor implementation of the agreement.

NOTES

1. 28 *Code of Federal Regulations* §36.303(c)
2. 45 C.F.R. §84.52(a).
3. 45 C.F.R. §84.21(f).
4. 45 C.F.R. §84.52(d)(1).
5. 45 C.F.R. §84.52(d)(3).
6. 45 C.F.R. §84.52(d)(2).
7. *Sumes v. Andres*, 938 F.Supp. 9 (D.D.C. 1996).
8. 28 C.F.R. §36.303(b)(1).
9. 42 U.S. Code §12181 *et. seq.*
10. See *Pennsylvania Department of Corrections, et. al. v. Yeskey*, 118 U.S. 1952 (U.S. 1998), *National Disability Law Reporter* 12: 195.
11. 42 U.S.C. §§12182, 12183.
12. 28 C.F.R. §36.301(c).
13. 56 *Fed. Reg.* 35,553 (July 26, 1991).
14. 28 C.F.R. §36.303(a).
15. Ibid.
16. See IRS publications 535 and 334, and IRS Form 8826.
17. In the HHS Section 504 regulations, these rules are in Subpart F, 45 C.F.R. §84.51 *et seq.*
18. 10 New York Hospital Codes, Rules, and Regulations §405.7(a)(7)(ii).
19. Maryland Human Relations Code Ann. §498; Maine Rev. Stat. Title 5 §4591.
20. Excerpted from the American Medical Association, Office of the General Counsel, Division of Health Law, *Legal Issues for Physicians: The Americans with Disabilities Act and Hearing Interpreters* [Available: http://www.ama-assn.org/physlegl/legal/ada.htm].

For an extended discussion of the AMA's policy regarding ADA requirements, see The American Medical Association in cooperation with The American Academy of Physical Medicine and Rehabilitation, *The Americans with Disabilities Act: A Practice of Accommodation* (Chicago: The American Medical Association, 1998).

21. "Position on the Provision of Auxiliary Aids for Hearing-Impaired Patients in Inpatient, Outpatient, and Emergency Treatment Settings," memorandum from Roma J. Stewart (Director, Office for Civil Rights, Department of Health, Education, and Welfare) to OCR regional directors, April 21, 1980.

22. Ibid.

23. Ibid.

24. DeVinney and United States of America v. Maine Medical Center, Civil No. 97–276–P–C (May 18, 1998). Portions of this policy have been reproduced in appendix E.

25. *Williams v. Jersey City Medical Center*, Sup. Ct. of New Jersey, Hudson County Law Division, No. HUD-L-5059-95 (June 23, 1998).

26. *Connecticut Association of the Deaf, et al.* and *United States of America v. Middlesex Memorial Hospital, et al.* No. 395-CV-02408 (AHN) D. Conn. (August 20, 1998).

27. *Lemonica v. Northshore University Hospital*, in *National Disability Law Reporter Highlights* 10 (September 11, 1997): 12.

28. Approximately 43,000 (10 percent) of the prevocationally deaf population need mental health services, but fewer than two percent receive them. Rehabilitation Services Administration, *Third Annual Conference on Deafness, RSA Region III, Ocean City, Md.* (Washington, D.C.: U.S. Department of Health, Education, and Welfare, 1977).

29. National Information Center on Deafness, "Residential Facilities for Deaf Adults" and "Residential Programs for Deaf/Emotionally Disturbed Children and Adolescents" (Washington, D.C.: Gallaudet University, 1993).

30. L. Raifman and M. Vernon, "Important Implications for Psychologists of the Americans with Disabilities Act: Case in Point, the Patient Who is Deaf," *Professional Psychology: Research and Practice* 27 (372): 376.

31. M. Vernon, "Techniques of Screening for Mental Illness Among Deaf Clients," *Journal of Rehabilitation of the Deaf* 2 (1969): 24.

32. S. Saperstein, "Deaf Woman Confined Wrongly, Suit Claims, Held 55 Years at D.C. Home for Retarded," *Washington Post*, Sept. 14, 1985, p. B1.

33. R. Myers, ed., *Standards of Care for the Delivery of Mental Health Services to Deaf and Hard of Hearing Persons* (Silver Spring, MD: National Association of the Deaf, 1995): 11.

34. Irene W. Leigh, ed., *Psychotherapy with Deaf Clients from Diverse Groups* (Washington, D.C.: Gallaudet University Press, 1999).
35. Ibid.
36. *Wyatt v. Stickney*, 325 F. Supp. 781 (M.D. Ala. 1970), 344 F. Supp. 373 (1972); aff'd. sub. nom. *Wyatt v. Aderholt*, 503 F. 2d 1305 (5th Cir. 1974).
37. R. Myers, ed., *Standards of Care for the Delivery of Mental Health Services to Deaf and Hard of Hearing Persons* (Silver Spring, MD: National Association of the Deaf, 1995).
38. See L. Raifman and M. Vernon, "New Rights for Mental Patients; New Responsibilities for Mental Hospitals," *Psychiatric Quarterly* 67 (1996): 209–220.
39. 43A Okla. Stat. §3-503, "Oklahoma Comprehensive Mental Health Services for the Deaf and Hard-of-Hearing Act."
40. For example, *Camenisch v. University of Texas*, 616 F.2d 127 (5ᵗʰ Cir. 1980), vacated as moot, 451 U.S. 390 (1981).
41. *North Carolina Association of the Deaf v. N.C. Department of Human Resources*, U.S. Department of Health and Human Services, Office of Civil Rights (OCR), Complaint No. 04-92-3150 (1992). Settlement Agreement and Release, Dec. 31, 1992.
42. *National Association of the Deaf Legal Defense Fund v. Ohio Department of Mental Health*, OCR Docket No. 05883054, Aug. 9, 1990.
43. Ibid., 2–3.
44. *Tugg v. Towey*, 864 F. Supp. 1201, 5 NDLR 311 (S.D. Fla. 1994).
45. *Doe v. Wilzack*, U.S.D.C.Md., Civ. No. HAR 83-2409 (Stipulated Judgment Order, Feb. 26, 1986).
46. *Handel et al. v. Levine et al.*, Ramsey County District Court File 468475.
47. *Snow v. State*, 469 N.Y.S., 2d 959 (A.D.2 Dept 1983), aff'd 485 N.Y.S. 2d 987 (1984).
48. *Wouri v. Zitnay,* No. 75-80-SD (S.D. Maine, July 14, 1978).

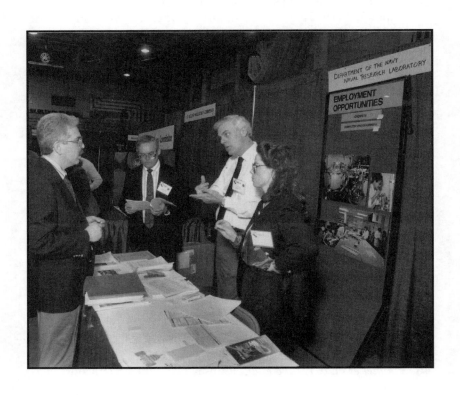

Chapter 7

Employment

Employer attitudes create the largest single barrier to employment opportunities. Employers often have stereotypical assumptions that underestimate the capabilities of an individual with disabilities. One early study indicated that individuals with disabilities must generally be more qualified or competent than individuals without disabilities in order to overcome negative attitudes and assumptions.[1] Employers often refuse to hire individuals with disabilities because of unjustified fears that these individuals cannot perform the job safely. However, other studies on the safety of people with mental and physical disabilities in the employment setting indicate that these fears are groundless.[2]

Employers have used communication barriers as the reason for limiting job opportunities for deaf applicants and employees. Communication difficulties, however, are "often exaggerated, and fairly effective substitutes for oral communication have been disregarded."[3] Inability to use the telephone is often given as a reason not to consider a deaf applicant, even when use of a telephone is not an integral part of the job. In jobs requiring only occasional telephone communication, minor changes in job responsibilities can accommodate the deaf worker. For example, a deaf worker could assume some of a hearing co-worker's responsibilities while the hearing person answers the phones. E-mail, fax transmissions, and use of the relay system can permit a deaf worker to handle many telephone duties.

If a job requires significant telephone contact with another office, a reasonable accommodation may be to install a telecommunications device in both offices, thus allowing the deaf employee to perform all job duties. In supervisory positions, a secretary or interpreter can answer the telephone and facilitate the conversation either through speechreading, notes, or sign language, whichever method the deaf person prefers.

The requirement of attendance at various meetings or conferences is also used as a reason not to consider deaf applicants. But reasonable accommodations—such as interpreters or computer-assisted, real-time transcription (CART) services—can enable deaf workers to participate fully in group meetings and training sessions.

Today, there are a variety of federal statutory remedies available to combat employment discrimination. Those remedies are found in Title I of the ADA and in Sections 501, 503, and 504 of the Rehabilitation Act. As mentioned in chapter two, Title I of the ADA is designed to remove barriers that prevent qualified individuals with disabilities from enjoying the same employment opportunities that are available to people without disabilities. Title I covers private employers with fifteen or more employees. The title also covers employment agencies, unions, and joint labor/management committees.

The ADA applies to employment practices such as recruitment, hiring, job assignments, firing, promotions, pay, layoffs, benefits, leave, training, and all other employment-related activities. Under the ADA, it is also unlawful for an employer to retaliate against an individual who asserts his or her rights under the statute. Likewise, the act also protects an individual who is a victim of discrimination because of family, business, social, or other relationships with someone with a disability.

The remedies available to employees with disabilities in Sections 501, 503, and 504 of the Rehabilitation Act are similar in many respects. These three sections, however, differ somewhat in application, scope, and quality. Each applies to different types of employers:

+ Section 501 to the federal government
+ Section 503 to companies that do business with the federal government (federal contractors)
+ Section 504 to recipients of federal financial assistance

Each section imposes varying levels of responsibility upon employers. Sections 501 and 503 require affirmative action, while Section 504 imposes a duty of nondiscrimination. Section 504 allows an aggrieved individual to go directly to federal court to enforce his or her statutory rights, while Section 501 requires the individual to first file an administrative complaint before seeking relief in court; Section 503 only permits an administrative remedy. The sections also differ in the procedures to be followed in filing an administrative complaint. When faced with employment discrimination based on a disability, one must determine which of the three sections applies.

QUALIFIED INDIVIDUALS WITH A DISABILITY

The ADA and the Rehabilitation Act do not guarantee jobs for people with disabilities. Instead, they prohibit discrimination in employment against individuals with disabilities who are "qualified" for a job. The ADA defines a qualified individual with a disability as someone who has a physical or mental impairment which substantially limits a major life activity but who can perform the essential functions of a job with or without reasonable accommodation.[4]

The definition of a qualified individual with a disability under the Rehabilitation Act differs slightly under the three parts of the act. The Section 501 regulation for federal employees describes a qualified individual with a disability as an individual who, with or without reasonable accommodation, can perform the essential functions of the position in question without endangering the health and safety of the individual or others.[5]

The Section 503 and 504 regulations refer to a qualified individual with a disability as one who is capable of performing a particular job, with reasonable accommodation to his or her disability.[6]

In all of these definitions, the two central questions in determining whether an individual with a disability is qualified for a specific position are (1) What are the essential functions of the job? and (2) Are there reasonable accommodations that will make it possible for the individual with a disability to perform the essential functions of the job?

ESSENTIAL FUNCTIONS

The regulations to the ADA and Sections 501, 503, and 504 suggest that a determination of the "essential functions" of a job must consider whether employees in the position are actually required to perform each of the job functions and, if so, whether the removal of the function fundamentally changes the job? A function may be considered essential if it is a necessary part of the job; there are a limited number of other employees available to perform the function; or a function is highly specialized, and the person in the position is hired for special expertise or ability to perform it.

The concept of "essential functions" is critical in making certain that employers do not disqualify people with disabilities just because these people have difficulty with a task that is only marginally related to the job. For example, a deaf person considered for a word processing position should not be disqualified because he or she may have difficulty using the telephone.

In practice, essential functions for a job must be determined on a case-by-case basis. This analysis is complicated by the employer's duty to restructure the job, including rewriting job descriptions, if necessary, to eliminate nonessential tasks that are barriers for workers with disabilities. This is part of the employer's duty to make reasonable accommodation to the needs of workers with disabilities. In judicial or administrative proceedings, the burden of showing what is an essential function rests with the employer.

As mentioned earlier, a determination of whether an individual can perform essential functions must include an assessment of whether or not a reasonable accommodation exists that would allow the individual to perform an essential function.

REASONABLE ACCOMMODATIONS

Failure to make reasonable accommodations "to the known physical or mental limitations of an otherwise qualified applicant or employee with a disability" is considered discrimination under both the ADA and the Rehabilitation Act. Under these laws, an employer must provide an employee with reasonable accommodations that will allow him or her to perform the essential functions of the job as long as it does not create an undue burden for the employer.

Reasonable accommodation includes modifications or adjustments to a job, the work environment, or the way things are customarily done that enable a qualified individual with a disability to perform the essential functions of a position. According to the ADA, reasonable accommodations may include:

+ making existing employee facilities readily accessible to and usable by individuals with disabilities
+ job restructuring, such as the creation of part-time or modified work schedules
+ reassignment to a vacant position
+ acquisition or modification of equipment or devices
+ appropriate adjustments or modifications of examinations, training materials or policies
+ the provision of qualified readers or interpreters.[7]

Reasonable Accommodations

The regulations to Sections 501, 503, and 504 of the Rehabilitation Act provide similar examples of possible reasonable accommodations:

+ making facilities such as work benches, parking lots, telephones, lavatories, and entrances readily accessible to and usable by people with disabilities
+ restructuring jobs in order to reassign nonessential tasks
+ arranging part-time or modified work schedules
+ acquiring or modifying equipment or machinery
+ providing readers for blind employees and interpreters for deaf employees.[8]

The Equal Employment Opportunity Commission (EEOC) Interpretive Guidance separates reasonable accommodations into three general categories:

1. those that are required to ensure equal opportunity in the application process,
2. those that enable the employees with disabilities to perform the essential functions of the job, and
3. those that enable employees with disabilities to enjoy the same benefits and privileges of employment as are enjoyed by employees without disabilities.

Accommodations may include making sure a kitchen facility provided for the convenience of the employees is accessible to individuals with disabilities or that employees with disabilities have access to the same insurance coverage as employees without disabilities.[9]

The regulations also require that the employer conduct an informal, interactive discussion with the applicant or employee who is in need of the accommodation. "This process should identify the precise limitations resulting from the disability and potential reasonable accommodations that could overcome those limitations."[10]

Reasonable accommodations are often a matter of common sense. For example, a deaf welder worked in an outdoor yard where trucks delivered fruit bins. His supervisor fired him because he believed the man could not work there safely because of the trucks coming in and out of the yard. Later the supervisor realized that the deaf employee could be stationed to see any danger from the trucks entering the yard. With this accommodation, and with fellow employees informed of his deafness, the man could safely perform his job in a fully satisfactory manner.

Another situation involved a bookkeeper who was hard of hearing who had difficulty working in one part of her office because background noise interfered with her hearing aid. When she was reassigned to a quieter part of the office, her difficulty was reduced and her productivity increased.

Sometimes employers do not wish to hire deaf workers because they claim that deaf workers will not be able to hear fire alarms and warning devices on machinery. These employers can make a simple accommodation by installing a visual alarm system.

In a recent case, *Bryant v. Better Business Bureau of Greater*

Maryland, a hard of hearing employee who worked in the membership department, brought an ADA claim alleging that her employer denied her a reasonable accommodation. The employer had transferred the employee to a different position instead of providing her with a better amplification device or a TTY, which would have enabled her to complete her duties. The court held that the reasonable accommodation question asks whether "the accommodation (1) would be effective, i.e., would it address the job-related difficulties presented by the employee's disability; and (2) would [the accommodation] allow the employee to attain an equal level of achievement, opportunity and participation, that a non-disabled individual in the same position would be able to achieve."[11]

In another case, *EEOC v. Pinnacle Holdings, Inc.*, the employer failed to provide or consider possible accommodations for an employee who was hard of hearing. The employer subsequently fired the individual because she could not hear the intercom. The jury found the employer's actions violated the ADA and awarded compensatory damages to the individual.[12]

In the federal workplace, the Civil Service Reform Act of 1978 and the *Federal Personnel Manual* also provide reasonable accommodations for deaf federal employees by specifically authorizing agency heads to employ or assign interpreters to deaf employees.[13] A federal employee won a lawsuit when the judge found that his supervisors had not considered Office of Personnel Management guidelines about reasonable modifications.[14]

EMPLOYER DEFENSES AND EXEMPTIONS

If an employer can demonstrate that an individual with a disability poses a direct threat to his or her health or safety or to others in the workplace, or if the employer can demonstrate that the reasonable accommodation is an undue hardship, then the employer may have a defense against liability under the ADA.

Direct Threat

An employer can sometimes defend against a charge of discrimination by showing that individuals pose a direct threat to their own health or safety or to that of others in the workplace. However, the ADA has a strict definition of "direct threat," which states that such a determination must be based on an individualized assessment of the person's present ability to safely perform the essential functions of the job. If a person poses a direct threat, the employer must see if a reasonable accommodation would either eliminate or reduce the risk to an acceptable level. In determining a direct threat, decisions must be made on a case-by-case basis based on objective, factual evidence rather than on fears or stereotypes.

The ADA legislative history and the EEOC refer to a federal case involving a hard of hearing person, *Strathie v. Department of Transportation,* as an example of the requirement that decisions on safety must be based on actual facts of risk. In the *Strathie* case, the state of Pennsylvania had a rule prohibiting hearing aid users from obtaining licenses to drive school buses. A Pennsylvania federal court had supported the ban on issuing such licenses to hearing aid users on the basis of general safety concerns. The federal appeals court reversed the lower court, finding evidence in the record rebutting the state's safety concerns and showing that an appropriate hearing aid would enable a hard of hearing person to drive a school bus without appreciable risk to passenger safety. This evidence had to be considered in determining whether a driver wearing a hearing aid actually would present a risk to the safety of school bus passengers.[15]

In another case, *Rizzo v. Children's World Learning Center,* a woman who was hard of hearing and used hearing aids was removed from her position as the driver of a van for a children's educational center because her employer was afraid that she would not be able to "hear a child choking in the back of the van."[16] The employer contended that the employee posed a direct threat to the children. A jury awarded the woman $100,000 in her ADA discrimination claim. The court of appeals affirmed the ruling, stating that the woman was qualified for her position and that there was no evidence that an essential element of the job was the ability to hear a choking child. The court said that the relevant inquiry was whether the person is able to safely drive the van and not present a direct threat to the children's safety.

Undue Hardship

Undue hardship means significant difficulty or expense for the business. In deciding whether an accommodation would be an undue hardship to the business, the following conditions should be considered:

1. the nature and net cost of the accommodation needed, taking into consideration the availability of tax credits and deductions, and/or outside funding;
2. the overall financial resources of the business site providing the accommodation, the number of employees, and the effect on resources;
3. the overall financial resources of the business, including its size in terms of number of employees and number and type of business sites;
4. the type of business operation and the relationship of the facility to the overall business.[17]

The analysis to the EEOC regulations gives the following example involving a deaf applicant. An independently owned fast-food franchise receives no money from the parent company that gives out the franchises. The franchise refuses to hire a deaf person because it says it would be an undue hardship to provide an interpreter for monthly staff meetings. Since the financial relationship between the local franchise and the parent company is only a franchise fee, only the financial resources of the local franchise would be considered in deciding whether providing the accommodation would be an undue hardship. However, a different fast food chain might be organized differently. If a factual determination shows that there is a financial or administrative relationship between the parent company and the local site providing the accommodation, then the parent company's resources should be considered in determining whether the hardship is undue.[18]

Under Sections 501 and 504 of the Rehabilitation Act, a recipient employer does not have to provide a reasonable accommodation if it would cause "undue hardship" on the program's operation. The factors that determine if there is an undue hardship are:

1. the overall size of the recipient's program with respect to number of employees, number and type of facilities, and size of budget;
2. the nature of the recipient's operation, including the composition and structure of the recipient's work force; and
3. the type and cost of the accommodation needed.[19]

The analysis to the Section 504 regulation gives some examples of factors to be weighed in determining if an accommodation causes undue hardship:

A small day-care center might not be required to expend more than a nominal sum, such as that necessary to equip a telephone for use by a secretary with impaired hearing, but a large school district might be required to make a teacher's aid available to a blind applicant for a teaching job.[20]

Section 503 has a similar defense for employers but uses the term "business necessity" instead of "undue hardship." The same factors apply in determining either business necessity or an undue hardship. Either one, if proven, excuses an employer from providing a reasonable accommodation.

QUALIFICATION STANDARDS, TESTS, AND OTHER CRITERIA

It is unlawful under the ADA for an employer to use qualification standards, employment tests, or other selection criteria that screen out or tend to screen out individuals with disabilities.[21] Tests may be given if they are job-related and required by business necessity. It would be discriminatory, for example, for an employer to require every applicant to pass a written test that measures language skills when the essential functions of the job in question do not require those skills. Too often such tests have excluded deaf people from being hired or promoted. In some situations, parts of written tests may be waived as an appropriate accommodation for a deaf person.

Under the ADA, an employer must select and administer tests to a person with a sensory, manual, or speech impairment that accurately reflect the test taker's skills or aptitude rather than his or her impairment. For example, it would be illegal to require an oral test for a person who does not have the ability to speak.

In Texas, an employer refused to hire an individual who had hearing and vision impairments on the basis of his disabilities. The employer had posed a disability-related inquiry to the applicant during the interview process. The jury awarded both compensatory and punitive damages to the individual because of the unlawful pre-offer inquiries about the nature and severity of the applicant's disability.[22]

Medical Examinations

Deaf people are sometimes denied particular jobs on the basis of medical criteria that disqualify any person with a hearing loss. Deaf people have been medically disqualified as bus mechanics or geologists solely on the basis of their hearing loss. These blanket medical exclusions can be challenged if they are not job related. In addition, under Section 504 regulations an employer may make offers of employment dependent upon the results of medical examinations only if such examinations are administered confidentially and in a nondiscriminatory manner to all employees.[23]

Prior to a job offer, an employer cannot conduct medical examinations or ask about an applicant's disability. However, an employer can ask about the person's ability to perform specific essential job functions with or without reasonable accommodation. An employer can also require a medical examination *after* an offer of employment has been made and before the start of employment. The employer may make the offer of employment contingent on the results of the examination if all entering employees take the examination and the information obtained during the examination is kept confidential.

However, supervisors and managers may be informed regarding necessary restrictions or accommodations to the work of the employee, and first aid and safety personnel may be informed if the disability might require emergency treatment. Government officials investigating ADA compliance may also be informed of the examination results. The employer cannot discriminate against an individual with a disability on the basis of the examination unless the reasons for rejection are job-related and necessary for the conduct of the employer's business. The employer also cannot refuse to hire an individual because of a disability, if that person can perform the essential functions of the job with an accommodation. Repeatedly, deaf and hard of hearing applicants have been excluded from consideration for jobs on the basis of medical examinations before jobs have been offered. This section of ADA prohibits such practices.

Once an employee has been hired and started work, an employer cannot require that he or she take a medical examination or ask questions about an employee's disability unless the questions are related to the job and necessary for the conduct of the employer's business.

The EEOC has issued a guidance on pre-employment inquiries under the ADA.[24] This guidance offers examples of permissible and impermissible questions and examinations. For example, the employer may ask about an applicant's ability to perform the physical requirements of a job, such as lifting a certain amount of weight or climbing ladders. Employers may ask applicants to demonstrate or describe how they would perform job tasks. The guidance also discusses what constitutes a medical examination and the types or procedures and tests that are permissible. An employer may ask applicants to perform physical agility or fitness tests in which the applicant demonstrates ability to perform actual or simulated job tasks.

AFFIRMATIVE ACTION

A substantive difference between the ADA and the three employment sections of the Rehabilitation Act is their mandate for affirmative action hiring policies. Affirmative action characteristically means special programs to actively recruit, hire, train, accommodate, and promote qualified disabled people. Nondiscrimination, on the other hand, usually means an obligation to treat disabled employees in the same manner as other employees and provide reasonable accommodations.

The ADA contains no affirmative action hiring provisions. Sections 501 and 503 of the Rehabilitation Act require the federal government and federal contractors to take affirmative action to hire, promote, and retain qualified people with disabilities. Section 504, however, does not require affirmative action; it simply requires nondiscrimination.[25]

With regard to disabilities, however, identical treatment may itself be discriminatory. An employer who holds a staff meeting for all employees has effectively excluded a deaf employee from participating if no interpreter is provided. The same is true of an employer who hires a person in a wheelchair to work in a building that does not have ramps. By treating the disabled employee precisely the same as the nondisabled employee, the employer has acted unfairly. In all situations in which identical treatment constitutes discrimination against disabled employees, Section 504 requires recipients of federal financial assistance to take specific steps to provide equal opportunity and *equally effective* means of taking advantage of that opportunity.

Federal Obligations

The federal government has established several policies and programs designed to fulfill its affirmative action obligations under Section 501. For example, the government will make special arrangements for applicants taking the Civil Service examination when applicants' disabilities prevent them from competing equally. These include waiving certain verbal tests for deaf applicants and providing readers for blind applicants, interpreters for deaf applicants, enlarged answer blocks for applicants with poor manual dexterity or motor coordination, taped and/or braille tests, and extended time limits for taking the tests.

The government also has special hiring programs designed to facilitate the appointment of disabled employees. One hiring program is the temporary trial appointment, which gives the disabled employee an opportunity to know what he or she can do and overcome the employer's anxieties about the person's capabilities. Under this program, individuals with physical and mental disabilities can be hired for a temporary period without going through the normal competitive hiring procedures. As soon as the employee has demonstrated his or her ability to do the job, the appointment can be made permanent.

Another program used to hire disabled individuals is known as the "excepted" or "Schedule A" appointment. It is available to applicants with severe disabilities. Under the excepted appointment program, people with disabilities can be hired for permanent jobs by federal agencies without having to take the Civil Service examination. The purpose of the program is to avoid the discriminatory effects of the examination.

Following its obligation under Section 501 and the Civil Service Reform Act of 1978, the federal government has authorized several methods of hiring interpreters for deaf employees in various work situations. Each federal agency has the option of either (1) hiring full-time interpreters, (2) using other employees who can interpret competently, or (3) contracting out with individual interpreters or interpreter referral agencies on an as-needed basis. The best method depends on the work situation involved. If a particular deaf employee's job requires frequent use of an interpreter, or if there are several deaf employees in one agency whose combined needs require frequent service, then a full-time interpreter on staff would be the best solution. If an interpreter is needed for an occasional or regular office meeting, it might be best to contract for services of a private interpreter.

FURTHER ASSISTANCE

More detailed information on the procedures for taking advantage of all these special federal programs and services can be obtained by contacting federal job information centers throughout the country. Also, the personnel office of each federal agency has a selective placement coordinator who is responsible for implementing these programs.

These federal selective placement coordinators want advice and need assistance from vocational rehabilitation counselors on all issues and problems involving recruitment, hiring, and accommodations for disabled employees. Rehabilitation counselors

> ### Guidance for Rehabilitation Counselors
>
> The federal government has suggested ways that rehabili-
> tation counselors can take the initiative to ensure that af-
> firmative action is implemented:
>
> - ✦ survey federal agencies to determine what types of jobs
>   are likely to be available and which of these are likely
>   to be in demand by disabled individuals
> - ✦ Work with other counselors and organizations to es-
>   tablish referral systems
> - ✦ Provide follow-up assistance to agency supervisors
>   after a disabled person has been hired
> - ✦ Arrange for selective placement coordinators, manag-
>   ers, and supervisors to tour rehabilitation and indepen-
>   dent living centers and to attend workshops and
>   consciousness-raising programs
> - ✦ Give recognition awards and publicity to agencies that
>   actively participate in employment programs for dis-
>   abled individuals
> - ✦ Share information about federal job vacancies and per-
>   sonnel needs with rehabilitation counselors in the area
> - ✦ Involve selective placement coordinators in the activi-
>   ties of rehabilitation agencies[26]

should develop contacts with federal personnel offices; they
should be thoroughly familiar with federal hiring practices and
job application procedures. Continuing interaction among counselors, selective placement coordinators, managers, and supervisors is essential.

REMEDIES

Individuals with disabilities have the same remedies available to
all other protected groups under Title VII of the Civil Rights Act
of 1964, as amended by the Civil Rights Act of 1991.[27] The Civil
Rights Act of 1991 provides the same remedies as those under
both Title I of the ADA and Section 501 of the Rehabilitation

Act. Before filing a discrimination complaint the Civil Rights Act provides that an individual must exhaust administrative remedies. Thus, before an individual can get into court, he or she must first file a complaint with the EEOC or the appropriate state or local fair employment practice agency.

An employer found in violation of the employment section of the ADA may be ordered to discontinue discriminatory practices, to correct policies and practices, to hire a qualified individual with a disability, or to rehire the person with back pay and provide the person with a reasonable accommodation. In addition, an employer may be required to provide compensatory and punitive damages for intentional discrimination.[28] Damages may not be awarded where the employer demonstrates "good faith efforts" to identify and make reasonable accommodations.[29] Employers who lose a specific case will be required to pay the disabled person's attorney's fees and costs.

There are various remedies available under Section 503 of the Rehabilitation Act. These sanctions include injunctive relief, withholding progress payments, terminating the contract, and debarring the violator from receiving future government contracts.[30] A court may impose sanctions for an employer's noncompliance with affirmative action mandates, failure to ensure protection for individuals filing complaints, or failure to comply with Section 503.[31]

ENFORCEMENT PROCEDURES

Procedures under the Americans with Disabilities Act

As mentioned earlier, the EEOC enforces Title I of the ADA. An individual who believes that he or she has been the victim of employment discrimination can file a complaint with the EEOC district office that services his or her area. A discrimination charge must be filed within 180 days of the alleged discriminatory act. If there is a state or local law that provides relief for discrimination on the basis of a disability, an individual may have up to 300 days to file a charge. It is best, however, to contact your local EEOC office promptly if discrimination is suspected.

After the EEOC concludes its investigation, it will either offer to conciliate, issue a "notice of a right to sue" letter to the individual alleging discrimination, or take legal action on behalf of the United States. Once the individual has received this letter from the EEOC, the individual may file a complaint in federal or state court. This complaint must be filed within 90 days of receiving the notice.

Procedures under the Rehabilitation Act

Section 501: Federal Employees

A federal employee or applicant with a disability who believes he or she has been discriminated against by a federal agency can file an administrative complaint with that agency under Section 501. There are strict time limits imposed for each step of the procedure. While waiver of the time limits is sometimes allowed for good cause, a complaint can be rejected for failure to meet the deadline. The person with a disability has the right to be represented by an attorney at all stages of the complaint process. If an interpreter is necessary to ensure effective communication at any stage of the proceedings, the agency must provide and pay for one. The administrative complaint process is as follows:

A. Informal Precomplaint Counseling
   1. An employee or applicant for employment must contact the agency's equal employment opportunity (EEO) office. The contact may be made in person or by letter. No form is required.
   2. The EEO office will assign an EEO counselor to the case. The person bringing the complaint (complainant) must provide all the information about the discriminatory policy or action to the EEO counselor.
   3. The role of the EEO counselor is to:
      a. make an inquiry into the complaint and discuss it with all the people involved;
      b. attempt an informal resolution within twenty-one days;
      c. not discourage the complainant from filing a formal complaint; and

        d. not reveal the identity of the complainant unless authorized to do so.

    4. If informal resolution cannot be achieved, the EEO counselor will send the complainant a "Notice of Final Interview" informing him or her of the right to file a formal complaint with the agency.

B. Formal Complaint

    1. If informed counseling is not successful, the complainant has a right to file a formal complaint with the agency's EEO office.

        a. The formal complaint is written on a form provided by the agency's EEO office and is filed with that office.

        b. The written complaint should discuss in detail all of the facts involved and should include copies of letters and other documents substantiating those facts.

        c. If there is a continuing pattern or policy of discrimination, the complainant should describe the discriminatory activity as "continuing" in order to avoid any time/deadline problems.

    2. Rejection of complaint

        a. The agency may reject the entire complaint or some of the issues raised if it is not filed on time, the complaint raises matters identical to another complaint of the employee, the complainant is not an employee or applicant of the agency, or the complaint is not based on disability discrimination.

        b. If the agency rejects the complaint, the complainant must be notified in writing. The employee may then appeal to the Equal Employment Opportunity Commission (EEOC) or file suit in federal district court.

    3. Investigation of complaint

        a. If the agency accepts the complaint the agency will appoint an EEO investigator, a person other than the EEO counselor.

        b. The investigator will conduct an in-depth inquiry, take sworn affidavits from the people involved, and gather documents and statistics.

        c. If the complainant believes that important witnesses have not been interviewed or that important evidence has not been explored, he or she should notify the investigator in writing.

4. Adjustment of complaint

When the investigation is completed, the investigator writes a report. The EEO office sends copies of the report to both the complainant and the employer and provides them an opportunity to informally adjust (settle) the matter on the basis of the results of the investigation. If the complaint is informally adjusted, the terms of the adjustment must be in writing.

5. Proposed disposition
   a. If the complaint cannot be adjusted, the agency will issue a proposed disposition (decision).
   b. If the complainant is satisfied with the proposed disposition, the agency must then implement the terms of the disposition.
   c. If the complainant is dissatisfied with the proposed disposition, he or she may request a hearing before the EEOC in writing or file suit in federal district court of receipt of the proposed disposition.

6. EEOC hearing
   a. At the hearing, as at all other stages in the process, the complainant has the right to be represented by an attorney and to have a qualified interpreter.
   b. On the basis of evidence submitted at the hearing, the examiner (judge) will issue a recommended decision that the agency can reverse.
   c. If the complainant is dissatisfied with the decision, he or she may appeal to the EEOC Office of Review and Appeals or file suit in federal court.

C. Right to Sue in Federal Court
   1. The complainant can file suit in federal district court at any time after 180 days from the date the formal EEO complaint was filed, if the agency has not yet issued a final decision.
   2. In addition, as noted above, the complainant can file suit within 30 days after completion of other stages of the administrative process (e.g., after receipt of the notice of proposed disposition or after receipt of final agency action).[32]

Section 503: Federal Contractors

Section 503 of the Rehabilitation Act requires employers who have contracts with the federal government for more than $2,500 to take affirmative action to hire and promote qualified disabled people. About 300,000 private businesses are subject to Section 503. The work performed under these contracts includes construction of government buildings, repair of federal highways, and leasing of government buildings. In addition to primary contractors, Section 503 covers companies that have subcontracted for more than $2,500 of federal business from a primary contractor.

The administrative complaint procedure under Section 503 differs significantly from that described under Section 501. Section 503 is enforced by the U.S. Department of Labor's Office of Federal Contract Compliance Programs (OFCCP). An applicant or employee who believes he or she has been discriminated against by a federal contractor can file a written complaint with the regional OFCCP office. The regional OFCCP is supposed to investigate promptly and attempt to resolve the complaint. If the regional OFCCP finds no violation of Section 503, then the complainant may appeal to the Washington, D.C. headquarters of the OFCCP. If the regional OFCCP finds that the employer has in fact violated Section 503, then an attempt is made to resolve the matter informally and provide the appropriate relief to the complainant.

If the employer refuses to provide the appropriate relief, OFCCP can then employ more formal enforcement mechanisms. These include having OFCCP bring suit in federal court, withholding payments due on existing federal contracts, termination of existing federal contracts, and/or barring the contractor from receiving future federal contracts. If OFCCP begins any of these enforcement methods, the employer can request a formal administrative hearing. While the complainant can participate in the administrative hearing, it is primarily a dispute between OFCCP and the employer. The complainant is a witness, but not a party, to the enforcement action. Like the Section 501 EEO complaint procedure, the OFCCP process is long and time-consuming.[33]

Section 504: Federal Financial Recipients

Unlike the ADA or the other sections of the Rehabilitation Act, individuals alleging a violation of Section 504 do not have to exhaust any administrative remedies before filing an action in court.

Employers are required to adopt grievance procedures that will facilitate prompt complaint resolution.[34] The procedures for enforcing Section 504 are discussed in chapter three. As noted there, Section 504 applies to all recipients of federal financial assistance. "Federal financial assistance" under Section 504 differs from a "federal contract" under Section 503. It can mean grants and loans of federal money, services of federal personnel, or the lease of federal buildings for less than fair market value. Because of widespread dependence on federal money, recipients of federal financial assistance are many and varied.

Before receiving such assistance, all recipients must sign an "assurance of compliance" form agreeing to obey Section 504. The U.S. government as well as advocacy groups for people with disabilities have always taken the position that Section 504 prohibits employment discrimination by all recipients of federal aid, regardless of the purpose for which their federal funds are to be used. In other words, if a hospital received federal funds to buy medical equipment, Section 504 covers that hospital's employment practices.

State Statutes

State laws sometimes provide a remedy for employment discrimination when federal laws do not apply. A number of states have included a category such as "physical or mental disability" to the list of classes protected by traditional human rights and employment discrimination laws. Formerly these laws covered only race, sex, and religion. These laws are useful because they often apply to all public and private employers, thereby prohibiting discrimination even by employers who do not have federal contracts or grants, or those who have fewer than fifteen employees.

There is no uniformity in state human rights laws. Some protect physically disabled workers but not mentally disabled ones. Some require reasonable accommodations to disabled workers, but many do not. Some allow private causes of action—the right of individuals to sue in state court; others are limited to administrative enforcement by underfunded public agencies. In most states the agency charged with enforcement is the state civil rights commission or state employment agency (see appendix B). Enforcement procedures and remedies vary widely, as do the definitions of protected disabilities and of covered employers.

NOTES

1. Richard, Triandis, and Patterson, "Indices of Employer Prejudice Toward Disabled Applicants," *Journal of Applied Psychology* 45 (1953): 52.
2. See Wolfe, "Disability Is No Handicap for Dupont," *The Alliance Review* (Winter, 1973–74): 13; and Kalenick, "Myths about Hiring the Physically Handicapped," *Job Safety and Health* 2 (1974): 9,11.
3. A. Crammatte, *The Formidable Peak, A Study of Deaf People in Professional Employment,* 118 (Washington, D.C.: Gallaudet College, 1965).
4. 42 U.S. Code §12111(8).
5. 29 *Code of Federal Regulations* §1613.702(f).
6. 41 C.F.R. §60.741.2(t), 29 C.F.R. §32.3.
7. 42 U.S.C. §12111(9).
8. 41 C.F.R. §60.741.2(v); 29 C.F.R. §1613.704(b).
9. 29 C.F.R. app. §1630.2(o).
10. 29 C.F.R. §1630.3.
11. 923 F. Supp 720 (D. Md. 1996).
12. No. CIV-95-0708 PHX RGS (D.Ariz).
13. 5 U.S.C. §5331.
14. *Crane v. Dole,* 617 F. Supp. 156 (D.D.C. 1985).
15. *Strathie v. Department of Transportation,* 716 F.2d 227 (3d Cir. 1983).
16. *Rizzo v. Children's World Learning Center,* 173 F.3d 254 (5th Cir. 1999).
17. 42 U.S.C. §12111(10).
18. 56 *Fed. Reg.* 35,745 (July 26, 1991).
19. 45 C.F.R. §84.12(c); 29 C.F.R. §1613.704(c).
20. 42 *Fed. Reg.* 22,688 (May 4, 1977).
21. 29 C.F.R. §1630.10.
22. *EEOC v. Community Coffee Co.,* No. H-94-1061(S.D. Tex. June 28, 1995).
23. 45 C.F.R. §84.14(c) and (d).
24. See "Enforcement Guidance on Pre-Employment Inquiries under

the ADA," National Disability Law Reporter Statutes and Regulations II (Horsham, Pa.: LRP Publications, 1994).

25. 29 U.S.C. §791, §793.
26. See Office of Personnel Management, "Handbook of Selective Placement of Persons with Physical and Mental Handicaps," OPM Doc. 125-11-3 (March 1979).
27. 42 U.S.C. §1981(a).
28. 42 U.S.C. §1981(b).
29. 42 U.S.C. §1981(a)(3).
30. 41 C.F.R. §60-741.
31. 41 C.F.R. §60-741.51.
32. For more detailed information, see 29 C.F.R. §§1613.201–1613.806.
33. For court rulings that there is no private right to sue under Section 503, see *Rogers v. Frito-Lay*, 611 F.2d 1074 (5th Cir. 1980); *Simpson v. Reynolds Metal Co.*, 629 F.2d 1226 (7th Cir. 1980); *Simon v. St. Louis County*, 656 F.2d 316 (8th Cir. 1981); and *Davis v. United Air Lines*, No. 81-7093 (2nd Cir. 1981). For court rulings that an individual may bring suit under Section 503, see *Hart v. County of Alameda*, 485 F. Supp. 66 (N.D. Cal. 1979); and *Chaplin v. Consolidated Edison of New York*, 482 F. Supp. 1165 (S.D. N.Y. 1980).
34. 45 C.F.R. §84.7(b).

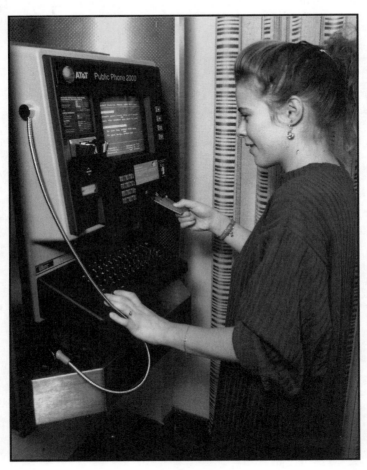

Chapter 8

Architectural Barriers

Inaccessible buildings pose barriers for many people with disabilities, including deaf people. Deaf people do not have equal use of buildings that have poor acoustics and voice-only intercom or entry systems, and buildings that do not have TTY payphones, visual smoke alarms, or visual notification systems.

Different federal and state laws establish standards of architectural accessibility for new and existing buildings. Enforcement is complicated by the overlapping standards and the need to identify the agency that has enforcement authority.

THE ACCESS BOARD

In 1973, Congress established an independent federal agency, the Architectural and Transportation Barriers Compliance Board (known as the Access Board). The Access Board enforces the Architectural Barriers Act of 1968, and it sets other federal accessibility standards.[1] Originally, the Access Board was made up of the representatives of nine federal agencies. It has since been enlarged several times. In 1998, the board had twelve federal agency members and thirteen public members appointed by the President. A majority of Access Board members must be people with disabilities.

In 1978, the Access Board was given increased authority to investigate communication barriers, including the absence of telecommunication devices; to provide technical assistance to make buildings and transportation vehicles accessible; and to adopt accessibility standards.

The Americans with Disabilities Act of 1990 (ADA) significantly expanded the role of the Access Board. The board has since developed accessibility guidelines for buildings and facilities covered by the (ADAAG), and it provides technical assistance to individuals and organizations on the removal of architectural, transportation, and communication barriers. Proposed changes to ADAAG are currently under review.

The most recent addition to the responsibilities of the Access Board was Section 255 of the Telecommunications Act of 1996, which requires the board to develop and to maintain accessibility guidelines for telecommunications and telecommunications equipment.[2] (See chapter twelve for a discussion of telecommunications standards and policy under the Telecommunications Act.)

ARCHITECTURAL BARRIERS ACT

The Architectural Barriers Act of 1968 requires most buildings and facilities designed, constructed, altered, or leased with federal money after 1968 to be accessible to individuals with disabilities.[3] This means that buildings cannot have barriers to people who are in wheelchairs, who use crutches, or who are blind or deaf. Everyone must be able to enter and use these buildings. The potential impact of this law is great.

Buildings covered by the Architectural Barriers Act must meet the Uniform Federal Accessibility Standards (UFAS) established by four federal agencies: the General Services Administration, the Department of Housing and Urban Development, the Department of Defense, and the U.S. Postal Service.[4]

If a person knows of a federal building that violates these accessibility standards, he or she may file a written complaint with the Access Board, which has the authority to conduct investigations and to attempt to achieve voluntary compliance. If voluntary compliance is not possible, the general counsel of the Access

Board can file a citation against the federal agency accused of violating the standards. A hearing is held before an administrative law judge to determine if there has been a violation of the barriers act. The judge can order the violating agency to obey the act or withhold or suspend its funding. The judge's order is final and binding on any federal department or agency. A complainant who remains unsatisfied with the findings of the administrative law judge may seek judicial review of an Access Board decision in federal court.

Questions or complaints about architectural, transportation, and communication barriers in federally owned or operated facilities may be submitted in writing to:

Architectural and Transportation Barriers
  Compliance Board
1331 F Street, NW, Suite 1000
Washington, DC 20001-1111
(202) 272-5434 (voice)
(202) 272-5449 (TTY)
http://www.access-board.gov

The letter of complaint should identify the person who is complaining (including address and telephone/TTY number), the barrier to which the person objects, the federal agency that is responsible for the building, and the building's owner and occupant.

ACCESSIBILITY GUIDELINES FOR NEW AND ALTERED BUILDINGS

The Access Board is responsible for developing ADA accessibility guidelines (ADAAG) to ensure that new and altered buildings are readily accessible to individuals with disabilities. Existing buildings must also be retrofitted to be architecturally accessible, but only if doing so would be "readily achievable," involving minimal expense. By contrast, the requirements for new or renovated buildings are far more explicit. They are also mandatory, requiring that all new buildings are accessible in the first place. The guidelines' goal is to assure that over time, all new places of public accommodation and commercial facilities will become accessible. The standards issued by the Access Board have been incorporated into regulations issued by the Department of Justice and the Department of Transportation under Titles II and III of the ADA.[5]

The Access Board initially issued the ADAAG Standards in 1991 and completed the guidelines for state and local government buildings and facilities in 1998.[6] These guidelines are far more explicit than the UFAS standards in the area of communication access for deaf and hard of hearing individuals. The guidelines contain requirements that must be satisfied in each facility and provide technical specifications for designing elements and spaces that are part of typical facilities (entrances and doorways, sleeping rooms, pay telephones, toilets and bathrooms, passageways, and assembly rooms). For the deaf and hard of hearing community, the most significant technical standards include telephones and TTY installations, visual smoke detectors, and assistive listening systems.

The Access Board occasionally updates the standards. For example, the ADAAG standards do not include provisions for minimum standards of acoustical design within buildings, even though background noise levels and reverberation are significant factors for successful speech communication. Organizations representing deaf and hard of hearing people have asserted that a poor acoustical environment is a significant barrier to individuals with hearing, speech, and/or language impairments. In April 1997, the Access Board received a petition for rulemaking from a parent of a child with severe hearing loss, asking that the board address the issue of acoustics in school facilities. The board responded by seeking public comment on acoustical standards that might be incorporated into an enforceable standard to be added to ADAAG.[7] Although the petition is still being considered, it may eventually be the basis for a new standard of acoustical design and acoustical performance characteristics in classrooms or related spaces used by children, such as day care facilities.

Public Telephones

The ADAAG standards apply to new or renovated state or local government facilities: arenas, convention centers, and secured areas of dentention and correctional facilities. If these facilities have at least one interior pay telephone, they must also provide at least one interior pay TTY. Convention centers must have one TTY on each floor level that has a pay phone.

The rules are slightly different for privately owned and operated buildings that are places of public accommodation. Any new or renovated site that has at least four public pay telephones (with at least one in an interior location) must provide at least one pay TTY. Where there is a bank of three or more pay telephones, at least one telephone in each bank must be equipped with a shelf and an outlet (for people to use their own portable TTYs). A pay TTY must also be provided at the following places, if they have at least one interior pay phone:

+ a stadium, arena, or convention center
+ a hotel with a convention center
+ a covered mall
+ a hospital emergency room, recovery room or waiting room
+ a transit facility
+ an airport

At an airport, there must be also be a public TTY if there are four or more public pay telephones in any of the following locations: a main terminal outside a security area, a concourse within a security area, or a baggage claim area in a terminal.

Assembly Areas

The ADAAG standards require assistive listening systems in certain "assembly areas." The guidelines define an assembly area as "a room or space accommodating a group of individuals for recreation, educational, political, social, civic, or amusement purposes." New or renovated assembly areas where audible communications are integral to the use of the space and that have fixed seating for at least fifty people or that have audio amplification systems must have a permanently installed assistive listening system.

The ADAAG standards define assistive listening systems as devices intended to augment standard public address and audio systems by providing signals that can be received directly by people with special receivers or their own hearing aids and which eliminate or filter background noise. The appropriate type of assistive listening systems for a particular location depends on the characteristics of the setting, the nature of the program, and the intended audience.

Alarm Systems

Visual alarm systems are necessary to alert deaf and hard of hearing people to emergencies involving smoke and fire, or other necessary evacuations. The ADAAG standards provide that, at a minimum, visual signal appliances shall be provided in buildings and facilities in restrooms and any other general usage areas, including hallways and lobbies. Visual alarm signal appliances must be integrated into the building or facility alarm system. Sleeping accommodations are to have a visual alarm connected to the building emergency alarm system or have a standard electrical outlet into which such an alarm can be connected. The ADAAG standards specify the minimum candela and strobe requirements so that visual alarms will be strong enough to attract attention.

BARRIER REMOVAL UNDER SECTION 504

Section 504 of the Rehabilitation Act of 1973 can be invoked to remove architectural barriers in structures used by recipients of federal financial assistance. Section 504 regulations at the Departments of Health and Human Services (HHS) and Education require each new facility or new part of a facility to be designed and constructed to be readily accessible to disabled people.[8] Alterations and new construction will comply with Section 504 if they meet the UFAS standards, as under the Architectural Barriers Act.

Most federal agencies have adopted the UFAS standards by referring to them in their own Section 504 regulations. If a building is constructed, altered, or leased by the federal government, complaints about architectural barriers can be filed with either the particular federal agency involved (under Section 504) or with the Access Board (under Section 502). If the federal financial assistance was given to a non-federal program for some purpose other than construction, alteration, or lease—such as programming—then, under Section 504, complaints about architectural barriers can only be filed with the particular agency providing the assistance.

REMOVING BARRIERS USING STATE LAWS

State architectural barrier laws can also be used to challenge architectural obstructions. Some of these laws are broader in application than the Rehabilitation Act because they are not limited to buildings that receive federal funding. For example, a state or local law may require all newly constructed places of public accommodation to be accessible. If so, this would include privately-owned restaurants and stores as well as state structures and facilities that receive federal assistance. Other state laws specifically deal with the problems of deaf people. Most states and counties require landlords of apartment buildings to install both auditory and visual smoke detectors and alarms.[9] If a state does not have such a law, deaf people might want to lobby for one.

AIR CARRIER ACCESS ACT

The Air Carrier Access Act of 1986 prohibits discrimination on the basis of disability in air travel and requires air carriers to accommodate the needs of passengers with disabilities.[10] The law applies to all U.S. air carriers providing air transportation. In 1990, the U.S. Department of Transportation issued a rule defining the obligations of air carriers and the rights of passengers with disabilities under this law.[11]

Under the Department of Transportation's rule, air carriers may not discriminate against an individual based on his or her disability. Additionally, air carriers may not require that a person with a disability accept specialized services, such as pre-boarding, if they are not requested by the passenger. An air carrier may not exclude a qualified individual with a disability from—or deny such individuals the benefit of—any air transportation or related services that are available to other people. Carriers may not refuse to provide transportation to people on the basis of disability unless there is some safety reason for doing so. If the air carrier believes that there is a safety issue involved, the carrier must provide the person with a written explanation of its decision within ten days. In addition, air carriers may not require advance notice that an individual with a disability is traveling on their carrier unless there is a request for a reasonable accommodation which requires preparation time. In these cases, an airline may require up to forty-eight hours advance notice.

An air carrier may not require that an individual with a disability travel with an attendant unless the air carrier has reason to believe the attendant is essential for safety. Although air carriers sometimes claim that they cannot communicate adequately with a deaf or deaf-blind passenger, the passenger can almost always establish essential communication. However, if the air carrier believes the passenger cannot establish effective communication, the carrier cannot charge for the transportation of the attendant.[12]

Air carriers must permit dogs and other service animals to accompany individuals with disabilities on a flight.[13] Air carriers should try to accommodate service animals by placing them at the seat location of the deaf or hard of hearing individual whom they are accompanying.[14] If this is not possible, the air carrier should "offer the passenger the opportunity to move to a seat location, if present on the aircraft, where the animal can be accommodated, as an alternative to requirement that the animal travel with checked baggage."[15]

Air carriers that have telephone reservation and information services available to the public must also have TTY services available for deaf and hard of hearing individuals.[16] Air carriers that make video presentations of safety briefings to passengers must ensure that the video presentations are accessible to deaf people. Thus, air carriers must use captioning or an inset of a sign language interpreter as part of the video presentation.

As with other passengers, an individual with a disability must conform to the Federal Aviation Administration's (FAA's) rules for carry-on luggage. Assistive devices, however, should not count against any limit imposed for the number of carry-ons allowed. Moreover, if the individual with a disability chooses to pre-board, wheelchairs and other assistive devices will receive priority for overhead storage space over other passenger items brought on board at the same airport. Likewise, assistive devices have priority over other items for storage in the baggage compartment. An air carrier cannot require an individual with a disability to sign waivers of liability for damage to or loss of wheelchairs or other assistive devices.

Airport facilities owned or operated by carriers must also meet the same accessibility standards that apply to federally-assisted airport operators. In particular, each terminal shall contain at least one TTY to enable deaf or hard of hearing passengers to make phone calls from the terminal. TTYs must be placed in a "clearly marked, readily accessible location, and airport signage shall clearly indicate the location" of the TTY.[17] In addition, the regulations require that the terminal information systems consider the needs of deaf individuals. "The primary information mode shall be visual words or letters, or symbols, using lighting and color coding."[18]

Carriers must designate one or more "complaints resolution officials" (CRO) to be available at each airport the carrier serves. If the CRO is not available at the airport, the carrier must make a CRO available via TTY. The CRO will respond to complaints from passengers and will also respond to written complaints. The CRO has the authority to make dispositive resolution on behalf of the carrier.

For further information on the Air Carrier Access Act, contact:

Office of General Counsel
Department of Transportation

400 7th St., SW, Room 10424
Washington, D.C. 20590
(202) 366-9306 (voice)
(202) 755-7687 (TTY)
http://www.dot.gov

FAIR HOUSING ACT

The Fair Housing Act has long prohibited discrimination in race or color, national origin, religion and sex. In 1988, Congress amended the Fair Housing Act (FHA) to protect people with disabilities from discrimination in the sale or rental of housing.[19] In addition to prohibiting discrimination, the FHA also included provisions that would eliminate architectural barriers in certain multi-unit dwellings available for first occupancy after March 13, 1991. The FHA incorporates the "reasonable accommodation" and "least restrictive environment" principles of the ADA, the Rehabilitation Act, and the Individuals with Disabilities Education Act (IDEA). The FHA protects people with disabilities as well as people who are associated with someone who has a disability.

The FHA covers most housing. In some circumstances, the act exempts owner-occupied buildings with not more than four units, single-family housing sold or rented without the use of a broker, and housing operated by organizations and private clubs that limit occupancy to members. Except for these limited situations, the FHA applies to all sales, rental, and financing of homes, apartments, and condominiums.

In general, landlords and sellers may not refuse to rent or sell housing, refuse to negotiate for housing, or set different terms and conditions or privileges for the sale or rental of a dwelling based on disability. Mortgage lenders may not refuse to make mortgage loans or impose different terms or conditions such as different interest rates, points, or fees, based on disability.

There are some additional protections. A landlord must let an individual with a disability modify the existing premises if such modifications would afford the individual the full enjoyment of the premises. Courts have generally held, however, that the expense of such modifications shall be paid for by the individual with a disability. Thus, landlords and builders must allow tenants or buyers to install visible alarms and doorbells, but the tenants must pay the additional cost. In the case of rental property, the landlord may condition his or her permission for modification upon the deaf individual's agreement to restore the premises to their original condition upon leaving the premises. Restoration is not required, however, where the modifications would not interfere with the next tenant's use and enjoyment of the premises.

Public housing projects have even greater obligations to their tenants with disabilities. Landlords in public housing projects or in buildings for which the landlord receives Section 8 funding may have to pay for the installation of flashing doorbell and visual notification systems and other modifications.[20]

The FHA also requires landlords, sellers, and condominium associations to make reasonable accommodations in rules, policies, practices, or services, when the accommodations may be necessary to allow a deaf individual equal opportunity to use and enjoy a dwelling. In analyzing this provision, courts have stated that individuals must be able to show that without the accommodation, they likely will be denied an equal opportunity to enjoy the housing of their choice.[21] While this provision has mainly been used to challenge state and local zoning practices, it has also been used to challenge "no pets" policies in dwellings where a deaf individual seeks to keep an assistance dog.[22]

In *Bronk v. Ineichen*, the court found that if a deaf tenant needed an assistance dog in order to live in a building, the FHA could require the building owner to relax the rule prohibiting animals. However, the deaf person has the responsibility of demonstrating that the dog was necessary to enable the tenant to live in the apartment. The court also stated that the landlord could not require an additional security deposit for an assistance dog. Deaf tenants or condominium owners can also challenge an intercom system or other security system that depends on responding to a voice intercom or buzzer for entry. If installing a visual system or TTY would be a "reasonable modification" of the security system, then the landlord should provide the alternative system.[23]

There are several mechanisms for filing complaints about housing discrimination under the FHA. You may file suit, at your expense, in a federal or state court. A complaint may be filed with a state or local agency for investigation. In addition, a complaint can be filed with the U.S. Department of Housing and Urban Development (HUD). HUD may refer the complaint to a state or local agency with Fair Housing Act powers, or it may accept the complaint for its own investigation. HUD will notify the alleged violator of the complaint and permit that person to submit an answer, investigate the complaint and determine whether there is reasonable cause to believe there is a violation of FHA, and notify you if it cannot complete the investigation. HUD will try to reach an agreement with the person you complained about. In some cases, HUD may ask the Attorney General to seek immediate injunctive relief, if it believes irreparable harm will be caused due to a serious violation of the FHA. If HUD finds reasonable cause to believe that discrimination occurred, the case will be heard in an administrative hearing or referred to federal court. Administrative law judges and federal judges may order the violator to compensate a victim for actual damages, provide injunctive relief, pay the government a penalty, and pay reasonable attorneys' fees and costs.

An administrative complaint must be filed with HUD within one year after the discriminatory practice occurred. When filing a complaint about an alleged discriminatory action, be prepared to tell HUD the following information:

+ your name and address
+ the name and address of the person your complaint is against (the respondent)
+ the address or other identification of the housing involved
+ a short description of why you believe your rights were violated
+ the date(s) of the alleged violation.

To find the name of the closest regional HUD office, call (800) 669-9777 (voice) or (800) 927-9275 (TTY). Every HUD regional office is equipped with TTYs or can be reached by relay service. You can also reach the central HUD office in Washington, D.C., or file a complaint using its web site, http://www.hud.gov.

NOTES

1. 29 U.S. Code §792.
2. 47 U.S.C. §153.
3. Architectural Barriers Act of 1968, as amended, 42 U.S.C. §4151, et seq.
4. 49 *Fed. Reg.* 31,528 (August 7, 1984). The UFAS standards follow the format and scoping requirements of the American National Standards Institute, known as ANSI A117.1
5. 28 C.F.R. §35.151; 28 C.F.R. §36.401–406.
6. 36 C.F.R. §1191. On January 3, 1998, the Access Board published ADAAG amendments for state and local facilities. The U.S. Department of Justice has not yet adopted these amendments as part of the enforceable standard under Title II of the ADA.
7. 36 C.F.R. Chapter XI, Docket No. 98-4, Petition for Rulemaking; Request for Information on Acoustics.
8. 45 C.F.R. §84.23(a).
9. See, for example, the Maine statute on visual smoke detectors, 25 M.R.S.A. §2464.
10. 49 U.S.C. §41705.
11. 14 C.F.R. Part 382.
12. 14 C.F.R. §382.35(c).
13. 14 C.F.R. §382.55(a).
14. 14 C.F.R. §382.37(c).
15. *Ibid.*
16. 14 C.F.R. §382.47.
17. 14 C.F.R. §382.23 (4).
18. 14 C.F.R. §382.23(5).
19. PL 100-430, approved September 13, 1988, the Fair Housing Amendments Act, amending Title VIII of the Civil Rights Act of 1968 (Fair Housing Act).
20. 42 U.S.C. §3601 et seq.
21. See *Smith & Lee Assoc. Inc. v. City of Taylor*, 102 F.3d. 781, 795 (6th Cir. 1996).
22. See *Alliance for the Mentally Ill v. City of Naperville*, 923 F. Supp. 1057 (N.D. Ill. 1996).
23. See *Bronk v. Ineichen*, 54 F.3d. 425 (7th Cir. 1995).

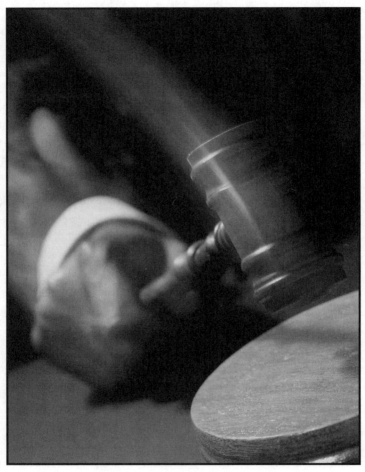

Chapter 9

The Legal System

In the absence of an interpreter, it would be a physical impossibility for the accused, a deaf [defendant], to know or understand the nature and cause of the accusation against him and . . . he could only stand by helplessly . . . without knowing or understand[ing], and all this in the teeth of the mandatory constitutional rights which apply. Mere confrontation would be useless.

U.S. SUPREME COURT (1925)[1]

The incident described above took place more than seventy years ago. Today, although the laws have changed, conditions for many deaf people dealing with the legal system are not much different. Deaf people experience numerous difficulties with the legal system because of communication barriers. They often cannot afford a lawyer; if they can, it may be difficult to locate one who is able to communicate with them and understand their needs. If they have to go to court, they often do not understand the proceedings and cannot adequately explain their side of the story.

In recent years considerable progress has been made at both federal and state levels to make courts more accessible to deaf people. The Americans with Disabilities Act (ADA) requires all state and local courts to be accessible to deaf individuals, and requires the provision of interpreters, transcription, or other appropriate auxiliary aids for deaf people in court.[2] The cost of these services cannot be assessed against deaf litigants.[3] State laws on interpreter services and qualifications for jury duty are slowly being rewritten to ensure necessary access.

Despite these advances, today's courts still deny equal access and due process to deaf or hard of hearing people. Even some judges are unfamiliar with the federal civil rights laws. Many state laws regarding the provision of sign language interpreters are either inadequate or clash with ADA and Section 504 of the Rehabilitation Act of 1973. They fail to ensure that deaf defendants understand fully the charges against them and participate effectively in their own defense. For example, a number of state interpreter laws fail to provide interpreters for arrest and civil and administrative proceedings. State laws that permit judges to assess the cost of interpreters as court costs violate both the ADA and Section 504.

ACCESS TO COURTS

In the United States, the ability of a deaf person to participate in court proceedings depends on whether the person is in state or federal court. Each state has its own laws to regulate its own court system, and the federal court system has different rules and policies. In federal courts, the Bilingual, Hearing, and Speech-Impaired Court Interpreter Act of 1979 governs to a large extent when an interpreter must be provided for a deaf defendant, party, or witness.[4] In state and local courts, deaf and hard of hearing people enjoy rights to equal access under the ADA and Section 504 that are much broader than the protections available in federal courts.

State and Local Courts

Deaf and hard of hearing people have the right to communicate effectively and to participate in proceedings conducted by all state and local courts. Specifically, they are entitled to have courts provide auxiliary aids to enable them to understand the proceedings. This right is based on two federal laws, the ADA and Section 504 of the Rehabilitation Act.[5] These federal laws protect *all* people participating in state and local court activities, including litigants, witnesses, jurors, spectators and attorneys.[6] They apply to proceedings in any state or local court, including civil, criminal, traffic, small claims, domestic relations, and juvenile courts.

The appropriate auxiliary aid depends on the individuals' amount of hearing, as well as their communication and literacy skills. For deaf people who use sign language, the most effective auxiliary aid a court can provide is usually the service of qualified sign language interpreters trained in legal procedure and terminology. For deaf people who do not use sign language and who have good levels of reading comprehension, the appropriate auxiliary aid may be the use of a computer-assisted, real-time transcription (CART) system. Through this system, a court reporter enters the words spoken during the proceeding into a computer, which simultaneously transcribes the words onto a computer screen which can be read by the deaf person. For other people, an oral interpreter may be needed to facilitate speechreading. For those who benefit from hearing aids, the appropriate auxiliary aid might be amplified or modified sound equipment or moving a trial to a small courtroom with good acoustics.

The U.S. Justice Department has issued regulations explaining the requirements of both the ADA and Section 504.[7] In 1980 the Justice Department noted that:

> Court systems receiving Federal financial assistance shall provide for the availability of qualified interpreters for civil and criminal court proceedings involving persons with hearing or speaking impairments. (Where a recipient has an obligation to provide qualified interpreters under this subpart, the recipient has the corresponding responsibility to pay for the services of the interpreters.)[8]

The Justice Department also noted that "court witnesses with hearing or speaking impairments have the right, independent of the right of defendants, to have interpreters available to them for their testimony."[9]

Court systems are not equally accessible to deaf individuals who cannot understand and participate effectively in court proceedings. In recognition of this fact, state and local courts are obligated to provide auxiliary aids, such as interpreters and CART services, at no cost to the deaf individual. In its ADA regulations, the Justice Department requires state and local courts to provide auxiliary aids to ensure effective communication with deaf and hard of hearing individuals in all court proceedings:

(a) A public entity shall take appropriate steps to ensure that communications with applicants, participants, and members of the public with disabilities are as effective as communications with others.

(b)(1) A public entity shall furnish appropriate auxiliary aids and services where necessary to afford an individual with a disability an equal opportunity to participate in, and enjoy the benefits of, a service, program, or activity conducted by a public entity.

(2) In determining what type of auxiliary aid and service is necessary, a public entity shall give primary consideration to the requests of the individual with disabilities.[10]

This law protects deaf parents of minors who are involved in court proceedings. Parents of a minor who is the subject of a juvenile proceeding are clearly "participants" in the proceeding even though the parents are not parties or witnesses, and they are entitled to qualified interpreting services during the proceeding.

The Justice Department regulation defines the term "auxiliary aids" for deaf and hard of hearing individuals to include qualified interpreters and CART services.[11] In its analysis of the regulation, the department uses the CART system as an example of an effective auxiliary aid or service in a courtroom for a person who is deaf and uses speech to communicate.[12] The Justice Department regulation also makes it clear that the individual with a disability cannot be charged for the auxiliary aid provided by a state or local court:

A public entity may not place a surcharge on a particular individual with a disability . . . to cover the costs of measures, such as the provision of auxiliary aids or program accessibility, that are required to provide that individual . . . with the nondiscriminatory treatment required by the Act or this part.[13]

Some state courts still have laws that permit state judges to assess the cost of interpreter services as "court costs." These state laws violate the ADA. In its analysis to the ADA regulation, the Justice Department explicitly addressed the issue of court costs:

> The Department [of Justice] has already recognized that imposition of the cost of courtroom interpreter services is impermissible under Section 504 . . . . Accordingly, recouping the costs of interpreter services by assessing them as part of court costs would also be prohibited."[14]

Complaints Against State and Local Courts

Despite the ADA and Section 504, some judges refuse to provide deaf people with the equal access promised by law. In these instances, lawsuits against the courts and the judges have been necessary to ensure compliance.

In Indiana, Cindy Clark filed a small claims action in a state court. She asked the judge to appoint a qualified interpreter at no cost. The judge refused, stating that "the court will hear evidence by way of written documents rather than verbal communication or signing." Clark sued the state of Indiana and the county court judge in a federal court, claiming discrimination under the ADA and Section 504. The case settled when the Indiana Supreme Court agreed to amend its own trial rules in order to comply with the ADA. The county court agreed to provide an interpreter for Clark's small claims court proceeding and further agreed that the fee would not be assessed against Clark regardless of the outcome of the case.[15]

In Ohio, a deaf man was a defendant in a criminal proceeding in a county court. A county judge ordered him to pay more than $200 for the interpreter who was present during his hearings. The man filed a complaint in an Ohio federal court, claiming violations of the ADA and Section 504. In response to the lawsuit, the county judge entered an order relieving the man of the obligation to pay for interpreter fees. The county court also adopted a new policy providing that, "All parties and witnesses who appear before the court, who are deaf, shall be afforded a properly certified and trained interpreter at County expense . . . No interpreter's fee shall be taxed as court costs against any deaf parties or witness."[16]

The repercussions of a court's or a judge's failure to provide auxiliary aids and equal access are, in many cases, the denial of justice. As a result of violations of the ADA and Section 504 in the courtroom, deaf parents have unfairly and needlessly lost their children. In one child custody case, a court refused to provide real-time captioning or a suitable alternative during trial for a father with a serious hearing loss.[17] In a case that truly gives meaning to the phrase "justice delayed is justice denied," the father did not see his daughter for five years. He brought a Title II ADA complaint against the county and the county court in a federal district court. The jury awarded him $400,000.

Despite advances, deaf individuals continue to be denied interpreter services or are assessed interpreter fees as court costs in blatant noncompliance with the ADA and Section 504. Sometimes, legal actions against states and individual judges are necessary to eradicate this discrimination.

Federal Courts

It is ironic that litigants in federal court have fewer rights to access than litigants in state courts. However, the ADA and Section 504 do not apply to the federal court system. Access to federal courts is governed by the Bilingual, Hearing, and Speech-Impaired Court Interpreter Act.[18] This law requires that, in any criminal or civil action initiated by the federal government, the court must appoint a qualified interpreter. The service is paid for by the government, whether or not the person needing the service is indigent. If, on the other hand, a deaf person files a suit, this law does not require the federal court to provide an interpreter.

In those suits where an interpreter must be provided, the director of the Administrative Office of the U.S. Courts determines the qualifications required of court appointed interpreters. Each district court must maintain a list of certified interpreters in the office of the clerk of the court. The director of court administration must consult organizations of and for deaf people in preparing such lists. These organizations include the National Association of the Deaf (NAD) and the Registry of Interpreters for the Deaf (RID).[19] If an interpreter is unable to communicate effectively with the defendant, party, or witness, the court's presiding officer must dismiss that interpreter and obtain the services of another.

The shortcoming of this law is that only criminal and civil cases initiated by the federal government require the appointment of interpreters. On April 12, 1996, the Administrative Office of the United States Courts addressed this shortcoming by extending interpreter services to *all* federal court proceedings. In a memorandum to all chief judges of the federal courts entitled "Services to Persons with Communication Disabilities,"[20] the guide was revised to read:

1. **General Policy.** As adopted in September 1995, it is the policy of the Judicial Conference that all federal courts provide reasonable accommodations to persons with communication disabilities.

2. **Sign Language Interpreters and Other Auxiliary Aids and Services.** Each federal court shall provide, at judiciary expense, sign language interpreters or other appropriate auxiliary aids and services to participants in federal court proceedings who are deaf, hearing impaired, or have other communication disabilities. The court shall give primary consideration to a participant's choice of auxiliary aid or service. "Auxiliary aids and services" includes qualified interpreters, assistive listening devices or systems, or other effective methods of making aurally delivered materials available to individuals with hearing impairments. "Participants" in court proceedings include parties, attorneys, and witnesses. . . "Court proceedings" include trials, hearings, ceremonies and other public programs or activities conducted by a court. "Primary consideration" means that the court is to honor a participant's choice of auxiliary aid or service, unless it can show that another equally effective means of communication is available, or that the use of the means chosen would result in a fundamental alteration in the

nature of the court proceeding or in undue financial or administrative burden.[21]

Notably, the services that must be provided for participants and jurors are not required for spectators under this federal policy. However, the federal courts could elect to do so in situations where they determine it to be appropriate, "for example, providing an interpreter to the deaf spouse of a criminal defendant so that the spouse may follow the course of the trial."[22] In addition, although a CART system may be provided, the policy only requires these services be provided the duration of that person's participation in the proceedings. For example, in a case with a deaf witness, CART services were provided "only for the duration of a deaf witness's testimony."[23] It remains to be seen whether these limitations can be justified.

ATTORNEYS' OBLIGATIONS TO DEAF CLIENTS

Another key element to equal access in the legal system is the difficulty many deaf and hard of hearing people have in retaining lawyers who are able to respond to their clients' specialized needs while also protecting their clients' rights. Few lawyers would question the importance of being able to communicate effectively with their clients. Title III of the ADA underscores the importance of effective communication and requires private attorneys to provide deaf and hard of hearing clients with sign language interpreters and other accommodations that are necessary for effective communication.

Section 504 requires courts to provide interpreters for indigent criminal defendants to confer with their court-appointed attorneys. Interpreters for communication between deaf defendants and their court-appointed counsel is specifically provided in addition to interpreters during the court proceedings:

> . . . in cases where the courts appoint counsel for indigents, the courts under this subpart are also required to assign qualified interpreters (certified, where possible, by recognized certification agencies) . . . to aid the communication between client and attorney. The availability of interpreting

services to the indigent defendant would be required for all phases of the preparation and presentation of the defendant's case. The courts may establish some reasonable guidelines on the use of interpreter services that would not adversely affect the ability of the defendant and the defendant's attorney to develop and present the defendant's case.[24]

Every state has adopted rules of professional conduct that obligate lawyers to represent their clients competently and zealously. It is difficult to imagine how a lawyer who fails to communicate effectively with a client could satisfy that duty of competent and zealous representation. In addition to this ethical responsibility, attorneys have a statutory duty to provide effective communication to deaf clients under Title III of the ADA, which grants people with disabilities the right to equal access to public accommodations.[25]

Title III of the ADA specifically includes lawyers' offices in the definition of public accommodations. Public accommodations are required to provide auxiliary aids and services to ensure effective communication; lipreading and writing notes back and forth are seldom effective methods of communication with sign language users. An attorney who relies on these methods cannot be assured of communicating effectively or accurately with his or her client.[26]

The analysis to this regulation makes it clear that both Congress and the Justice Department expect "that public accommodation(s) will consult with the individual with a disability before providing a particular auxiliary aid or service."[27] The analysis further states that, "It is not difficult to imagine a wide range of communications involving areas such as health, legal matters, and finances that would be sufficiently lengthy or complex to require an interpreter for effective communication."[28]

The Department of Justice also noted:

The Department wishes to emphasize that public accommodations must take steps necessary to ensure that an individual with a disability will not be excluded, denied services, segregated or otherwise treated differently from other individuals because of the use of inappropriate or ineffective auxiliary aids. In those situations requiring an interpreter, the public accommodations must secure the services of a qualified interpreter, unless an undue burden would result.[29]

A public accommodation may avoid provision of an auxiliary aid or service only if it can demonstrate that providing the aid or service would fundamentally alter the nature of the service, or would constitute an undue burden or expense. However, if the attorney's office is able to demonstrate that there is a fundamental alteration or an undue burden in the provision of a particular auxiliary aid, the lawyer is not off the hook altogether. The attorney must nevertheless be prepared to provide an alternative auxiliary aid.[30]

Whether or not the provision of a particular auxiliary aid would constitute an "undue burden" is not always a simple matter. The undue burden standard is applied on a case-by-case basis. Undue burden is not measured by the amount of income the lawyer or other private business is receiving from that particular deaf client. Instead, undue burden is measured by a number of factors, including the financial resources of the law firm as a whole.[31] Therefore, it is possible for a lawyer to be responsible for providing auxiliary aids even for pro bono clients, if the cost of the aid would not be an undue burden.

The Justice Department does not permit an attorney or other place of public accommodation to charge a person with a disability for the cost of the auxiliary aid. Therefore, billing the deaf client for interpreter services as a "client cost" is not permissible. It is clear from Title III of the ADA and the Justice Department's ADA regulations and analysis that attorneys must be responsible for ensuring effective communication with their deaf clients, and that costs may not be passed on to the client.

EQUAL ACCESS IN LAW ENFORCEMENT AND THE COURTS

Without effective communication when dealing with law enforcement, deaf and hard of hearing people are subject to gross violations of their personal and constitutional liberties. This area, almost more than any other, has the potential to instantly and irrevocably alter a person's life. A deaf person who is arrested for a crime he or she did not commit can face serious barriers when it comes to expressing innocence. A deaf victim who is asked to tell the story of a rape or assault without an interpreter has been twice victimized. Unlike other arrestees, a deaf person might not be permitted to contact legal counsel or family. Although the ADA and Section 504 offer protection so that the deaf person will have equal access in each of these situations, that protection is meaningless if deaf people and law enforcement agencies are unaware of deaf people's rights.

Regulations for Police Departments Receiving Federal Assistance

The Justice Department's Section 504 regulation is specific in its requirements for police departments that receive financial assistance:

> A recipient that employs fifteen or more persons shall provide appropriate auxiliary aids to qualified handicapped persons with impaired sensory, manual, or speaking skills where a refusal to make such provision would discriminatorily impair or exclude the participation of such persons in a program receiving Federal financial assistance. Such auxiliary aids may include . . . qualified interpreters. . . . Department officials may require recipients employing fewer than fifteen persons to provide auxiliary aids when this would not significantly impair the ability of the recipient to provide its benefits or services.[32]

The department's analysis of the regulation explains this requirement in more detail:

> Law enforcement agencies should provide for the availability of qualified interpreters (certified, where possible, by a recognized certification agency) to assist the agencies when dealing with hearing-impaired persons. Where the hearing-impaired person uses American Sign Language for communication, the term "qualified interpreter" would mean an interpreter skilled in communicating in American Sign

Language. It is the responsibility of the law enforcement agency to determine whether the hearing-impaired person uses American Sign Language or Signed English to communicate.

If a hearing-impaired person is arrested, the arresting officer's Miranda warning should be communicated to the arrestee on a printed form approved for such use by the law enforcement agency where there is no qualified interpreter immediately available and communication is otherwise inadequate. The form should also advise the arrestee that the law enforcement agency has an obligation under Federal law to offer an interpreter to the arrestee without cost and that the agency will defer interrogation pending the appearance of an interpreter.[33]

Neither the regulation nor its analysis limits the provision of interpreters to arrested deaf people. Victims and complainants are also entitled to interpreters for effective communication. In addition, deaf or hard of hearing people who attend programs and functions sponsored by a law enforcement agency, such as informational workshops and educational programs, must be provided qualified interpreters upon request.

The analysis stresses the critical importance of the interpreter's qualifications. Quality can be ensured by contacting the NAD or the RID for a list of certified and qualified interpreters. If the interpreter is inadequate—as judged by either the deaf person, the interpreter, or a law enforcement or court official, another interpreter must be secured. The analysis places specific responsibility on the recipient agency to ascertain what kind of sign language the deaf person feels most comfortable with and then to secure an interpreter who is competent in that language.

Effective Communication under the ADA

Title II of the ADA prohibits discrimination against people with disabilities in state and local government services, programs, and activities. Law enforcement agencies are covered under the ADA because they are programs of state or local governments. The

ADA affects how police officers and deputies receive citizen complaints; question witnesses; arrest, book, and hold suspects; and operate telephone emergency (911) services.

Police officers need to ensure effective communication with individuals who are deaf or hard of hearing. Whether a qualified sign language interpreter or other communication is required depends on the nature of the communication—if a deaf person was asking a police officer for traffic directions, a notepad and pencil would be sufficient. It also depends on the needs of the individual—for example, some deaf people do not sign, and may prefer to use speechreading.

The length, importance, or complexity of the communication will help determine whether an interpreter is necessary for effective communication, i.e., during interrogation and arrests, where the legality of a conversation will be questioned in court. The Justice Department cautions that, "Police officers should be careful about miscommunication in the absence of a qualified interpreter—a nod of the head may be an attempt to appear cooperative in the midst of a misunderstanding, rather than consent or a confession of wrongdoing."[34]

In the ADA Title II regulation, the Justice Department defines the term "qualified interpreter" to mean "an interpreter who is able to interpret effectively, accurately and impartially both receptively and expressively, using any necessary specialized vocabulary."[35] The department also cautions against using family members or friends as interpreters, because "factors such as emotional or personal involvement or considerations of confidentiality may adversely affect the ability to interpret 'effectively, accurately, and impartially.'"[36]

INTERPRETER COMPETENCE

Securing qualified interpreters in law enforcement and court environments is critical. In its analysis to both the Section 504 and the ADA regulations, the Justice Department notes that recipients of federal funds and state and local governments (including court systems and the police) must use qualified interpreters to ensure a defendant is advised of his or her rights and the trial is deemed fair. The Justice Department has not required interpreters to be certified under Section 504 and the ADA, due to the difficulty in some areas of the nation to secure certified interpreters. However, it is doubtful that any individual who has not been formally trained or educated as an interpreter can perform the functions of an interpreter in this type of setting.

The mere existence of a federal or state law providing interpreters is no guarantee that they are actually provided and that they function appropriately. Some police departments may attempt to use a staff member "who knows sign language" to interpret. However, a person who can only fingerspell or a person who has taken a class or two in sign language will not be qualified. It is impossible for a person with such limited sign language to communicate the important rights that are at stake.

In Virginia, where state law requires the appointment of qualified interpreters, an unskilled and uncertified interpreter was provided to a deaf rape victim testifying at a preliminary hearing. Although the interpreter told the court that he was not skilled at reading sign language, the judge proceeded with the hearing. When the prosecutor asked the victim what had happened, she gave the sign for "forced intercourse." The interpreter said that her reply was "made love," an altogether different sign and certainly a different concept. The legal effect of the interpreter's mistake was devastating. Later, when she answered, "blouse," to the prosecutor's question of what she was wearing, the interpreter told the court, "short blouse," creating the impression that she had dressed provocatively.[37] A better interpreter was provided at the trial before the jury.

Effective enforcement of the right to a qualified interpreter is extremely important. It will require a continuing effort to raise the awareness of judicial and administrative judges and court clerks about relevant laws and the communication patterns of deaf people.

The obligation of law enforcement agencies to provide interpreters is founded not only in regulations and statutes, but in constitutional law as well. Courts have suppressed evidence obtained from deaf defendants when it was found that the *Miranda* advice of rights was not adequately communicated.[38] In some cases where confessions were suppressed, the *Miranda* warnings had been conveyed in sign language beyond the defendant's level of comprehension. In other cases, the *Miranda* warnings were given in written form that was well beyond the defendant's reading level. Sometimes, confessions and other pieces of evidence were suppressed because the *Miranda* warnings were not given at all.

Securing an interpreter with an NAD or RID legal skills certificate allows for a timely explanation of rights, that includes careful explanation of every legal term and sign. Providing qualified interpreters is one way police departments can both prevent objections to the adequacy of the communication and comply with the Justice Department's ADA and Section 504 rules. Presentation of a printed advice of rights form without providing interpretation will seldom if ever be sufficient. Some police departments videotape all communications with deaf defendants in order to verify for the court that the rights warning was effectively communicated and that the interpreter acted properly.

MIRANDA ADVICE OF RIGHTS

In the landmark decision *Miranda v. Arizona,* the U.S. Supreme Court recognized that questioning by police in the stationhouse or jail is inherently coercive and undermines the privilege against self-incrimination.[39] As a result of this decision, police are now required to "effectively inform" accused people of their constitutional rights before any questioning can take place. Without use of a qualified interpreter, most deaf people would not be able to fully understand their rights, and any waiver of their rights would not meet the Court's standard of being voluntary, knowing, and intelligent.

The standard written advice of rights form given to suspects before questioning requires a sixth- to eighth-grade reading comprehension level. Hearing people's ability to understand the rights set forth in this form is not seriously impaired by a reading deficiency, because they can be told out loud what is written on the form. The listening comprehension level of people with normal hearing and of people with reading problems usually exceeds their reading comprehension level.[40] However, the reading level required by the *Miranda* warnings and advice of rights forms remains far above the reading comprehension of many deaf people for whom English is a second language. Police officers need to ensure that deaf people receive a careful explanation of their rights by a qualified sign language interpreter.

The conceptual and linguistic difficulties posed by the *Miranda* requirement cannot be overcome by a direct translation into sign language. Sign language uses everyday rather than formal concepts. Critical concepts that may be unfamiliar to many deaf people include "right" and "Constitution." Some deaf people would not understand the term "lawyer" in the full sense of understanding a lawyer's function.

There are not many signs to express legal terms. The sign for "Constitution" is newly created; most American Sign Language users would be unfamiliar with either the sign or the English word, let alone the concept behind it.

Fingerspelling important legal terms will not generally increase understanding, especially if the accused deaf person has a low reading level.[41] To be understood, the terms and their meanings must be carefully explained in clear concepts. A qualified interpreter is fundamental at this point. Acting out and other demonstrative approaches by a qualified interpreter might allow deaf defendants to understand the rights familiar to many hearing defendants.

Examples of the Problem

One case illustrates the problem of communicating the *Miranda* advice of rights to a deaf defendant. David Barker, a deaf man with a reading comprehension level of grade 2.8, was charged with murder. The charges were dropped, but when Barker was in custody for unrelated charges a year later, police questioned him extensively about the murder by means of written notes. They did so without providing him either a sign language interpreter or advice of counsel. After several hours of questioning, Barker signed the *Miranda* waiver of rights and then a confession.

When Barker was interrogated a month later with an interpreter, he showed confusion in answering questions. Asked if he had understood the *Miranda* advice of rights, he replied in sign language, "a little bit." He also referred to promises allegedly made by the police guaranteeing hospitalization.

The court suppressed the first confession as being involuntary and suppressed a second confession on the grounds that the original promise of hospitalization continued to influence him, making the second confession involuntary. The court wrote:

> There was additionally offered testimony by experts in the field of sign language for the deaf that the expression "Constitutional rights," being an abstract idea, is extremely difficult to convey to the deaf, especially, as in this case, when the educational level of the individual is so curtailed. There was testimony that the warning, "Do you understand that you have the right to have an attorney present at all times during the questioning?," may well have been signed, and understood as "Do you understand it is all *right* to have an attorney present?," which obviously is far from the actual portent of the warning.[42]

Two other cases illustrate that without the assistance of an interpreter at the time of an arrest, a deaf person may often spend excessive time in jail and be unaware of a right to counsel and to post bail. Sometimes, a deaf person may even be unaware of the charges.

For example, Oklahoma state law requires that interpreters be provided to deaf defendants upon arrest.[43] In one instance, however, a deaf man arrested for a misdemeanor was in jail for two days without being given an interpreter. The Oklahoma Supreme Court found that the state law applies to city police departments and that because the deaf man could not understand his rights or communicate with those who could help him, he was forced to stay in jail longer than a hearing person would have stayed in the same situation. The city was found to be in violation of Section 504.[44]

In another case, Joseph Serio alleged that the city of Milwaukee and its police officers violated Section 504 by failing to provide an interpreter throughout the course of his arrest and subsequent processing. The officers were investigating Serio's alleged violation of an anti-harassment restraining order that had been secured by his former girlfriend. When the officers went to Serio's home, they unsuccessfully attempted to communicate with him through his hearing son. The officers then attempted to communicate with Serio through the use of written notes. This also proved unsuccessful. Serio asked for an interpreter, but the request was denied. The police officers arrested him for violating the restraining order and took him to jail. He made at least one written request for an interpreter, but an interpreter was never provided.

Serio was released on bail the next day. He sued the City of Milwaukee and the officers, claiming that they violated Section 504 by failing to provide an interpreter. A jury awarded Serio $65,000 for compensatory damages and $90,000 for punitive damages. A Wisconsin appeals court affirmed, finding "credible evidence was presented to the jury that at several points during his arrest and processing Serio requested an . . . interpreter [and] the City never provided one." The court specifically rejected the city's arguments that it was entitled to a new trial. The city had contended that interpreters were present during the trial, making the jury unfairly sympathetic to Serio and that the excessive punitive damage award was not "in the interest of justice."[45]

ACCESS TO PRISON PROGRAMS AND ACTIVITIES

Once in jail to serve their terms, deaf people are frequently denied basic due process rights and access to rehabilitation programs simply because prison staff cannot communicate with them. The Justice Department's Section 504 regulation sought to remedy this problem. The regulation specifically states that prisons should provide qualified interpreters "to enable hearing-impaired inmates to participate on an equal basis with nonhandicapped inmates in the rehabilitation programs offered by the correctional agencies (e.g., educational programs)."[46]

Nevertheless, there have been a number of important discrimination complaints brought by deaf inmates. For example, a deaf and blind prisoner in a state prison in Arizona could not communicate effectively with prison guards and other prison personnel. He could not talk to prison counselors or medical staff when he was ill. He was charged with breaking a prison rule, but he could not understand the testimony against him at the disciplinary hearing or explain his version of what had happened. When he sued the state prison system, the case was dismissed by an Arizona federal court. The U.S. Court of Appeals for the Ninth Circuit held that the prisoner could bring his complaint in court under Section 504 and the Fourteenth Amendment of the Constitution. The court upheld the Justice Department's Section 504 regulations, which require prison systems to provide auxiliary aids for deaf individuals to give them equal access to prison programs and activities.[47]

In another case, a deaf inmate in Maryland's prison system was denied an interpreter at a disciplinary hearing and was therefore unable to present a defense. The disciplinary board took away "good time" days that would have led to earlier release, and it transferred him for psychological evaluation from a minimum-security camp to a maximum-security house of corrections. The state psychologist there could not communicate with him and, therefore, could not competently evaluate him. The prisoner filed a lawsuit in a Maryland federal court requesting a court order requiring the state to provide an interpreter to any deaf inmate who faces administrative charges. The suit argued that, without a qualified interpreter, a deaf inmate who uses sign language cannot testify or question witnesses and is thereby denied his or her constitutional right to a fair hearing.

The federal court approved a consent decree that provided interpreters for deaf prisoners in many situations of prison life:

- ✦ at adjustment team hearings
- ✦ when officials give notice that a disciplinary report is being written

+ whenever a deaf inmate is provided counseling or psychiatric, psychological, or medical care
+ in any on-the-job or vocational training or any educational program

This consent decree is an excellent model of how to provide deaf prisoners both their basic due process rights and access to needed counseling, medical services, and rehabilitation programs.[48]

In response to the discrimination complaints brought by prisoners with disabilities, state and local governments began challenging these lawsuits on the ground that neither the ADA nor Section 504 applied to prisons. In 1998, a unanimous U.S. Supreme Court held that the ADA did in fact apply to prisons and that the prisons had to make their services, programs, and activities accessible to inmates with disabilities.[49] Immediately after that decision, a Texas federal court applied the case to a deaf person who had been arrested. The arrestee alleged that city police officers failed to provide an interpreter at the time of his arrest, that he appeared before two different judges for probable cause and bond hearings without interpreter services, and that he remained in a county lock-up for two weeks without interpreter services. The defendants contended that the ADA and Section 504 did not apply to pre-trial arrest and detention, but the court disagreed, holding that the ADA applies to all programs, activities, and services of state and local governments.[50]

Interpreter Privilege

States have begun to recognize that interpreters in a confidential attorney-client situation are covered by the attorney-client privilege. The privilege means that interpreters cannot be forced to reveal any information based on that confidential interview. The privilege exists to ensure that clients will freely discuss their problems with their lawyer without fear of disclosure. Some states have laws explicitly applying this privilege to sign language interpreters. For example, Texas law states:

A qualified interpreter or relay agent who is employed to interpret, transliterate, or relay a conversation between a person who can hear and a person who is hearing impaired or speech impaired is a conduit for the conversation and may not disclose or be compelled to disclose through reporting or testimony or by subpoena the contents of the conversation.[51]

In states that have not explicitly addressed this issue, laws and precedents pertaining to the status of translators should be applied to sign language interpreters.

A Maryland circuit court ruled that interpreters could not be ordered to disclose statements that a deaf suspect made to his attorney. An interpreter with legal-specialist certification had been subpoenaed to testify before a grand jury about a jailhouse interview between a deaf defendant, his attorney, and the defendant's relatives. The judge stated: "When both attorney and client depend on the use of an interpreter for communicating to one another, the interpreter serves as a vital link in the bond of the attorney-client relationship."[52] The judge also stated that the presence of close relatives at such interviews may be helpful in aiding the accuracy of the communication, thereby "enabling the attorney to provide meaningful assistance to his client." The case was appealed. The Maryland Court of Special Appeals did not deal with the question of whether the communication was confidential. It reversed the decision, saying that the lower court lacked the jurisdiction to issue the decree.[53]

Telephone Access

The Justice Department's ADA and Section 504 regulations require installation of TTYs in all state and local government agencies with which the public has telephone contact. In the analysis of its Section 504 regulation, the department refers specifically to the obligation of police departments: "Law enforcement agencies are also required to install TTYs or equivalent mechanisms . . . to enable people with hearing and speaking impairments to communicate effectively with such agencies."[54] The Justice Department has also determined that arrestees who are deaf or hard of hearing should be provided with a TTY for making outgoing calls. TTYs must be available to inmates with disabilities under the same conditions as telephone privileges are offered to all inmates.

The installation of TTYs at police stations can help protect the lives and property of deaf citizens. Moreover, the general public benefits from an additional segment of the local population's ability to make police reports by telephone. Many cities across the country have already installed TTYs in their police departments and other offices.

Similarly, deaf individuals must have direct access to 911 or similar emergency telephone services, including emergency response centers which must be equipped to receive calls from TTYs and computer modem users without relying on third parties or state relay services. Operators must be trained to use the TTY when the caller is silent and when the operator recognizes the TTY tones on the other end of the line.

EQUAL JUSTICE: CONSIDERATIONS FOR THE FUTURE

Although recent state and federal legislation has greatly advanced the rights of deaf people involved with the legal system, much remains to be done if they are to achieve full access and equal justice.

First, states without interpreter laws or with laws that clash with federal law should adopt model statutes that provide qualified interpreters to any deaf party or witness in any judicial action. In criminal cases, interpreters should be provided to the deaf person during any police interrogation. Civil and administrative proceedings must also require interpreters paid for by the government.

Second, laws such as the ADA and Section 504 must be fully enforced. The Justice Department must ensure full compliance with its regulations if the rights of deaf people involved with the legal system are to be protected.

Third, judges, court administrators, lawyers, and law enforcement officers must become more aware of the communication issues affecting them and deaf people.

Good laws, thorough enforcement, and enlightened attitudes will ensure that deaf people obtain equal justice under law.

NOTES

1. *Terry v. State of Alabama*, 105 U.S. 386 (1925).
2. 28 *Code of Federal Regulations* §35.160(b).
3. 28 C.F.R. §35.130(f). See analysis by the U.S. Department of Justice at 56 *Fed. Reg.* 35,705 (July 26, 1991) Imposition of the cost of courtroom interpreter services as court costs is impermissible under Section 504.
4. 28 U.S. Code §1827.
5. 42 U.S.C. §12131; see also 29 U.S.C. §794.
6. Neither the Americans with Disabilities Act nor Section 504 applies to federal courts.
7. See "U.S. Department of Justice Final Rule: Nondiscrimination on the Basis of Disability in State and Local Government Services," 28 C.F.R. Part 35, 56 *Fed. Reg.* 35,694 (July 26, 1991). See also "U.S. Department of Justice Final Rule: Nondiscrimination on the Basis of Handicap in Federally Assisted Programs—Implementation of Section 504 of the Rehabilitation Act and Executive Order 11914," 28 C.F.R. Part 42, 45 *Fed. Reg.* 37,820 (June 3, 1990).
8. 45 *Fed. Reg.* at 37,630.
9. 45 *Fed. Reg.* at 37,631.
10. 28 C.F.R. §35.160.
11. 28 C.F.R. §35.104.
12. 56 *Fed. Reg.* at 35,712.
13. 28 C.F.R. §35.130(f).
14. 56 *Fed. Reg.* at 38,705–38,706.
15. *Clark v. Hon. Douglas R. Bridges, in his official capacity as Judge of the Monroe County Circuit Court, and the State of Indiana*, No. IP93-877-C (S.D. Ind. Sept. 23, 1994).
16. *Shafer v. Hon. Robert J. Judkins, in his official capacity as Judge of the Highland County Court, the State of Ohio, et al.*, No. C-193-887 (S.D. Ohio Aug. 16, 1994).
17. *Popavich v. Cuyahoga County Court of Common Pleas, et al.* No. 1:95, CV 684 (E.D. Ohio, 1998).
18. 28 U.S.C. §1827.
19. National Association of the Deaf, 814 Thayer Ave., Silver Spring,

MD 20910-4500, (301) 587-1789 (TTY), (301) 587-1788 (Voice), NADinfo@nad.org, www.nad.org; Registry of Interpreters for the Deaf, 8630 Fenton Ave., Suite 324, Silver Spring, MD 20910, (301) 608-0050 (Voice/TTY), www.rid.org.

20. See the memorandum from Leonides Ralph Mechamy, Director, Administrative Office of the United States Courts, Washington, D.C. (April 12, 1996).

21. Judicial Conference Policy and Procedures, General Management and Administration, Chapter III, Part G. (Guidelines For Providing Services to the Hearing-Impaired and Other Persons with Communication Disabilities.)

22. Ibid.

23. Ibid., fn. 1.

24. 45 *Fed. Reg.* at 37,630.

25. 42 U.S. Code §§12181–12183.

26. According to 28 C.F.R. §36.303(c), "A public accommodation shall furnish appropriate auxiliary aids and services where necessary to ensure effective communication with individuals with disabilities."

27. See 56 *Fed. Reg.* at 35,567, quoting H.R. 485, 101st Cong., 2d Sess., pt. 2, at 107 (1990).

28. 56 *Fed. Reg.* at 35,567.

29. Ibid.

30. 28 C.F.R. §36.303(f).

31. 28 C.F.R. §36.104.

32. 28 C.F.R. §42.503(f).

33. 28 C.F.R. §42, subpart G.

34. See U.S. Department of Justice, Civil Rights Division, Disability Rights Section, "Commonly Asked Question About the Americans with Disabilities Act and Law Enforcement." Available: http://www.usdoj.gov/.

35. 28 C.F.R. §36.104; 28 C.F.R. §35.104.

36. 56 *Fed. Reg.* at 35,553.

37. *Commonwealth v. Edmonds*, Cir. Ct., Staunton, Va. (1975).

38. See, for example, *State of Maryland v. Barker*, Crim. Nos. 17,995 and 19,518 (Md. Cir. Ct. Dec. 8, 1977); *State of Oregon v. Mason*, Crim. No. C-80-03-30821 (Or. Cir. Ct. May 27, 1980).

39. *Miranda v. Arizona*, 384 U.S. 436 (1966).

40. M. Vernon, L. Raifman, and S. Greenberg, "The Miranda Warnings and the Deaf Suspect," *Behavioral Sciences and The Law* 14 (1996):121–35; M. Vernon, "Violation of Constitutional Rights: The Language-Impaired Person and the Miranda Warnings," *Journal of Rehabilitation of the Deaf* 11 (4): 1–8.

41. M. Vernon, "Violation of Constitutional Rights: The Language-Impaired Person and the Miranda Warnings," *Journal of Rehabilitation of the Deaf* 11 (4): 1–8.
42. *State of Maryland v. Barker*, Crim. Nos. 17,995 and 19,518 (Md. Cir. Ct. Dec. 8, 1977).
43. 63 Oklahoma St. T. §2410.
44. *Kiddy v. City of Oklahoma City*, 576 P.2d 298 (Okla. Sup. Ct. 1978).
45. *Serio v. City of Milwaukee*, 522 N.W.2d 36 (Wisc. Ct. App. 1993).
46. *45 Fed. Reg.* at 37,360.
47. *Bonner v. Lewis*, 857 F.2d 559 (9th Cir. 1988).
48. *Pyles v. Kamka*, 491 F. Supp. 204 (D. Md. 1980); See also *Clarkson v. Coughlin*, 898 F. Supp. 1019 (S.D.N.Y. 1995); *Duffy v. Riveland*, 98 F.3d 447 (9th Cir. 1996).
49. *Pennsylvania Department of Corrections, et al. v. Yeskey*, 118 U.S. 1952 (U.S. 1998).
50. *Gordon v. City of Houston, Harris County, and State of Texas*, No. 98-0394 (S.D. Tex. June 18, 1998).
51. Texas Code, Section 82.002; Added by Acts 1991, 77nd Legislation, ch. 333, section 1.
52. *"Touhey v. Duckett,"* in *Criminal Law Reporter* 19 (1976): 2,483 (Cir. Ct. Anne Arundel, Cty., Md.).
53. *Duckett v. Touhey*, 36 Md. App. 238 (Md. Ct. Spec. App., 1977).
54. *45 Fed. Reg.* 37,630 (1980).

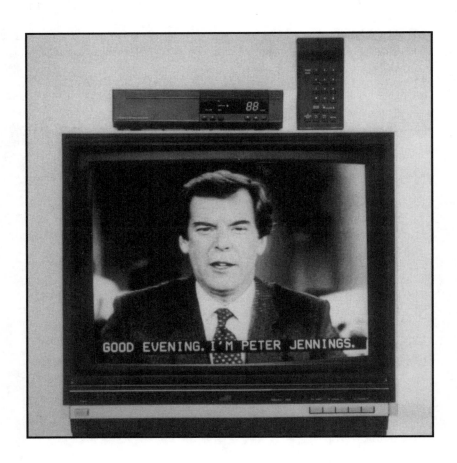

Chapter 10

Television

Television has become our major source of entertainment, news, and information. The Federal Communications Commission (FCC) reports that U.S. households watch television an average of over seven hours each day.[1] Without captioning, however, television provides little benefit or enjoyment for individuals who are deaf or hard of hearing. Captions provide essential access to national and worldwide current events, local and community affairs, and entertainment, bringing deaf and hard of hearing individuals into the cultural and political mainstream of our society. New federal captioning legislation is gradually making it possible for deaf and hard of hearing viewers to have access to nearly all forms of television programming.

THE BENEFITS OF CAPTIONING

Captioned television has made it possible for millions of people who are deaf or hard of hearing to see what television has to say. Captioning has taken two forms: *open captioning*, which involves broadcasting captions on a regular television signal to all receivers and which cannot be turned off by the viewer, and *closed captioning*, which involves transmitting the captions on a special television signal that requires the use of a decoder-adapter on the receiver. Today, almost all television captions are closed.

The potential audience that can benefit from closed captioning is quite significant. The National Captioning Institute (NCI) estimates that nearly 100 million Americans can directly benefit from closed captioned TV.[2] This estimate includes 28 million deaf and hard of hearing persons, 30 million Americans for whom English is a second language,[3] 12 million young children learning to read, 27 million illiterate adults,[4] and 3.7 million remedial readers.

Studies have consistently demonstrated the benefits of captioning for children and adults who are learning English or learning to read. A report commissioned by the Pew Charitable Trust in Philadelphia found that closed captioning has "a startling effect" on non-English-speaking children's ability to learn English words.[5] Most of the students in the study were from Southeast Asia. Similarly, results of a study at the University of Maryland showed that captioning improved word recognition for students with learning disabilities.[6] In addition, a Los Angeles English teacher turned off the sound on closed captioned programs to force her high school students to read the captions in order to understand the television shows. She reported marked improvement in the students' literacy skills.[7]

The number of senior citizens with hearing disabilities who are taking advantage of closed captions is also growing. It is well established that the population of the United States as a whole is aging. In the Washington, D.C. area, for example, the population of individuals older than 65 increased by more than sixteen percent between 1990 and 1996, nearly four times the rate of growth for the under-sixty-five population during that time.[8] Researchers from the Center for Assessment and Demographic Studies at Gallaudet University have estimated that more than thirty percent of people over the age of 65 will have a hearing loss by the year 2015.[9] A significant number of these individuals will require closed captioning to benefit from television programming.

THE HISTORY OF TELEVISED CAPTIONING

In 1972, the Public Broadcasting Service (PBS), a nonprofit, noncommercial television network, first introduced captioning with the nationally-broadcast cooking show, *The French Chef.* The captioning was done by WGBH, the PBS station in Boston, Massachusetts. This program, and a few others available only on public television, had open captions. By late 1973, WGBH was also providing open captions for the *ABC Evening News,* a half-hour program that daily took five staff people five hours to caption.

In 1972, PBS began developing a closed captioning system.[10] In 1975, PBS filed a petition with the FCC to reserve a segment of the television broadcast signal known as "Line 21" for transmitting closed captions. Line 21 is the last line in the vertical blanking interval (VBI) before the actual television picture begins. Closed captions are included in this video signal as invisible data. The captions are then decoded and generated into visual characters which are displayed on the television screen through a television set with a built-in decoder chip or a separate decoding device.

Since 1976, the FCC has reserved Line 21 for closed captioned transmissions. In 1979, Congress created the nonprofit National Captioning Institute (NCI) to offer closed captioning services to the broadcast television industry using Line 21.[11] Closed captioned television services began the following year when the NCI entered into a cooperative agreement with ABC, NBC, PBS, and Sears, Roebuck and Co.[12] Under this agreement, NBC, ABC, and PBS each captioned sixteen hours of programming per week, and Sears manufactured and sold decoders. In 1984, CBS also began transmitting closed captions using both Line 21 and its own teletext technologies.[13] Over the next decade, the number of television programs with captions grew dramatically, and by 1989 the entire prime time schedule on CBS, NBC, and ABC was captioned.[14] In all, by 1990 approximately 290 hours of programming were closed captioned each week.[15]

FEDERAL LEGISLATION

Despite the significant growth in captioned programming in the 1980s, the vast majority of cable programming, local news programming, late-night programming, and daytime programming remained without captioning as late as 1990. In 1991, approximately 72 percent of all Americans listed television as their primary news source.[16] However, only 150 out of 1,450 broadcast affiliates closed captioned their local news programs that year.[17]

Many attributed the resistance by networks to increase captioning hours to the fact that only a limited number of Americans owned devices that could decode captions on their television sets. In fact, in order to decode captions in the 1980s, individuals were required to purchase expensive and cumbersome external decoder equipment, which connected to their television sets. The cost and difficulties of installing these decoders kept sales down, and as of June, 1990, only 300,000 decoders had been sold to the American public.[18] With so small a viewing public, many networks did not have the commercial incentive to fund new captioned programs. For example, in proceedings held before the Commission on Education of the Deaf (COED) in the 1980s, ABC claimed that increased decoder usage would be necessary for captioning to become self-sustaining.

> "[If] decoders were more widely used and viewership to grow, the marketplace can be relied upon to increase captioning because more viewers would be reached at a decreased per capita cost. Increased decoder ownership—not just more captioning—is required for a strong, self-sustaining captioning service.[19]

In response, the COED recommended that Congress pass a law requiring all new televisions to have built-in decoder circuitry capable of receiving and displaying closed captions.[20]

TELEVISION DECODER CIRCUITRY ACT

In an effort to expand the caption viewing audience, and thereby create the necessary economic incentives for networks to caption more of their programs, Congress heeded the COED recommendation. In 1990, Congress enacted the Television Decoder Circuitry Act (TDCA).[21] The new law required all television sets with screens thirteen inches or larger, manufactured or imported into the United States after July 1, 1993, to be capable of displaying closed captioned television transmissions without the aid of external equipment.[22] This meant that television sets of this size would have to be equipped with internal decoder circuitry, which came to be known as a "decoder chip." In part, the law was patterned after the All Channel Receiver Act of 1962, which had mandated the inclusion of UHF tuners in all television sets.[23] Prior to that law, UHF transmissions also had been available to consumers only through a special adapter attached to their television sets.

Pursuant to the TDCA, the FCC has adopted display standards for built-in closed captioning decoder circuitry.[24] These standards are intended to enable the television viewer to enjoy the benefits of the latest innovative technologies for high quality closed captioning. For example, the FCC requires the use of technology that allows captions to appear anywhere on the screen. This feature allows for better identification of who is speaking during a television program. Additionally, several features that had proven effective in the separate decoder, such as a black background, are now required in new televisions containing the decoder circuitry.[25]

Because of the rapid changes in television technology, the drafters of the TDCA were concerned that any new television technologies, such as high definition and other forms of digital TV, be capable of transmitting closed captions. A section was included in the TDCA requiring the FCC to take appropriate action to ensure that as new technologies are developed, closed captioning will continue to be available to television viewers without the need of a separate decoder.[26]

On July 14, 1999, the FCC heeded this legislative directive and adopted a Notice of Proposed Rulemaking to adopt technical standards for the display of closed captions on digital television receivers.[27] In addition, the FCC proposed a rule that would require closed captioning decoder circuitry to be included in all digital television receivers. In releasing these proposals, the FCC explained that its intent was to fulfill its continuing obligations under the TDCA. These FCC proposals remained pending at the time this book went to print.

Passage of the TDCA did in fact result in the growth of the captioning audience. By 1995, twenty-five million television sets equipped with decoder circuitry had been sold in the United States, providing closed captioning to as many as sixty million American homes.[28] After passage of the TDCA, the number of captioned programs also increased somewhat. In the early 1990s, captioning was added to some children's programming, late-night talk shows, national sports programming, and premium cable stations.

However, the significant increase in captioning on cable programming that was expected to result from the market incentives created by the TDCA did not occur. Most basic cable networks continued to caption few or none of their programs, leaving deaf and hard of hearing people with only minimal access to television programs. Consumers decided that they would need to return to Congress to obtain a captioning law.

TELECOMMUNICATIONS ACT OF 1996

Congressional Action

In the early 1990s, Congress decided to revisit federal requirements for the provision of cable services to the American public. Deaf and hard of hearing consumers seized this opportunity to secure a provision in the pending bill to expand television captioning requirements. Consumers successfully pointed to the cable industry's consistent failure to caption more of its programs. In response, Congress enacted Section 305 of the Telecommunications Act in 1996, establishing extensive requirements for the provision of closed captions on television programming.[29]

The 1996 Telecommunications Act applied the new captioning mandates to all programming providers and owners that transmit video programming to customers' homes, including broadcasters, cable operators, satellite operators, and other programming distributors. It directed the FCC to set up a transition schedule for captioning two categories of television programming: (1) *new programming*—programming first published or exhibited after the effective date of the FCC's captioning rules, and (2) *pre-rule programming*—programming first published or exhibited prior to the effective date of such FCC rules. Congress set different access standards for these two categories, requiring television programmers to make all new programming "fully accessible" through the provision of closed captions, and requiring programmers to "maximize" the accessibility of pre-rule programming. This latter category includes, for example, old re-runs, as well as new made-for-TV movies that were shown before the FCC's rules became effective. As noted below, the FCC's captioning rules became effective on January 1, 1998, setting the dividing line for the new and pre-rule categories.

Section 305 authorized the FCC to exempt certain types of programming from the captioning requirements. Specifically, Congress gave the FCC permission to exempt programs under the following three conditions:

1. The FCC may exempt, by rule, closed captioning on programs, classes of programs, or services if the provision of captions would be economically burdensome to the video programming provider or owner of that programming;
2. The FCC may exempt closed captioning where the provision of captions would be inconsistent with contracts in effect on February 8, 1996; and
3. The FCC may grant individual exemptions from the closed captioning requirements, in response to petitions for such exemptions, where the provision of captions would result in an undue burden for a video programming provider or owner.

FCC Captioning Order

On August 22, 1997, the FCC established an elaborate schedule of deadlines by which compliance with the captioning mandates is to be achieved, together with permissible exemptions from the captioning rules.[30] Dissatisfied with many of the possible exemptions, the National Association of the Deaf and several other consumer groups challenged the rules, asking the FCC to strengthen the requirements for captioning access. Among other things, these groups asked the FCC not to limit captioning to only 95 percent of new programming, and not to exempt Spanish-language programming, overnight programming, and short advertisements. Yet at the same time, several television stations requested that the FCC impose even more exemptions than were contained in the 1997 Order. For example, networks sought exemptions for home shopping programming, all instructional programming on public television stations, and interactive game shows.

On September 17, 1998, the FCC rejected virtually all requests by networks for new exemptions, and granted several of the consumer requests for enhanced captioning access.[31] The final FCC rules concern new, pre-rule, and Spanish-language programming.

New Programming

The FCC requires that 100 percent of all new non-exempt programming must be captioned over an eight-year period, beginning January 1, 1998.[32] The FCC has explained that, in order to meet this obligation, each channel must caption (during each calendar quarter): 450 hours of programming within the first two years (by December 31, 2001), 900 hours within four years, and 1,350 hours within six years. The remaining programming that is not exempt must be captioned within eight years.[33]

If a station already captions more programming than is required by the transition schedule, it is *not* permitted to reduce the amount of captioning in accordance with the above schedules. Rather, programming providers must continue to provide captioning "at a level substantially the same" as the average level they provided captioning during the first six months of 1997.[34]

Pre-Rule Programming

The FCC rules direct programmers to caption 75 percent of all pre-rule programming over a ten-year transition period;[35] at least 30 percent of such programming must be captioned by January 1, 2003.[36] The FCC has indicated that it will re-evaluate its decision to require captioning for only 75 percent of this type of programming after four years.

Spanish-Language Programming

The FCC rules direct programmers to caption 100 percent of their new, non-exempt Spanish-language programs over a twelve-year period, and 75 percent of their non-exempt, pre-rule programs over a fourteen-year period.[37] The FCC adopted benchmarks for this type of programming as follows: 450 hours of *new, non-exempt* programming per channel must be captioned during each calendar quarter by the end of 2003, 900 hours must be captioned by the end of 2006, and 1,350 hours must be captioned by the end of 2009. Thirty percent of *pre-rule non-exempt* programming must be captioned beginning January 1, 2005.

Exemptions

To avoid imposing an economic burden upon program providers, the FCC has exempted the following types of programming from all of the captioning requirements:

- all advertisements under five minutes in duration
- late night programming shown between the hours of 2 A.M. and 6 A.M. local time
- programming in a language other than English or Spanish
- primarily textual programming, such as program channel schedules and community bulletin boards
- promotional programming and brief programming used as a bridge between full-length programs
- public service announcements (PSAs) under ten minutes in duration; however, all federally-funded PSAs, regardless of length, must be captioned as mandated under the ADA
- locally produced and distributed non-news programming with limited repeat value, such as parades and high school sports
- video programming produced for the instructional television fixed service, which is distributed to individual educational institutions, and locally produced instructional programming that is narrowly distributed to individual educational institutions
- non-vocal musical programming such as a symphony or ballet
- new networks during the first four years of their operation[38]

Small programming providers that have annual gross revenues of up to $3 million are exempted altogether from the closed captioning rules.[39] And all programming providers are permitted to limit their expenditures on captioning to 2 percent of their annual gross revenues.[40]

As noted above, in addition to the above exemptions, other programming providers may petition the FCC for individual exemptions from the captioning requirements if they can prove that compliance with these requirements would result in an undue burden.

Lastly, re-runs of a captioned program must be shown with the captions intact only if the program has not been edited before it is re-shown. Editing, typically done for new commercial breaks, disrupts the timing of captions. The consequence is that the captions on an edited program must be reformatted for the captions to make sense. The FCC has decided not to require reformatting of captions for the time being, but has indicated a willingness to review this decision in the future.

Quality Standards

Although the Telecommunications Act is silent on the issue of ensuring high standards of captioning quality, many consumer groups urged the FCC to promulgate quality standards to ensure *full access* to television programming. Among other things, these groups sought standards to ensure comprehensive captioning of background sound effects, real-time captioning for live news broadcasts, accuracy in spelling and typing, proper synchronization of captions with audio content, and no obstruction of other textual messages (such as emergency warnings and names of speakers that appear on the screen).

The FCC has also decided, for the time being, not to issue standards for the nontechnical aspects of quality. However, the rules do require programming distributors to deliver closed captions intact and to monitor their equipment in order to ensure the technical quality of the closed captions transmitted.[41] Previously, no such requirements existed, and often captions were unintentionally stripped during the transmission of programming, to the dismay and frustration of caption viewers.

In addition, the FCC has established special rules for the captioning of live news broadcasts. There are two ways of providing textual information for live news programs: *real-time captioning* and the *electronic newsroom captioning technique* (ENCT). Real-time captioning uses live individuals to simultaneously caption the entire audio portion of a program. ENCT uses special equipment to convert pre-scripted news materials transmitted via a teleprompter into closed captions. Because ENCT is tied to what comes over the teleprompter, typically this method does not provide captioning for live interviews, banter among anchor persons, field reports, sports and weather updates, and other late-breaking stories which are not pre-scripted.

Consumer groups representing the interests of people who are deaf or hard of hearing have long complained that ENCT is not an adequate method of providing television access. In its original 1997 captioning order, the FCC issued rules that would have permitted the use of ENCT for all television programmers. When consumers challenged this part of the FCC's 1997 Order, the FCC revised its requirements for access to live new shows. The FCC now will not allow the four major national television broadcast networks (CBS, Fox, NBC, and ABC) and their affiliates in the top twenty-five television markets (i.e., typically the largest cities) to count programs captioned with ENCT toward compliance with the FCC's captioning transition schedule.[42] National non-broadcast networks (e.g., HBO, CNN and other cable or satellite networks) that serve at least 50 percent of the total number of households subscribing to television programming services will also not be permitted to count ENCT toward their captioning requirements.[43] The FCC has promised to periodically review its rules on access to live news programming, and if necessary extend its requirements for real-time captioning to other television program providers in the future.

EMERGENCY CAPTIONING

In 1977, the FCC adopted a rule requiring television broadcasters to present emergency bulletins both visually and aurally when using the Emergency Broadcasting System.[44] Prior to this time, during emergencies, the television station would interrupt the sound portion of the television signal to make oral announcements, but the picture would continue without any indication that something was wrong. Sometimes the words "Emergency Bulletin" would appear on the screen, and an off-camera announcer would read the details of the emergency. The deaf viewer, unable to hear what was said, could not make realistic plans for safety. For example, when fires ravaged wide sections of California in 1970, officials used loudspeakers and radio and television broadcasts to warn residents to evacuate threatened areas. Several deaf people burned to death because they could not hear the loudspeakers or the radio bulletins and because the television announcements gave no visual information about the danger. Their deaths might have been prevented if the warnings had also been provided visually.

This and similar tragedies prompted appeals to the FCC. Thousands of letters from people all over the country convinced the FCC to adopt a visual warning rule. The rule now states:

> Any emergency information transmitted in accordance with this Section shall be transmitted both aurally and visually or only visually. Television broadcast stations may use any method of visual presentation which results in a legible message conveying the essential information. Methods which may be used include, but are not limited to, slides, electronic captioning, manual methods (e.g., hand printing) or mechanical printing processes. However, when emergency operation is being conducted under a National, State, or Local Level Emergency Broadcast System (EBS) Plan, emergency announcements shall be transmitted both aurally and visually.[45]

In 1997, the FCC expanded its requirements for access to emergency information to cable television networks, establishing what is called the "Emergency Alert System."[46] The requirement to create this system comes from the Cable Television Consumer Protection and Competition Act of 1992. The act directed the FCC to ensure that viewers of video programming on cable systems are provided with the same emergency information as is

provided by the EBS.[47] The FCC's rules require all cable operators serving 5,000 or more customers to provide the full EAS
message in both audio and visual formats on *all* channels. Systems with 10,000 or more subscribers began meeting this obligation on December 31, 1998. Systems with 5,000 to 10,000
subscribers must comply by October 1, 2002.[48]

Systems with fewer than 5,000 subscribers have a slightly different obligation. By October 1, 2002, these systems may either
provide the full EAS audio and visual message on all channels *or*
provide a video interrupt and audio alert on all channels and the
full EAS audio and video messages on at least one programmed
channel.[49] The video interrupt must flash a blank or black television screen simultaneously with, and for the same amount of time
as, the full EAS message. Cable systems that use this method of
alerting the public (as opposed to transmitting the actual message
on every channel), must distribute public service announcements
telling viewers which channel will contain the full audio and
video message. Cable owners may use billing statements to fulfill
this distribution requirement. The FCC adopted this more lenient
requirement for smaller cable systems because operators of such
systems raised concerns about the financial hardships they would
suffer were they required to transmit the full EAS message on all
of their channels.[50] However, the FCC has left open the possibility that consumers and industry may develop alternative solutions for disseminating EAS messaging in systems serving fewer
than 5,000 customers.[51]

Although the EBS and EAS requirements for visual access to
televised emergency information are intended to ensure access by
deaf and hard of hearing individuals, these systems are required
only for national emergencies, and are merely voluntary for local
emergencies. As a result, televised information about emergencies
often remains uncaptioned. For example, even though the EBS visual warning rule had been in effect for several years, in 1989
during the San Francisco and Los Angeles earthquakes and Hur-
ricane Hugo, local stations failed to provide captions to accompany their reports. Similarly, information about bombings,
tornadoes, blizzards, and other emergencies throughout the nation commonly have not been captioned.

To remedy this situation, in 1998 the FCC initiated a proceeding to ensure that all televised emergency information is captioned.[52] This proceeding is an extension of the FCC's closed captioning proceeding, and addresses the need to provide real-time captioning for *all* live emergency news information, regardless of whether the EBS or EAS is used. Real-time captioning would provide simultaneous text for all televised information provided through audio. Consumers are hopeful that the rules that result from this proceeding will close all remaining gaps regarding access to televised emergency information.

NOTES

1. *In the Matter of Closed Captioning and Video Description of Video Programming, Implementation of Section 305 of the Telecommunications Act of 1996, Video Programming Accessibility,* Report, MM Dkt. No. 95-176 (July 29, 1996) at ¶29, citing *Nielson Media Research* (1994). The report is hereafter cited as FCC Captioning Report. The report provides a comprehensive source of information on the benefits, availability, funding, and costs of closed captioning through 1996.
2. National Captioning Institute (NCI), "Nearly 100 Million Americans Can Benefit from Watching Captioned TV." [NCI FYI Fact Sheet] 1996.
3. NCI has reported that "forty percent of the 60,000 closed captioning decoders sold in 1989 were to people for whom English is a second language." See "TV Closed Captions Fight Illiteracy," *USA Today,* July 11, 1990, at 6D.
4. Studies have shown that closed captioning is an effective tool in teaching literacy skills. Wilson,"Using Closed Captioned Television to Teach Reading to Adults," *Reading Research and Instruction* 28(4)(1989): 27-37; See also F. Chisman, *Jump Start, The Federal Role in Adult Literacy, Final Report on the Project of Adult Literacy,* Southport, Ct.: Southport Institute for Policy Analysis, (1989).
5. "TV Closed Captions Fight Illiteracy," *USA Today,* July 11, 1990, at 6D.
6. Koskinen, Wilson, Gambrell, & Jensema, "Closed Captioned Television: A New Technology for Enhancing Reading Skills of Learning Disabled Students," *E.R.S. Spectrum, Journal of Scholarly Research & Information* (1986).

7. "TV Closed Captions Fight Illiteracy," *USA Today,* July 11, 1990, at 6D.

8. *The Washington Post,* Sec. A, p. 1 (March 8, 1996).

9. D. Hotchkiss. "Hearing Impaired Elderly Population: Estimation, Projection and Assessment," [pamphlet] Gallaudet Research Institute, Gallaudet University, Washington, D.C., 1989; Brown, Hotchkiss, Allen, Schein & Adams, "Current and Future Needs of the Hearing Impaired Elderly Population," [pamphlet] Gallaudet Research Institute, Gallaudet University, Washington, D.C., 1989.

10. In the early 1980s the Greater Los Angeles Council on Deafness, Inc., brought a class action suit against Community Television of Southern California to mandate open captioning. *Greater Los Angeles Council on Deafness, Inc. v. Community Television of Southern Calif.,* 719 F. 2d 1017, 1019 (9th Cir. 1983), *cert. denied Gottfried v. United States,* 467 U.S. 1252 (1984). The council argued that because Community Television received federal funds, it should provide open captioning under Section 504 of the Rehabilitation Act of 1973. Both the U.S. District Court and the U.S. Court of Appeals for the Ninth Circuit ruled that Section 504 of the Rehabilitation Act does not mandate that federally funded television programs be produced and broadcast with open captions rather than closed captions. The courts both noted that the U.S. Department of Education helped originate closed captioning and required all programs it funded to be produced with closed captions. Further, as a condition of its grants, the department required that public stations transmit closed captions on all programs that had been produced with closed captions. See also *Community Television v. Gottfried,* 459 U.S. 498 (1983), which states that Section 504 does not require the FCC to impose a greater obligation on public licensees than on commercial licensees to provide special programming for individuals with hearing disabilities.

11. Commission on Education of the Deaf, *Toward Equality: Education of the Deaf,* Commission on Education of the Deaf (1988) at 113. The COED was a temporary federal commission created in the 1980s to study and make recommendations on improving educational opportunities for deaf Americans.

12. Ibid.; *See also* Sy DuBow, "The Television Decoder Circuitry Act—TV for All," *Temple Law Review ADA Symposium Issue,* 64 (1991): 609, for a general discussion on the history of closed captioning.

13. Ibid.

14. S. Rep. No. 393, 101st Cong., 2d Sess. 2 (1990).

15. H. Rep. No. 767, 101st Cong., 2d Sess. 5 (1990).

16. FCC Captioning Report ¶29, citing Roper Starch Worldwide,

America's Watching: Public Attitudes Toward Television 17 (1995).

17. S. Rep. No. 393, 101ˢᵗ Congress, 2d Sess. 2 (1990), citing Caption Center Survey, WGBH, Boston, Mass. (1990).

18. *TV Decoder Circuitry Act: Hearings on S. 1974 Before the Senate Subcommittee on Communications*, 101st Cong., 2d Sess. (1990) p. 67 (Statement of John Ball, president of the National Captioning Institute).

19. Commission on Education of the Deaf, *Toward Equality*, 119.

20. Ibid., 120.

21. Television Decoder Circuitry Act of 1990, PL101-431, 104 Stat. 960 (1990) (TDCA), 47 U.S.Code §303(u), 330(b).

22. In 1988, ninety-six percent of new television sets had thirteen-inch or larger screens. *TV Digest* (September 11, 1989): 12.

23. 47 U.S. Code §303(s).

24. *In the Matter of Amendment of Part 15 of the Commission's Rules to Implement the Provisions of the Television Decoder Circuitry Act of 1990, Report and Order*, Gen. Dkt. No. 91-1 (adopted April 12, 1991; released April 15, 1991). The standards cover the use of color characters, italics, upper and lower case characters, smooth scrolling, caption size, and compatibility with cable scrambling technology.

25. The FCC pointed out that "it is essential that television receivers display captions that are readable. By providing a black background, the legibility of the caption is assured."

26. 47 U.S. Code §330(b).

27. *In the Matter of Closed Captioning Requirements for Digital Television Receivers*, Notice of Proposed Rulemaking, ET Dkt. No. 99-254 (July 14, 1999).

28. FCC Captioning Report, ¶12.

29. Telecommunications Act of 1996, PL 104-104, 110 Stat. 56 (1996) (Feb. 8, 1996). Section 305 of the act added a new Section 713, Video Programming Accessibility, to the Communications Act of 1934, 47 U.S.C. §713.

30. *In the Matter of Closed Captioning and Video Description of Video Programming, Implementation of Section 305 of the Telecommunications Act of 1996, Video Programming Accessibility*, Report and Order, FCC 97-279, MM Dkt. No. 95-176 (August 22, 1997).

31. *In the Matter of Closed Captioning and Video Description of Video Programming, Implementation of Section 305 of the Telecommunications Act of 1996, Video Programming Accessibility*, Order on Reconsideration, FCC 98-236, MM Dkt. No. 95-176 (October 2, 1998).

32. 47 C.F.R. §79.1(b)(1)(iv).
33. The FCC divides the year into three-month blocks; each channel must meet these captioning requirements during each quarter.
34. 47 C.F.R. §79.1(b)(5).
35. Any programming produced or shown before January 1, 1998 falls into this "pre-rule" category.
36. 47 C.F.R. §79.1(b)(2).
37. 47 C.F.R. §79.1(b)(3), (b)(4).
38. 47 C.F.R. §§79.1(a)(1), (d), *et.seq.*
39. 47 C.F.R. §79.1(d)(12).
40. 47 C.F.R. §79.1(d)(11).
41. 47 C.F.R. §79.1(c).
42. 47 C.F.R. §79.1(e)(3).
43. Ibid. As an example, the FCC explains that if the combined national subscribership of all multichannel programming providers (cable, satellite and wireless cable) is eighty million households, then nonbroadcast networks that serve at least forty million households would be covered by this rule.
44. 47 C.F.R. §73.1250(h).
45. Ibid.
46. *In the Matter of Amendment of Part 73, Subpart G, of the Commission's Rules Regarding the Emergency Broadcast System,* Second Report and Order, FCC 97-338, FO Dkt 91-301, FO Dkt. 91-171, (Sept. 29, 1997) (EAS 2nd R&O).
47. Cable Television Consumer Protection and Competition Act of 1992, PL No. 102-385 §16(b), 106 Stat. 1460, 1490 (1992), adding subsection (g) to Section 624 of the Communications Act of 1934, 47 U.S.Code §544(G).
48. EAS 2nd R&O ¶¶7–22.
49. Ibid. at ¶22.
50. Ibid. at ¶26.
51. Ibid.
52. *In the Matter of Closed Captioning and Video Description of Video Programming, Implementation of Section 305 of the Telecommunications Act of 1996, Video Programming Accessibility (Further Notice of Proposed Rulemaking),* FCC 97-279, MM Dkt. No. 95-176 (Jan. 14, 1998). At the time of printing, this proceeding was still pending.

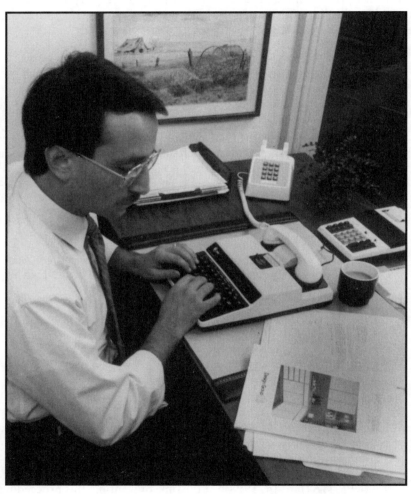

Chapter 11

Telephone Service

Historically, deaf and hard of hearing people have been unable to access the majority of our nation's telecommunications products and services; even today, a considerable number of these products and services depend on auditory and verbal input and output. Rapid and efficient telecommunications services, readily available to almost all hearing Americans, have been largely denied to those who cannot hear. The telephone network has placed unnecessary barriers of expense and difficulty on deaf people, limiting their ability to communicate with family, friends, businesses, government, and social service providers. However, numerous developments over the past decade have begun to erode the telecommunications barriers that have existed for most of this century.

A recent federal law, the Telecommunications Act of 1996, now requires manufacturers of telecommunications products and providers of telecommunications services to ensure that their products and services are accessible to individuals with disabilities, if doing so would be readily achievable.[1] Additionally, telecommunications relay systems are now in full operation throughout the country, TTY users have access to more public pay phones, and expanded mandates for hearing aid compatible telephones and telephones with volume control are being implemented. The new developments promise to improve the way in which deaf and hard of hearing individuals can enjoy telecommunications in their home, workplace, school, and the community.

REGULATION OF TELECOMMUNICATIONS

Telephone companies are public utilities whose rates and practices are regulated by federal and state agencies. The federal agency that regulates interstate telephone practices is the Federal Communications Commission (FCC). Each state also has its own agency that regulates the operations of telephone companies within its state. The state agencies are usually called public utility commissions (PUCs). The FCC and PUCs work to ensure that telephone companies operate in the public interest by providing adequate and nondiscriminatory service to the public for a fair price.

Telecommunications Relay Services

Telecommunications relay services enable people who use TTYs or other non-voice terminal devices to have conversations with people who use conventional voice telephones. The call is relayed back and forth by a third party who reads what the TTY user types and types what the voice telephone user speaks. In the early 1980s, private relay systems began to develop around the country, linking TTYs to the public telecommunications network. Most of these private programs were funded with donations and staffed with volunteers. Unfortunately, funding shortages caused most of these state and private programs to impose restrictions on relay users. Few programs relayed interstate calls, and many placed limitations on the length, number, and time of day that calls could be made. Even with these restrictions, the demand for relay services was overwhelming. The tremendous need for relay services eventually resulted in the passage of two federal laws requiring relay services.

Telecommunications Accessibility Enhancement Act

The first of these laws is the Telecommunications Accessibility Enhancement Act (TAEA).[2] Enacted in 1988, the TAEA requires the federal government to provide relay services for calls to, from, and within the federal government. The federal relay system has been in existence since 1986. It was originally established by the Architectural and Transportation Barriers Compliance Board (Access Board) and operated by the U.S. Treasury Department. Before the passage of the TAEA, however, the federal relay system had been poorly publicized and understaffed. The TAEA transferred authority for its operations to the General Services Administration and added staff to accommodate many more users. In addition to enlarging the federal relay program, the TAEA ordered the publication of federal TTY numbers in a government-wide directory and directed both houses of Congress to develop a policy about placing TTYs in members' offices.

Title IV of the Americans with Disabilities Act

The second piece of legislation requiring relay services is Title IV of the Americans with Disabilities Act (ADA). Title IV has required all telephone companies to provide intrastate (within the state) and interstate (across state lines) relay services throughout the United States since July 26, 1993.[3] The FCC's Title IV rules require relay services to be functionally equivalent to conventional voice telephone services. Functional equivalence is defined as follows:

+ Relay services must be provided twenty-four hours a day/ seven days a week for all local and long distance calls.
+ Relay systems must accept calls in both the Baudot and ASCII computer formats.
+ Relay calls must be relayed verbatim, unless one of the relay parties requests that the messages be summarized.
+ Individuals using relay services may not be charged any more for their calls than voice telephone users are charged for calls with the same points of origination and destination.
+ No restrictions may be placed on the type, length, or number of calls made by any relay user. This means that relay systems must be capable of handling third-party number, calling card, collect, and all other calls normally handled by telephone companies. The burden of proving that relaying a particular kind of call is not technologically possible rests on

the telephone companies. This requirement also allows relay callers to request relay operators—commonly referred to as communication assistants (CAs)—to make several calls for them each time they call into a relay center.[4]

There is one exception to the requirement that relay programs handle all types of calls. Telephone companies have proven to the FCC that it is technically impossible for relay centers to handle telephone calls made with coins from payphones. Specifically, relay centers are unable to handle the collection of coins or to notify callers of the number of coins necessary to complete these "coin sent–paid" calls. As a result, the FCC has suspended the requirement to handle coin sent-paid relay calls. In place of handling these calls, consumers and industry have worked out an "alternative plan" for handling local and long distance payphone relay calls. The plan has three components: (1) local relay calls may be made at payphones at no charge to consumers; (2) long distance (toll) payphone relay calls may be charged to a calling card or deducted from a pre-paid (debit) telephone card at rates no greater than coin call rates; and (3) the telephone industry must conduct a consumer education program to advise TTY users about the alternative plan and the methods of making local and long distance relay calls at payphones.

✦ CAs may not consider the content of a particular call in determining whether to relay that call. In other words, CAs cannot decide that they do not want to relay a call because they do not like the legal, moral, or ethical nature of the call. The FCC's prohibition against refusing calls based on their content is critical to the proper and effective operation of relay services. Without such a prohibition, practices regarding call content would vary from state to state, or CA to CA, resulting in inconsistent practices throughout the nation. For example, what one operator might consider light-hearted humor, another might find extremely offensive. Never knowing when their calls could be terminated or refused, both deaf and hearing people would quickly lose all trust in the relay system were this requirement not in place. (Note that CAs cannot be held criminally liable for relaying unlawful conversations unless they are knowingly involved in the illegal transactions or have actual notice of the illegality of the telephone transmissions.)

✦ CAs must also maintain the complete confidentiality of relayed conversations. They are prohibited from keeping records of relayed conversations beyond the length of the telephone call. However, under Section 705(a) of the Communications Act of 1934, CAs may be required to disclose interstate or foreign conversations when directed to do so by a court-issued subpoena or upon the demand of some other lawful authority.

✦ CAs are required to have competent skills in grammar, typing, spelling, and relay etiquette. In addition, CAs must be sufficiently acquainted with American Sign Language and with the cultures of the various communities that their relay systems are intended to serve.

✦ Relay systems must have very low "blockage" rates. This means that relay users should not receive busy signals when calling relay services at rates that are higher than those confronted by voice telephone users over the conventional telephone network. In addition, relay systems must be capable of answering eighty-five percent of all incoming calls within ten seconds. After receiving dialing information from the caller, CAs then have thirty seconds to dial the requested number.

✦ Relay users must be given their choice of long distance telephone companies.

✦ Relay users must have the same access to telephone operator services that are available to voice telephone users.

Relay Service Providers

Under the ADA, telephone companies (otherwise known as common carriers) are responsible for providing relay services wherever they provide conventional telephone services. In addition, individual states may take on this responsibility by having their state relay programs certified by the FCC. Both telephone companies and states are permitted to provide relay services individually, through a competitively selected vendor, or together with other telephone companies or states.

A state that wishes to receive certification to operate its own relay system must submit documentation to the FCC that proves that its program will (1) meet or exceed all of the operational, technical, and functional minimum standards contained in the FCC's regulations; (2) provide adequate procedures and remedies to enforce the state program; and (3) not conflict with federal law where its program exceeds the minimum standards contained in the FCC regulations.

When a state requests certification, the FCC must give the public notice and an opportunity to comment on that request. Once it is granted, certification remains in effect for a five-year period. A state may apply to the FCC for recertification one year before its certification expires. Alternatively, the FCC may revoke or suspend a state's certification if that state's practices do not follow the FCC's minimum guidelines.

Currently, all fifty states and Puerto Rico have individual, state-certified relay programs. With the exception of California, each of these states have selected single relay providers to handle local relay calls. Some of these states have their own relay centers physically located within their own states; others share regional centers centrally located among three or four states. California is presently the only state that allows its residents to choose among several relay providers for local calls. In addition, consumers in all states have their choice of several relay providers to handle long distance (toll) calls.

7-1-1 Uniform Dialing

Since the relay mandates took effect, each of the state relay programs have had their own relay access telephone numbers. In October of 1993, the National Center for Law and Deafness (NCLD), formerly of Gallaudet University, filed a petition for rule-making with the FCC, requesting the Commission to allocate the digits 7-1-1 for nationwide relay access. NCLD complained that access to relay services was confusing and difficult for individuals who traveled across state boarders. The petition sought a single nationwide access number to make relay access "convenient, fast, and uncomplicated," and to reduce the number of digits that needed to be dialed. Sometime after NCLD filed this petition, Hawaii and Canada independently began using 7-1-1 for relay access.[5] In February 1997, the FCC ultimately granted NCLD's petition, and directed 7-1-1 to be reserved for relay access on a nationwide basis.[6]

The FCC's action reserves the 7-1-1 code; however, it does not mandate that every state use these numbers for access to their relay programs. It is now up to each of these states, or the telephone companies in those states, to actually adopt the 7-1-1 code for their own customers. In July 1998, Bell Atlantic announced that it would start using 7-1-1 for TTY relay access in its states within approximately two years.[7]

Enforcement

Consumers who are not satisfied with a relay service should first file their complaints with the state agency responsible for implementing the local relay program. The state then has 180 days to resolve the complaint. If the consumer is still not satisfied, he or she may then bring the complaint to the FCC.

A telephone company that violates the ADA's relay provisions may be ordered to begin compliance immediately and may have to pay damages to the complaining party. Willful violations of the relay section may be subject to criminal penalties, including fines of up to $10,000.

New Relay Developments

In May of 1998, the FCC began a proceeding to expand its minimum standards for relay services. In that proceeding, the Commission issued a Notice of Proposed Rulemaking which suggested ways to broaden the definition of "telecommunications relay services."[8] Historically, the FCC interpreted Title IV of the ADA to require only TTY-to-speech and speech-to-TTY services. Under this definition, companies that provided relay services were only able to receive payment (reimbursement) for calls relayed between TTY and voice telephone users. However, technology advancements have made other types of relay services possible. The FCC does not want to stifle new innovative developments. It believes that relay service should be an evolving service that encourages use of these new technologies. Accordingly, the FCC has proposed two new types of relay services to be eligible for reimbursement: speech-to-speech (STS) and video relay interpreting (VRI).[9]

STS relay services use specially-trained individuals to relay conversations for persons with severe speech disabilities. The FCC's new regulations will require all telephone companies to provide STS services throughout their service areas within one year after it issues its final Report and Order regarding this new relay method.

VRI services use sign language interpreters, desktop video conferencing computers, and high speed transmission services to enable individuals who use sign language to make calls through interpreters. VRI works in the following manner: A VRI caller signs to an interpreter at a remote location. The interpreter interprets the conversation to the hearing person receiving the call and signs responses back to the VRI caller. Because VRI uses relatively new technology and because the costs of using VRI have not yet been fully established, the FCC has tentatively decided that it is not ready to require VRI at this time. However, VRI is already provided on a voluntary basis by the telephone companies in North Carolina, and several VRI trials continue to take place in other locations.[10] Even though VRI will not be required, the FCC's new rules will allow relay providers that do provide VRI to be reimbursed for these services.

Relay services have taken a significant step toward increasing independence and expanding opportunities for persons who are deaf and hard of hearing. However, consumers believe new technologies that would vastly improve the quality of relay services need to be integrated into existing and future telecommunications networks. These technologies include higher speed transmission protocols and voice recognition software programs. In the coming years, these and other technological innovations may increase the speed and accuracy of relay transmissions so that relay calls will truly be functionally equivalent to voice telephone calls.

Equipment Distribution Programs

The cost of owning a TTY can be prohibitive for deaf people, many of whom have below-average incomes. In addition to the initial cost, which can range from $300 to $600, the TTY user must also pay for repair, maintenance, and a signaling device. Expense is the main reason why many people who need TTYs do not have them. The cost of TTYs and other specialized telephone equipment has prompted more than half of the fifty states to develop equipment distribution programs.[11] These programs distribute specialized equipment to deaf and other disabled individuals free of charge or at a discount. Some states set income qualifications for individuals wishing to receive such equipment; other states merely require certification that the individuals have a hearing loss or are otherwise disabled.

HEARING AID COMPATIBILITY

Hearing-aid-compatible telephones enable individuals who use hearing aids with a telephone switch to block out background sounds and high-pitched squeals that can occur with incompatible telephones. The hearing aid switch enables the wearer to pick up sound waves generated by the electromagnetic field of the telephone receiver. Telephones with the required amount of electromagnetic leakage are considered to be compatible with hearing aids.

Until the early 1980s most telephones were hearing aid compatible. Before that time, most Americans rented their phones from AT&T; these rented phones had strong electromagnetic fields. In the 1980s new equipment companies began manufacturing and selling telephones directly to consumers. Many of these telephones did not have enough electromagnetic leakage to be compatible with hearing aids.

Telecommunications for the Disabled Act

In 1982, Congress took steps to rectify this situation. It passed the Telecommunications for the Disabled Act, which made clear that compatibility between telephones and hearing aids was necessary to accommodate the needs of individuals with hearing loss.[12] The Telecommunications for the Disabled Act directed the FCC to establish uniform technical standards for hearing aid compatibility. It created a mandate for all "essential telephones" to be equipped for use with hearing aids. Congress defined "essential" phones as coin-operated phones, phones for emergencies, and phones frequently needed by individuals with hearing disabilities. Finally, it directed that telephone equipment be labeled so that consumers would be aware of the compatibility between telephones and hearing aids.

Hearing Aid Compatibility Act

In the years following passage of the Telecommunications for the Disabled Act, consumers insisted that the definition of essential telephones was far too narrow to meet the needs of hearing aid users. Spearheaded by a group called the Organization for Use of the Telephone (OUT), consumers succeeded in obtaining passage of the Hearing Aid Compatibility Act in 1988 (HAC Act).[13] The HAC Act required that all telephones manufactured after August 16, 1989, be compatible for use with hearing aids. On May 18, 1989, the FCC promulgated regulations directing compliance with the new law.[14]

After the HAC Act was passed, hearing aid wearers were still concerned that the FCC had not taken steps to reduce the number of incompatible telephones that had been installed in workplaces and other institutions prior to the 1989 manufacturing deadline. As a result of consumer persistence in this area, in 1990 the FCC issued a rule to again expand the availability of HAC telephones. The new rule changed the definition of essential telephones to require that telephones located in common areas of the workplace and all credit-card-operated telephones be compatible with hearing aids by May 1, 1991.[15] In 1992 the FCC again broadened its rules to require HAC telephones in *all* areas of the workplace and in *all* hotel, motel, and hospital rooms.[16] These rules, set to go into effect on May 1, 1993, were indefinitely suspended by the FCC at the last minute as a result of hundreds of last-minute complaints from businesses around the country. The businesses complained that compliance with the 1992 rules would be too difficult.[17]

In 1995, the FCC gathered together various representatives from consumer organizations, industry, and the government to revise the HAC rules. After extensive deliberations, the Hearing Aid Compatible Negotiated Rulemaking Committee recommended various ways for the FCC to strengthen its HAC mandates. On July 3, 1996, the FCC released rules that adopted these recommendations.[18]

The FCC's hearing aid compatibility rules now contain the following mandates:

+ All workplace telephones (other than those in common areas, which are subject to the requirements noted above) were required to be HAC by January 1, 2000, with two exceptions: telephones purchased between January 1, 1985 and December 31, 1989 and telephones in workplaces with fewer than fifteen employees must be HAC by January 1, 2005.
+ All telephones in hotels and motels were required to be HAC by January 1, 2000, except hotels and motels that must replace telephones purchased between January 1, 1985 and December 31, 1989 may delay compliance until the years 2001 and 2004, depending on the number of guest rooms they have.
+ All telephones needed to signal emergency situations in confined settings, such as hospitals and residential health care facilities, were required to be HAC since November 1, 1998.
+ All telephones, including cordless telephones, that are manufactured in or imported into the United States after January 1, 2000, must have volume control.[19] Telephones which have volume control allow the telephone user to control the loudness of the other person's voice.[20]

TELECOMMUNICATIONS ACT OF 1996

In the 1990s, our nation entered a new era of telecommunications advances. Talk of the information superhighway and the release of new telecommunications devices, including wireless services, pagers, and interactive telephone systems, alerted consumers with disabilities to the need for a law that would ensure access to all of these new technologies.

After several years of negotiating with federal legislators, consumers got their wish. On January 8, 1996, Congress enacted Section 255 of the Telecommunications Act of 1996 which, for the first time in our nation's history, requires telecommunications manufacturers and service providers to make their equipment and services accessible to individuals with disabilities where it is readily achievable to do so.[21] The new law also requires manufacturers and service providers to make their products and services compatible with peripheral devices and specialized customer premises equipment, such as TTYs, where it is readily achievable to do so. Readily achievable is defined as "easily accomplishable and able to be carried out without much difficulty or expense."[22] In determining whether an access feature is readily achievable, the FCC will balance the costs and nature of the access feature against the resources available to a company on a case-by-case basis. Often it is readily achievable to provide access if such access is incorporated during the research and development stages of creating a product or service. Section 255 is expected to make a profound difference in the ability of new technologies and services to reach Americans with disabilities.

Congress directed the Access Board, in conjunction with the FCC, to issue guidelines for achieving compliance by telecommunications equipment manufacturers. To obtain assistance in creating these guidelines, in June, 1996 the Access Board developed a federal advisory committee comprised of consumer and industry representatives, called the Telecommunications Access Advisory Committee (TAAC). TAAC presented its recommendations to the Access Board in January of 1997. The Access Board used these recommendations to develop its Section 255 guidelines, which were released on February 3, 1998. Approximately one and a half years later, the FCC issued its own rules, designed to enforce compliance with Section 255 by both equipment manufacturers and service providers. For the most part, these rules mirror the Access Board's guidelines.

The FCC's rules require telecommunications manufacturers and service providers to identify and address the accessibility needs of individuals who are deaf and hard of hearing throughout the product design, development, and fabrication of their products, as early and consistently as possible. The rules recognize the need to incorporate access early in design processes, to avoid expensive and burdensome retrofits later on. In developing processes to identify accessibility barriers, manufacturers and service providers may engage in a number of actions. If, for example, a company conducts market research, product testing, or pilot demonstrations for a particular product, it should include individuals with disabilities in these activities to help it identify the needs of these individuals. By consulting with deaf individuals, manufacturers will get a better idea of the need to provide visual cues or vibrations for products (e.g., pagers) that may otherwise provide only aural cues.

The FCC's rules also require new telecommunications equipment and services to be compatible with peripheral devices and specialized equipment that are commonly used by individuals with disabilities. Examples of such devices are TTYs, visual signaling devices, and amplifiers. Under this mandate, products that offer voice communication (such as wireless phones) must provide a standard connection point for TTYs. In addition, these products must have a feature that enables users to alternate between using speech and TTY signals. The compatibility requirement also requires that there be a connection point on telecommunications devices so that they can effectively hook up to audio processing devices (such as amplifiers) that are used for telecommunications functions.

In addition to requiring *access* to telecommunications products and services, the FCC's rules require that people with disabilities be able to *use* products and services. The new rules define "usability" as access to product information (such as user manuals, bills, and technical support) that is functionally equivalent to information available to individuals without disabilities. For example, when a product is accompanied by an instructional video, the video should be provided with captions. Similarly, the appendix to the Access Board's Section 255 guidelines suggests that manufacturers should provide direct TTY access for their customer service lines so that deaf people can ask questions about products like everyone else. Companies that comply with Section 255 may not impose any additional charges for providing such access.

The FCC's Section 255 rules are broad in scope. The rules cover virtually every type of telecommunications equipment, including telephones, pagers, wireless devices, fax machines, answering machines, telecommunications software, and business systems. Similarly, the rules cover all types of telecommunications services, including call waiting, speed dialing, call forwarding, computer-provided directory assistance, call monitoring, caller identification, call tracing, and repeat dialing.

Enforcement of the Section 255 rules will primarily be through informal and formal consumer complaints filed at the FCC. To monitor the industry's progress in making equipment accessible, the Access Board will compile periodic "market monitoring reports" that will identify problem areas and solutions that have been used to achieve access to telecommunications products throughout the telecommunications market. The first of these reports is expected to be released in the spring of 2000.

Notice of Inquiry on Internet Telephony

At the same time that the FCC issued its final rules implementing Section 255, it also issued a Notice of Inquiry to gather information about access to Internet telephony. Internet telephony provides real-time transmissions using something called a packet-switched communications protocol. At the time this book goes to print, the FCC will be gathering information on the ways in which Internet telephony services will impact the disability community, and the steps that are needed by the FCC to guarantee access to this new technology.

Interactive Voice Systems and Voice Mail

Also included within the FCC's mandates are interactive voice response (IVR) systems and voice mail. IVR systems are phone systems that allow callers to select from a menu of choices by pressing numbers on their phones, in response to "prompts" from recordings. It has become increasingly common for government agencies, businesses, and educational institutions to use these systems to conduct their telephone business. However, IVR systems are not typically accessible to TTYs. Nor are they accessible to relay users because the speed of the messages used in these systems are too fast and the times given for responses are too short. Similarly, IVR systems are often difficult to navigate for people who have only mild hearing loss, but who have trouble hearing the prompts.

Although both IVR systems and voice mail services technically fall into the category of *information services*, rather than the *telecommunications services* which are covered under Section 255, the FCC has brought these services within the scope of its Section 255 rules through a legal doctrine known as "ancillary jurisdiction." This doctrine allows the FCC to extend its jurisdiction beyond the literal language of a statute when such jurisdiction is needed to meet the objective of that statute. The FCC has concluded that the access barriers that are created when IVR and voice mail services are inaccessible make it very difficult for people with disabilities to reach their parties or obtain the information they need by telephone. The FCC has determined that coverage of these services is necessary to fulfill the true intent of Section 255.[23]

LONG DISTANCE RATE REDUCTION

The charge for a long distance call is usually based on the number of minutes the telephone line is used, the distance between the callers, the day of the week, and the time of day the call is placed. Because TTY calls take much longer than voice calls to communicate the same message, long distance TTY calls and relayed calls are very expensive. Basic TTYs can transmit at a maximum speed of sixty words per minute. By contrast, the estimated average speaking rate for English is 165 words per minute. Thus, a typical TTY user may pay $6.50 to have the same long-distance telephone conversation that a hearing person could have for only $2.50.

AT&T, Sprint, and MCI all offer some type of rate reduction for TTY or relay users. Additionally, some states have laws or regulations directing the telephone companies of those states to offer TTY rate reductions. Some of these states require deaf customers to submit a statement from a doctor, audiologist, or public agency certifying that they have a hearing disability. Other states merely ask TTY users to apply for the reduced rate. In some states a reduction applies to the customer's entire household; in other states the discount is only applied to calls made with a TTY.

Most consumer advocates believe telephone charges should be based on the value of the service to the customer, rather than on the cost to the telephone company of providing the service. For example, if homes in rural or mountainous areas were charged the actual cost to the telephone company of running telephone lines and installing equipment, their rates would be very high. Yet all residential telephone customers, urban and rural, are charged the same fee for basic telephone service. This is done because the value of that service is the same for everyone and because the telephone system is more useful for everyone if it reaches as many people as possible. The cost of providing service to all households is averaged, and the cost is spread among all customers. Similarly, reduced rates for TTY calls help to ensure that deaf people have access to the telephone system on the same basis as other telephone users.

TTY-Equipped Pay Telephones

Public telephones have an important communication function. Deaf people who cannot afford a TTY or who are away from home need to use pay phones. Most deaf individuals do not own TTYs that are truly portable. Even people with portable TTYs are unable to use them at pay phones that do not have electrical outlets to supply the necessary power.

Guidelines issued by the Access Board pursuant to the ADA are gradually increasing the availability of TTY-equipped public telephones.[24] These guidelines apply to new construction and alterations in places of public accommodations and commercial facilities, as covered by Title III of the ADA. The requirements are as follows:

1. If the total number of pay phones at a given location is four or more, and at least one of these phones is located inside a building at that location, a TTY-equipped pay phone must be provided inside the building.
2. If even one public pay telephone is provided in a stadium or arena, a convention center, a hotel with a convention center, or a covered mall, at least one public TTY-equipped pay phone must be provided in the facility.
3. If even one public pay phone is located in or next to a hospital waiting room, recovery room, or emergency room, one public TTY-equipped pay phone must be provided at each location.

The Access Board rules also require that TTY-equipped pay phones be identified by the international TTY symbol. In addition, if a facility has a TTY-equipped pay phone, it must place a sign (using the international symbol) directing individuals to that phone next to banks of pay phones that are not equipped with TTYs. If a facility has no banks of telephones, it must place the directional sign at the main entrance to the facility.

In addition to requiring the installation of TTY-equipped telephones, the Access Board rules require some public pay telephones to accommodate portable TTYs. Specifically, the regulations require that new or altered places of public accommodations include at least one public pay telephone that can accommodate portable TTYs in each bank of three or more telephones.[25] These telephones must have a shelf for the TTY, an electrical outlet, and a telephone handset cord long enough to reach the TTY.

WIRELESS SERVICES AND OTHER NEW TECHNOLOGIES

Dramatic advances in technology have already begun to change the way Americans communicate with each other. For example, wireless technologies offer freedom to individuals in our society who wish to have access to a telephone, but who have mobile lifestyles. There are two types of wireless telecommunications devices: analog and digital. The wireless telecommunications industry is actively working on solutions to make these wireless devices compatible with TTYs and with hearing aids.

Use of the Internet, pagers, answering machines, fax machines, messaging services, and other technologies will continue to alter the means by which people stay in contact with one another. Consumers now have more choices than ever when selecting from among these products to meet their business and recreational needs. Competition in the telephone manufacturing and service industries will continue to adjust the cost of these new technologies and make them affordable to increasing numbers of Americans. It is critical for deaf and hard of hearing people to become knowledgeable about these telecommunications developments in order to take advantage of these changes as they occur.

NOTES

1. PL 104–104, 110 Stat. 56 (1996), codified at 47 U.S. Code §255.
2. PL 100–542, 102 Stat. 2721 (1988), codified at 40 U.S.C. §762 (1988).
3. Americans with Disabilities Act of 1990, Title IV, PL 101–336, 104 Stat. 327, codified at 47 U.S.C. §225 (1990).
4. *In the Matter of Telecommunications Services for Individuals with*

Hearing and Speech Disabilities, and the Americans with Disabilities Act of 1990, Report and Order and Request for Comments, CC Dkt. No. 90-571, FCC 91-213 (July 26, 1991).

5. For technical reasons, Hawaii requires dialing a "1" before the three-digit code.

6. *In the Matter of the Use of 711 Codes and Other Abbreviated Dialing Arrangements*, First Report and Order and Further Notice of Proposed Rulemaking, CC Dkt. No. 92-105, FCC 97-51 (February 19, 1997).

7. "Bell Atlantic To Make Calling Easier for Customers Who Are Deaf, Hard of Hearing," Bell Atlantic Press Release (July 8, 1998). Bell Atlantic provides telephone service to residents of the following states: Connecticut, Delaware, Maine, Maryland, Massachusetts, New Hampshire, New Jersey, New York, Pennsylvania, Rhode Island, Vermont, Virginia, Washington, D.C., and West Virginia.

8. *In the Matter of Telecommunications Relay Services and Speech-to-Speech Services for Individuals with Hearing and Speech Disabilities*, Notice of Proposed Rulemaking, CC Dkt. No. 98-67, FCC 98-90 (May 20, 1998).

9. Ibid. at ¶¶ 19–34.

10. Texas and Maryland are two other states that have conducted VRI trials.

11. Additional information about the various state equipment distribution programs may be obtained by contacting the State of Maryland Department of Budget and Management, 301 W. Preston Street, Baltimore, Maryland 21201.

12. PL 97–410, 96 Stat. 2043, codified as amended at 47 U.S.C. §610.

13. PL 100–394, 102 Stat. 976 (1988), codified at 47 U.S.C. §610 (1988).

14. *In the Matter of Access to Telecommunications Equipment and Services by the Hearing Impaired and Other Disabled Persons*, First Report and Order, CC Dkt. No. 87-124, FCC 89-137 (May 11, 1989), 54 *Fed. Reg.* 21,429 (May 18, 1989), codified at 47 C.F.R. Part 68.

15. *In the Matter of Access to Telecommunications Equipment and Services by the Hearing Impaired and Other Disabled Persons*, Memorandum Opinion and Order and Further Notice of Proposed Rulemaking, CC Dkt. No. 87-124, FCC 90-133 (June 7, 1990), 55 *Fed. Reg.* 28,762 (July 13, 1990), codified at 47 C.F.R. Part 68.

16. *In the Matter of Access to Telecommunications Equipment and Services by the Hearing Impaired and Other Disabled Persons*, Report and Order, CC Dkt. No. 87-124, FCC 92-217 (June 4, 1992), 57 Fed. Reg. 27,182 (June 18, 1992), codified at 47 C.F.R. Part 68.

17. *In the Matter of Access to Telecommunications Equipment and Services by the Hearing Impaired and Other Disabled Persons*, Order, CC Dkt. No. 87-124, FCC 93-191 (April 15, 1993).

18. *In the Matter of Access to Telecommunications Equipment and Services by Persons with Disabilities*, Report and Order, CC Dkt. No. 87-124 (July 3, 1996).

19. In its 1996 order, the FCC had set November 1, 1998 as the date by which these telephones were required to have volume control. The date was subsequently moved back to January 1, 2000, after the Consumer Electronics Manufacturers Association complained that the earlier date was not feasible. *In the Matter of Access to Telecommunications Equipment and Services by Persons with Disabilities*, Order on Reconsideration, CC Dkt. No. 87-124 (July 11, 1997).

20. 28 C.F.R. Part 36, ADAAG §4.l.3(17)(b). Accessibility guidelines promulgated by the Access Board to implement the ADA also contain requirements for volume control. Additionally, these guidelines require that twenty-five percent of all public pay telephones in newly constructed and altered buildings and facilities be hearing aid compatible. The guidelines further require that these telephones be identified by a sign containing a telephone handset radiating sound waves. ADAAG §4.30.7.

21. *supra* n.1.

22. 63 Fed. Reg. 5607 (February 3, 1998), codified at 36 C.F.R. Part 1193.

23. *In the Matter of Implementation of Sections 255 and 251(a)(2) of the Communications Act of 1934, as Enacted by the Telecommunications Act of 1996, Access to Telecommunications Service, Telecommunications Equipment and Customer Premises Equipment by Persons with Disabilities,* Report and Order and Further Notice of Inquiry, WT Dkt. No. 96-198, FCC 99-181 (September 29, 1999).

24. ADAAG §4.1.3(17).

25. ADAAG §4.1.3(17)(d).

Publications on Deafness and Education

The following books and journal articles may provide useful information for parents, teachers, and advocates for students who are deaf or hard of hearing. Please consult your local library or the Library of Congress for additional resources.

Adams, J. W. *You and Your Deaf Child*, 2d ed. Washington, D.C.: Clerc Books, Gallaudet University Press, 1997.

Autin, D. "Inclusion and the New Idea." *Exceptional Parent* 29 (May 1999): 66-70.

Banks, J. *All of Us Together: The Story of Inclusion at the Kinzie School*. Washington, D.C.: Gallaudet University Press, 1994.

Benderly, B. *Dancing Without Music*. Washington, D.C.: Gallaudet University Press, 1990.

Berg, F. S. *Acoustics and Sound Systems in Schools*. San Diego: Singular Publishing, 1993.

Burch, D., F. Caccamise, and S. Herald. *Signs for Legal and Social Work Terminology*. Rochester, N.Y.: Educational Resources Department, National Technical Institute for the Deaf, and Washington, D.C.: U. S. Department of Education, 1998.

Chow, P., L. Blais, and J. Hemingway. "An Outsider Looking In: Total Inclusion and the Concept of Equifinality." *Education* 119 (Spring 1999): 459-464.

Cokely, D., and C. Baker. *American Sign Language: A Teacher's Resource Text on Curriculum, Methods, and Evaluation*. Silver Spring, Md.: T.J. Publishers, 1980.

DuBow, S. "Application of Rowley by Courts and SEAs." *Education of Handicapped Law Reporter*, SA-107 (1983).

———. "Mainstreaming or Residential Schools for Deaf Students." *Gallaudet Today* (Spring 1985).

———. "Into the Turbulent Mainstream—A Legal Perspective on the Weight to be Given to the Least Restrictive Environment in Placement Decisions for Deaf Children." *Journal of Law and Education* 18 (1989): 215–228.

DuBow, S., and S. Geer. "Special Education Law Since Rowley." *Clearinghouse Review* 1001 (January 1984).

First, P., J. L. Curcio, J. J. Herman, and Janice L. Herman (Eds.). *Individuals with Disabilities: Implementing the Newest Laws*. Thousand Oaks, Calif.: Corwin Press, 1993.

Gorn, S. *What Do I Do When . . ." The Answer Book on Special Education Law*. 2d ed. Philadelphia: LRP Publications, 1997.

Higgins, P. C. *The Challenge of Educating Together Deaf and Hearing Youth: Making Mainstreaming Work*. Springfield, Ill.: Charles C. Thomas, 1990.

Jacobs, L. M. *A Deaf Adult Speaks Out*. 3d ed. Washington, D.C.: Gallaudet University Press, 1989.

Lane, L. G. *Gallaudet Survival Guide to Signing*. Rev. ed. Washington, D.C.: Gallaudet University Press, 1990.

Lantzy, M. L. *Individuals with Disabilities Education Act: An Annotated Guide to its Literature and Resources, 1980-1991*. Littleton, Colo.: F.B. Rothman & Co., 1992.

Leutke-Stahlman, B. "Providing the Support Services Needed by Students who are Deaf or Hard of Hearing." *American Annals of the Deaf* 143(5), 388–391.

Marschark, M. *Raising and Educating a Deaf Child*. New York: Oxford University Press, 1997.

Mindel, E. D., and M. Vernon. *They Grow in Silence*. Silver Spring, Md.: National Association of the Deaf, 1971.

Moores, D. F. *Educating the Deaf: Psychology, Principles and Practices*, 3d ed. Boston: Houghton Mifflin, 1987.

Ogden, P. *The Silent Garden: Raising Your Deaf Child*. Rev. ed. Washington, D.C.: Gallaudet University Press, 1996.

Prickett, H. T. *Advocacy for Deaf Children*. Springfield, Ill.: Charles C. Thomas, 1989.

Prinz, P. M., M. Strong, M. Kuntze, J. Vincent, et al. "A Path to Literacy Through ASL and English for Deaf Children," in *Children's Language*, vol. 9 (pp. 235–51), ed. by C. E. Johnson and J. H. V. Gilbert, et al. Mahwah, N.J.: Lawrence Erlbaum Associates.

Ramsey, C. L. *Deaf Children in Public Schools: Placement, Context, and Consequences*. Washington, D.C.: Gallaudet University Press, 1997.

Siegel, Lawrence M. *Least Restrictive Environment: The Paradox of Inclusion.* Horsham, Pa.: LRP Publications, 1994.

Spradley, J. P., and T. S. Spradley. *Deaf Like Me.* New York: Random House, 1978. Washington, D.C.: Gallaudet University Press, 1985.

Stewart, D. A., and B. Luetke-Stahlman. *The Signing Family: What Every Parent Should Know about Sign Communication.* Washington, D.C.: Gallaudet University Press, 1998.

Strong, M. "A Review of Bilingual/Bicultural Programs for Deaf Children in North America." *American Annals of the Deaf* 140(2) (April 1995): 84–94.

Strong, M., E. S. Charlson, and R. Gold. "Integration And Segregation in Mainstreaming Programs For Children And Adolescents With Hearing Impairments." *Exceptional Child* 34(3) (Nov. 1987): 181–195.

Tucker, B. P. *Federal Disability Law in a Nutshell.* 2d ed. St. Paul, Minn.: West Group, 1998.

———. *IDEA Advocacy for Children Who Are Deaf or Hard-of-hearing: A Question and Answer Book for Parents and Professionals.* San Diego, Calif.: Singular Publishing Group, 1997.

Turnbull, H. R., III, and A. Turnbull. *Free Appropriate Public Education: The Law and Children with Disabilities.* 5th ed. Denver: Love Publishing, 1998.

Underwood, J. K., and D. A. Verstegen. *The Impacts of Litigation and Legislation on Public School Finance: Adequacy, Equity, and Excellence.* New York: Ballinger, 1990.

Underwood, J. K., and J. F. Mead. *Legal Aspects of Special Education and Pupil Services.* Boston: Allyn and Bacon, 1995.

Underwood, J., J. A. Dodge, C. Weatherly, J. Weatherly, and J. Houton. *Individuals with Disabilities Education Act: A Legal Primer.* Alexandria, Va.: National School Boards Association, 1996.

Yell, M. L. "The Legal Basis of Inclusion." *Educational Leadership* 56(2) (Oct. 1998): 70–73.

Zapien, C. "Education and Deafness." *The Exceptional Parent* 28(9) (Sept. 1998): 40–48.

State Services

ALABAMA
Department of Rehabilitation Services
2129 East South Blvd.
P.O. Box 11586
Montgomery, AL 36111-0586
(334) 281-8780 Voice
(334) 613-2249 TTY
(800) 441-7607 V/TTY (in AL)
(334) 281-1973 FAX
elindsey@sovrs.rehab.state.al.us
www.rehab.state.al.us

ALASKA
Division of Vocational Rehabilitation
3600 S. Bragaw
Anchorage, AK 99508-4688
(907) 561-4466 V/TTY
(907) 562-7746 FAX
dmayes@educ.state.ak.us

ARIZONA
Arizona Council for the Hearing Impaired
1400 West Washington Street
Room 126
Phoenix, AZ 85007
(602) 542-3323 V/TTY

(800) 352-8161 V/TTY (in AZ)
(602) 542-3380 FAX
www.state.az.us/achi

Communication Disorders Office
Rehabilitation Services Administration
1789 West Jefferson
2nd Floor NW
Phoenix, AZ 85007
(602) 542-3332 Voice
(602) 542-6049 TTY
(602) 542-3778 FAX

ARKANSAS
Arkansas Rehabilitation Services
Office of the Deaf and Hearing Impaired
1616 Brookwood
P.O. Box 3781
Little Rock, AR 72203
(501) 296-1691 Voice
(501) 296-1670 TTY
(501) 296-1675 FAX
KWMusteen@ars.state.ar.us

CALIFORNIA
State Office of Deaf Access
Department of Social Services
744 P Street, MS 19-91
Sacramento, CA 95814
(916) 229-4573 Voice
(916) 229-4577 TTY
(916) 229-4198 FAX
deaf.access@dss.ca.gov

Deaf and Hard of Hearing Services
Department of Rehabilitation
2000 Evergreen Street
Sacramento, CA 95815
(916) 263-8938 Voice
(916) 263-7481 TTY
(916) 263-7480 FAX
Tbeatty@rehab.cahwnet.gov

COLORADO
Colorado Vocational Rehabilitation Services
600 Grant Street, Suite 302

Denver, CO 80203
(303) 894-2515 x222 Voice
(303) 894-2650 TTY (Krista)
(303) 894-2519 TTY (Jim)
(303) 894-2656 FAX

CONNECTICUT
Connecticut Commission on the Deaf and Hearing Impaired
1245 Farmington Avenue
West Hartford, CT 06107
(860) 561-0196 V/TTY
(860) 561-0162 FAX
cdhi@po.state.ct.us
www.state.ct.us/cdhi/index.htm

Bureau of Rehabilitation Services
25 Sigourney Street
Hartford, CT 06106-2055
(860) 424-4858 Voice
(860) 424-2231 TTY

DELAWARE
Delaware Office for the Deaf and Hard of Hearing
Division of Vocational Rehabilitation
4425 N. Market St., 3rd Fl.
Wilmington, DE 19802-1307
(302) 761-8275 Voice
(302) 761-8336 TTY
(302) 761-6611 FAX
LSarro@dvr.state.de.us

Division of Vocational Rehabilitation
4425 N. Market St., 3rd Fl.
Wilmington, DE 19802-1307
(302) 761-8275 Voice
(302) 761-8336 TTY
(302) 761-6611 FAX
LSarro@dvr.state.de.us

DISTRICT OF COLUMBIA
Rehabilitation Services Administration
810 First Street, NE
Suite 9055
Washington, DC 20002

(202) 442-8496 V/TTY
(202) 442-8725 FAX

FLORIDA
Deaf and Hard of Hearing Services Program
Division of Vocational Rehabilitation
2002 Old St. Augustine Road,
Building A
Tallahassee, FL 32399-0696
(850) 488-8380 Voice
(850) 413-9629 TTY
(850) 921-7217 FAX
bradlec@vr.fdles.tl.us

GEORGIA
Georgia Council for the Hearing Impaired, Inc.
4151 Memorial Drive, #103B
Decatur, GA 30032
(404) 292-5312 V/TTY
(800) 541-0710 V/TTY
(404) 292-3642 FAX
www.gachi.net

Georgia Department of Human Resources
Division of Rehabilitation Services
2 Peachtree Street Northwest
35th Floor
Atlanta, GA 30303-3142
(404) 657-3034 V/TTY
(404) 463-6425 FAX
mcgillka@dhr.state.ga.us

HAWAII
Hawaii State Coordinating Council on Deafness
Commission on Persons with Disabilities
919 Ala Moana Blvd., Room 101
Honolulu, HI 96814
(808) 586-8131 V/TTY
(808) 586-8130 TTY
(808) 586-8129 FAX
cpdppp@aloha.net
www.hawaii.gov/health/cpdindx.htm

Vocational Rehabilitation and Deaf Services Section
707 Richard Street, PH5
Honolulu, HI 96813

(808) 692-7723 V/TTY
(808) 692-7727 FAX
cyoung@dhs.state.hi.us

IDAHO
Idaho Council for the Deaf and Hard of Hearing
1720 Westgate Drive
Boise, ID 83704
(208) 334-0879 Voice
(208) 334-0803 TTY
(800) 433-1323 V (in ID)
(800) 433-1361 TTY (in ID)
(208) 334-0828 FAX
cooperp{dhtowers/dhw04/
cooperp}@dhw.state.id.us
ww2.state.id.us/cdhh/cdhhl.htm

Division of Vocational Rehabilitation
3350 Americana Terrace
Suite 210
Boise, ID 83706-2502
(208) 334-3650 Voice
(208) 334-3670 TTY
(800) 856-2720 [information]
(208) 334-3661 FAX
bdarcy@idvr.state.id.us

ILLINOIS
Commission for the Deaf and Hard of Hearing
618 E. Washington
Springfield, IL 62794
Exec. Dir.: Gerald Covell
(217) 557-4495 V/TTY
(217) 557-4492 FAX

Division of Services for Persons who are Deaf or Hard of Hearing
Dept. of Human Services
Office of Rehabilitation Service
100 West Randolph Street, Suite 8-100
Chicago, IL 60601
(312) 814-2939 Voice
(312) 814-3040 TTY
(312) 814-2923 FAX
(312) 814-5849 FAX
eroth@dors.state.il.us

INDIANA
Deaf and Hard of Hearing Services
Division of Disability, Aging, and Rehabilitative Services
402 West Washington Street, Room W-453
P.O. Box 7083
Indianapolis, IN 46207-7083
(317) 232-1143 V/TTY
(800) 962-8408 V/TTY (in IN)
(317) 232-6478 FAX
jfreeman@fssa.state.in.us

Division of Disability, Aging, and Rehabilitative Services
Vocational Rehabilitation Services
402 West Washington Street, Room W-453
P. O. Box 7083
Indianapolis, IN 46207-7083
(317) 232-1427 V/TTY
(317) 232-6478 FAX
dshaffer@fssa.state.in.us

IOWA
Deaf Services Commission of Iowa
Iowa Department of Human Rights
Lucas State Office Building
Des Moines, IA 50319
(515) 281-3164 V/TTY
(515) 242-6119 FAX

Division of Vocational Rehabilitation Services
510 East 12th Street
Des Moines, IA 50319
(515) 281-4151 Voice
(800) 532-1486 V/TTY
(515) 281-4703 FAX
rchilders@dvrs.state.ia.us

KANSAS
Kansas Commission for the Deaf and Hard of Hearing
3640 Southwest Topeka Blvd.
Suite 150
Topeka, KS 66611
(785) 276-5301 Voice
(785) 267-0532 TTY
(785) 267-0263 FAX
(800) 432-0698 V/TTY (in KS)
rja@srkrspo.wpo.state.ks.us

Rehabilitation Services
Department of Social and Rehabilitation Services
401 W. Frontier Lane
Olathe, KS 66061-7221
(913) 768-3304 Voice
(913) 768-3381 TTY
(913) 768-3583 FAX
skxn@srolathe.wpo.state.ks.us

KENTUCKY
Kentucky Commission on the Deaf and Hard of Hearing
632 Versailles Road
Frankfort, KY 40601
(502) 573-2604 V/TTY
(800) 372-2907 V/TTY (in KY)
(502) 573-3594 FAX
bobbie.scoggins@mail.state.ky.us
www.kcdhh.org

Department of Vocational Rehabilitation
209 Saint Clair Street
Frankfort, KY 40601
(502) 564-5440 V/TTY
(502) 564-6742 TTY
(502) 564-6745 FAX
Patty.Conway@mail.state.ky.us
www.ihdi.uky.edu/projects/
dvr/dvrhome.htm

LOUISIANA
Louisiana Commission for the Deaf
8225 Florida Boulevard
Baton Rouge, LA 70806-4834
(504) 925-4175 Voice
(800) 256-1523 Voice
(800) 543-2099 TTY
(504) 925-1708 FAX
jfaulkne@lrs.dss.state.la.us

Louisiana Rehabilitation Services
8225 Florida Boulevard
Baton Rouge, LA 70806-4834
(504) 925-4131 V/TTY
(504) 925-4184 FAX
rstarks@lrs.dss.state.la.us
www.dss.state.1a.us

MAINE
Division of Deafness
Bureau of Rehabilitation Services
150 State House Station
Augusta, ME 04333-0150
(207) 287-5145 Voice
(207) 287-5146 TTY
(800) 698-4440 V/TTY (in ME)
(207) 287-5166 FAX
alice.c.johnson@state.me.us

MARYLAND
Governor's Office of Individuals With Disabilities
One Market Center
300 W. Lexington Street, Box 10
Baltimore, MD 21201
(410) 333-6304 TTY
(410) 333-3098 Voice
(410) 333-6674 Fax

Maryland Division of Rehabilitation Services
2301 Argonne Drive
Baltimore, MD 21218
(410) 554-9404 Voice
(410) 554-9411 TTY
(410) 554-9412 FAX
dors@msde.state.md.us

MASSACHUSETTS
Massachusetts Commission
for the Deaf and Hard of Hearing
210 South Street, 5th Floor
Boston, MA 02111
(617) 695-7500 Voice
(617) 695-7600 TTY
(800) 882-1155 Voice (in MA)
(800) 530-7570 TTY (in MA)
(617) 695-7599 FAX
(800) 249-9949 V/TTY (in MA) (after hours-interpreter emergencies)
MCDHH.OFFICE@state.ma.us (not for interpreter requests)

Massachusetts Rehabilitation Commission
Fort Point Place
27-43 Wormwood Street

Boston, MA 02210-1606
(617) 204-3855
ext. 3734 (Voice)
ext. 3835 (TTY)
(617) 727-2793 FAX
Diane.C.Kendrick@MRC.state.ma.us

MICHIGAN
Division on Deafness
Michigan Family Independence Agency
320 N. Washington Sq., Ste. 250
Box 30659
Lansing, MI 48909
(517) 334-8000 V/TTY
(517) 334-6637 FAX
hunterc2@state.mi.us
http://www.mfia.state.mi/mcdc/dod.htm

Michigan Jobs Commission Rehabilitation Services
608 West Allegan St.
P.O. Box 30010
Lansing, MI 48909
(517) 335-6745 Voice
(517) 373-4035 TTY
(517) 373-4479 FAX
faulknerg@state.mi.us

MINNESOTA
Minnesota Commission Serving Deaf and Hard of Hearing People
Human Services Building
444 Lafayette Road
St. Paul, MN 55155-3814
(612) 297-7305 V/TTY
(612) 297-7155 FAX
curt.micka@state.mn.us or mike.cashman@state.mn.us

Rehabilitation Services Branch
Dept. of Economic Security
390 N. Robert St., First Floor
St. Paul, MN 55101-1812
(612) 297-8269 Voice
(612) 296-9141 TTY
(612) 297-5159 FAX
Rubin.Latz@state.mn.us
www.des.state.mn.us

MISSISSIPPI
Office of Vocational Rehabilitation Services
P.O. Box 1698
Jackson, MS 39215
(601) 853-5310 V/TTY
(800) 443-1000 V/TTY (in MS)
(601) 853-5325 FAX
rwebber@mdrs.state.ms.us

MISSOURI
Missouri Commission for the Deaf
1103 Rear Southwest Blvd.
Jefferson City, MO 65109
(573) 526-5205 V/TTY
(800) 796-6499 V/TTY
(573) 526-5209 FAX
MCD@mail.state.mo.us
www.oa.state.mo.us/deaf/mcd.shtml

Division of Vocational Rehabilitation
Department of Elementary and Secondary Education
3024 West Truman Rd.
Jefferson City, MO 65109
(573) 882-9110 Voice
(573) 882-9117 TTY
(573) 884-5250 FAX
smantoot@vr.dese.state.mo.us

MONTANA
Montana Vocational Rehabilitation
1818 10th Avenue S., Suite 5
Great Falls, MT 59405
(406) 454-6060 Voice
(406) 454-6080 TTY
(406) 454-6084 Fax
rellesch@mt.gov

NEBRASKA
Nebraska Commission for the Deaf and Hard of Hearing
4600 Valley Road, Suite 420
Lincoln, NE 68510
(402) 471-3593 V/TTY
(800) 545-6244 (in NE)
(402) 471-3067 FAX
twendel@ncdhh.state.ne.us
www.ncd.org/home/NCDHH

Division of Vocational Rehabilitation
301 Centennial Mall So.
P.O. Box 94987
Lincoln, NE 68509
(402) 471-3644 V/TTY
(402) 471-0788 FAX

NEVADA
Rehabilitation Division
711 South Stewart Street
Carson City, NV 89710
(702) 687-4452 Voice
(702) 687-3388 TTY
(888) 337-3839 ext. 4452 (in NV)
(702) 687-3292 FAX
scotapott@aol.com

NEW HAMPSHIRE
Program for the Deaf and Hard of Hearing
Division of Adult Learning and Rehabilitation
78 Regional Drive, Building 2
Concord, NH 03301-8530
State Coord.: Mr. H. Dee Clanton
(603) 271-3471 V/TTY
(603) 271-7095 FAX
(800) 299-1647 (in NH)
hdclanton@ed.state.nh.us

NEW JERSEY
Division of the Deaf and Hard of Hearing
New Jersey Department of Human Services
P.O. Box 074
Trenton, NJ 08625-0074
Director: Richard Herring
(609) 984-7281 V/TTY
(800) 792-8339 V/TTY (in NJ)
(609) 984-0390 FAX
RichardHerring@dhs.state.nj.us

Division of Vocational Rehabilitation Services
New Jersey Dept of Labor
P.O. Box 398
Trenton, NJ 08625-0398
(609) 292-9339 Voice

(609) 292-2919 TTY
(609) 292-8347 FAX
jcronin@dol.state.nj.us

NEW MEXICO
New Mexico Commission for the Deaf and Hard of Hearing
1435 St. Francis Drive
Santa Fe, NM 87505
(505) 827-7584 V/TTY
(505) 827-7588 TTY
(800) 489-8536 V/TTY (in NM)
nmcdhh@doh.state.nin.us
www.nmcdhh.org

State Department of Education
Division of Vocational Rehabilitation
435 St. Michael's Drive
Bldg. D
Santa Fe, NM 87505
(505) 954-8510 V/TTY
(505) 954-8562 Fax
tbrigance@state.nm.us

NEW YORK
Office of Vocational and Educational Services for Individuals with
    Disabilities
State Education Department
One Commerce Plaza, Room 1601
Albany, NY 12234
(518) 474-5652 V/TTY
(800) 222-5627 V/TTY
(518) 473-6073 FAX
dsteele@mail.nysed.gov

NORTH CAROLINA
Division of Services for the Deaf and Hard of Hearing
Department of Health and Human Resources
319 Chapanoke Road, Suite 108
Raleigh, NC 27603
(919) 773-2963 Voice
(919) 773-2966 TTY
(919) 773-2993 FAX
sbell@dhr.state.nc.us

Division of Vocational Rehabilitation Services
P.O. Box 26053
Raleigh, NC 27611
(919) 733-3364 Voice
(919) 733-5924 TTY
(919) 733-7968 FAX
tfish@dhr.state.nc.us
www.dhr.state.nc.us/dhr/dvrfmtranet/home.htrn

NORTH DAKOTA
Office of Vocational Rehabilitation
Dept. of Human Services
600 S. 2nd Street, Suite 1B
Bismarck, ND 58504-5729
(701) 328-8950 Voice
(701) 328-3975 TTY
(800) 755-2745 Voice (in ND)
(701) 328-8969 FAX
sogiew@ranch.state.nd.us

OHIO
Rehabilitation Services Commission
400 East Campus View Blvd.
Columbus, OH 43235-4604
(614) 785-5085 TTY
(614) 438-1325 Voice
(800) 282-4536 V/TTY (in OH)
(614) 438-1289 FAX
rsc-skp@ohio.gov
www.state.oh.us/rs

OKLAHOMA
Services to the Deaf and Hard of Hearing
Department of Rehabilitation Services
5813 South Robinson
Oklahoma City, OK 73109
(405) 634-9937 V/TTY
(800) 833-8973 V/TTY (in OK)
(405) 631-8815 FAX

OREGON
Deaf and Hard of Hearing Access Program
Oregon Disabilities Commission
1257 Ferry Street, SE

Salem, OR 97310
(503) 378-3142 V/TTY
(800) 358-3117 V/TTY (in OR)
(800) 521-9615 V/TTY (in OR)
(503) 378-3599 FAX
tj.x.davis@state.or.us
www.odc.state.or.us/dhhap.htm

Vocational Rehabilitation Division
North Portland Branch
4744 N. Interstate Avenue
Portland, OR 97217
(503) 280-6940 V/TTY
(503) 280-6960 FAX
sheila.r.hitchen@state.or.us
www.vrd.hr.state.or.us

PENNSYLVANIA
Office for the Deaf and Hard of Hearing
1110 Labor & Industry Bldg.
7th and Forster Streets
Harrisburg, PA 17120-0019
(717) 783-4912 V/TTY
(800) 233-3008 V/TTY (in PA)
(717) 783-4913 FAX

Office of Vocational Rehabilitation
1310 Labor & Industry Bldg.
7th and Forster Streets
Harrisburg, PA 17120
(800) 442-6351 Voice (in PA)
(717) 787-4885 TTY
(717) 772-1659 Voice
(717) 783-5221 FAX

PUERTO RICO
Vocational Rehabilitation Administration
Department of the Family
Box 924
Guaynabo, PR 00970
(809) 782-0011 V/TTY
(809) 783-4570 FAX

RHODE ISLAND
Commission on the Deaf and Hard of Hearing
Dept. of Administration Building
One Capitol Hill, Ground Level
Providence, RI 02908-5850
(401) 222-1204 Voice
(401) 222-1205 TTY
(401) 222-5736 FAX
slane@doa.state.ri.us
www.state.ri.us/ricdhh

Office of Rehabilitation Services
40 Fountain Street
Providence, RI 02903
(401) 421-7005, ext. 363 (Voice)
(401) 421-7016 TTY
(800) 752-8088, ext. 2608 (Voice)
(401) 421-9259 FAX
dcook@dhs.state.ri.us
www.org.state.ri.us

SOUTH CAROLINA
Vocational Rehabilitation Dept.
P.O. Box 15
West Columbia, SC 29171
(803) 896-6637 V/TTY
(803) 896-6877 FAX
scvrd@scsn.net

SOUTH DAKOTA
Communication Services for the Deaf
102 N. Krohn Place
Sioux Falls, SD 57103
(605) 367-5760 V/TTY
(800) 642-6410 V/TTY
(605) 367-5958 FAX
bjsoukup@mcimail.com

Division of Rehabilitation Services
Dept. of Human Services
Hillsview Plaza
East Highway 34
c/o 500 East Capitol
Pierre, SD 57501-5070

(605) 773-3195 V/TTY
(605) 773-5483 FAX
clarke.christianson@state.sd.us
www.state.sd.us/state/executive/dhs/drs/deaf.htm

TENNESSEE
Tennessee Council for the Hearing Impaired
400 Deaderick Street, 11th Floor
Nashville, TN 37248
(615) 313-4913 V/TTY
(800) 270-1349 TTY (in TN)
(615) 741-6508 FAX

Tennessee Division of Rehabilitation Services
Dept. of Human Services
400 Deaderick Street, 15th Floor
Nashville, TN 37248-0060
(615) 313-4714 V/TTY
(615) 741-4165 FAX
KSteede@mail.state.tn.us
www.state.tn.us/humanserv

TEXAS
Texas Commission for the Deaf and Hard of Hearing
P.O. Box 12904
Austin, TX 78711-2904
(512) 407-3250 Voice
(512) 407-3251 TTY
(512) 451-9316 FAX
dmyers@tcdhh.state.tx.us

Deaf, Hard of Hearing and Communication Disorders
Texas Rehabilitation Commission
4900 North Lamar Boulevard
Austin, TX 78751-2399
(512) 424-4176 Voice
(512) 424-4523 TTY
(512) 424-4982 FAX
jack.clifton@rehab.state.tx.us
www.trcnet/welcome.html

UTAH
Utah Community Center of the Deaf and Hard of Hearing
Utah State Office of Rehabilitation

5709 South 1500 West
Salt Lake City, UT 84123
(801) 263-4860 V/TTY
(800) 860-4860 V/TTY (in UT)
(801) 263-4865 FAX
wwales@usor.state.ut.us

Division of Services for the Deaf and Hard of Hearing
Utah State Office of Rehabilitation
5709 South 1500 West
Taylorsville, UT 84123-5217
(801) 263-4860 V/TTY
(801) 263-4865 FAX

VERMONT
Division of Vocational Rehabilitation
Department of Aging and Disabilities
103 South Main Street
Waterbury, VT 05671-2303
(802) 241-2186 V/TTY
(802) 241-3359 FAX
rene@dad.state.vt.us/dvr/
www.dad.sate.vt.us/dvr/

VIRGINIA
Department for the Deaf and Hard of Hearing
Ratcliffe Building
1602 Rolling Hills Drive
Richmond, VA 23229-5012
(804) 662-9502 V/TTY
(800) 552-7917 V/TTY (in VA)
(804) 662-9718 FAX
DDHHinfo@DDHH.state.va.us
www.cns.state.va.us/vddhh

Department of Rehabilitation Services
8004 Franklin Farms Dr.
P.O. Box K300
Richmond, VA 23288-0300
(804) 662-7614 V/TTY
(800) 552-5019 Voice
(800) 464-9950 TTY
(804) 662-7663 FAX
nunnalmc@drs.state.va.us
www.cns.state.va/us/drs

VIRGIN ISLANDS
Division of Disabilities and Rehabilitation Services
Virgin Islands Department of Human Services
3011 Golden Rock
St. Croix, VI 00820-4355
(800) 774-0930 Voice (in VI)
(340) 773-2323 Voice
(340) 773-3641 FAX

WASHINGTON
Office of Deaf and Hard of Hearing Services
Department of Social and Health Services
P.O. Box 45300
Olympia, WA 98504-5300
(360) 902-8000 V/TTY
(360) 753-0699 TTY
(360) 902-0855 FAX
Message only lines:
(800) 422-7930 Voice
(800) 422-7941 TTY
curtigl@dshs.wa.gov

Division of Vocational Rehabilitation
P.O. Box 45340
Olympia, WA 98504-5340
(360) 438-8048 V/TTY
(800) 637-5627 (in WA)
(360) 438-8007 FAX
jannia@dshs.wa.gov

WEST VIRGINIA
West Virginia Commission for the Deaf and Hard of Hearing
4190 Washington Street West
Charleston, WV 25313
(304) 558-2175 V/TTY
(304) 558-0026 TTY
(304) 558-0851 FAX
krussell@wrdhhr.org

Division of Rehabilitation Services
Box 50890
State Capitol Complex
Charleston, WV 25305-0890
(304) 766-4965 V/TTY

(800) 642-8207 Voice (in WV)
(304) 766-4690 FAX
barbara@wvdrs.wvnet.edu
www.wvdrs.wvnet.edu

WISCONSIN
Wisconsin Office for the Deaf and Hard of Hearing
Department of Health and Family Services
2917 International Lane
P.O. Box 7852
Madison, WI 53704
(608) 243-5625 Voice
(608) 243-5717 TTY
(608) 243-5680 FAX
hammeri@dwd.state.wi.us
VOSSMe@dwd.state.wi.us

Division of Vocational Rehabilitation
Department of Workforce Development
2917 International Lane
Madison, WI 53704
(608) 243-5600 Voice
(608) 243-5634 TTY
(608) 243-5681 FAX

WYOMING
Division of Vocational Rehabilitation
1100 Herschler Bldg.
Cheyenne, WY 82002
(800) 452-1408 V/TTY
(307) 777-5939 FAX
lcieli@missc.state.wy.us

Non-Governmental Organizations

Each organization was asked to identify up to four descriptors that best describe the organization's focus. The codes are:

C   Consumer and/or Advocacy

E   Educational

F   Funding Source

I   Information and/or Referral

M   Medical

P   Professional

Rc   Recreational

R   Religious

Rs   Research

S   Self-help/Support

So   Social

ABLEDATA
8455 Colesville Road, Suite 935
Silver Spring, MD 20910
Voice: (301) 608-8998

TTY: (301) 608-8912
Voice: (800) 227-0216
FAX: (301) 608-8958
Email: ABLEDATA@macroint.com
Web Page: http://www.abledata.com
ABLEDATA is an information and referral project that maintains a database of 25,000-plus assistive technology products. The project also produces fact sheets on types of devices and other aspects of assistive technology. (I)

ADARA: Professionals Networking for Excellence in Service Delivery
    with Individuals Who are Deaf or Hard of Hearing (formerly
    American Deafness And Rehabilitation Association)
P.O. Box 6956
San Mateo, CA 94403-6956
Voice/TTY: (650) 372-0620
FAX: (650) 372-0661
Email: ADARAorgn@aol.com
Web Page: http://www.adara.org
Publications: *JADARA* and the *ADARA UPDATE* (quarterly
    newsletter)
Promotes and participates in quality human service delivery to deaf and hard of hearing people through agencies and individuals. ADARA is a partnership of national organizations, local affiliates, professional sections, and individual members working together to support social services and rehabilitation delivery for deaf and hard of hearing people. (P)

Alexander Graham Bell Association for the Deaf, Inc.
3417 Volta Place NW
Washington, DC 20007
Voice/TTY: (202) 337-5220
FAX: (202) 337-8314
Email: agbell2@aol.com
Web Page: http://www.agbell.org
Publications: *The Volta Review* (journal), *Volta Voices* (magazine)
Gathers and disseminates information on hearing loss, promotes better public understanding of hearing loss in children and adults, provides scholarships and financial and parent-infant awards, promotes early detection of hearing loss in infants, publishes books on deafness, and advocates for the rights of children and adults who are hard of hearing or deaf. (F,I,P,S,C,E)

American Academy of Audiology
8201 Greensboro Drive, Suite 300
McLean, VA 22102
Voice/TTY: (703) 610-9022

Voice/TTY: (800) 222-2336
FAX: (703) 610-9005
Email: molek@audiology.org
Web Page@ http://www.audiology.com
Publications: *Audiology Today* (magazine), *Journal of AAA* (journal), *Audiology Express* (newsletter)
A professional organization of individuals dedicated to providing high quality hearing care to the public. Provides professional development, education, and research and promotes increased public awareness of hearing disorders and audiologic services. (E,P,I)

American Academy of Otolaryngology—Head and Neck Surgery
1 Prince Street
Alexandria, VA 22314-3357
Voice: (703) 836-4444
TTY: (703) 519-1585
FAX: (703) 683-5100
Email: entnews@aol.com
Web Page: http://www.entnet.org/
Publications: *Otolaryngology—Head and Neck Surgery* (journal), *The Bulletin* (magazine)
Promotes the art and science of medicine related to otolaryngology-head and neck surgery, including providing continuing medical education courses and publications. Distributes patient leaflets relating to ear, nose and throat problems and makes referrals to physicians. (M,P)

American Association of the Deaf-Blind
814 Thayer Avenue, Room 302
Silver Spring, MD 20910-4500
TTY: (301) 588-6545
FAX: (301) 588-8705
Email: aadb@erols.com
Publication: *Deaf-Blind American*
Promotes better opportunities and services for deaf-blind people. Mission is to assure that a comprehensive, coordinated system of services is accessible to all deaf-blind people, enabling them to achieve their maximum potential through increased independence, productivity, and integration into the community. The biennial conventions provide a week of workshops, meetings, tours, and recreational activities. (C, I)

American Hearing Research Foundation
55 E. Washington St., Suite 2022
Chicago, IL 60602
Voice: (312) 726-9670

FAX: (312) 726-9695
Publication: Newsletter
Supports medical research and education into the causes, prevention, and cures of deafness, hearing losses, and balance disorders. Also keeps physicians and the public informed of the latest developments in hearing research and education. (Rs)

American Society for Deaf Children
1820 Tribute Road, Suite A
Sacramento, CA 95815
Voice/TTY: (800) 942-ASDC (Parent Hotline)
Voice/TTY: (916) 641-6084 FAX: (916) 641-6085
Email: ASDC1@aol.com
Web Page: http://www.deafchildren.org
Publication: *The Endeavor*
ASDC is a nonprofit parent-helping-parent organization promoting a positive attitude toward signing and deaf culture. Also provides support, encouragement, and current information about deafness to families with deaf and hard of hearing children. (C, I, S, E)

American Speech-Language-Hearing Association
10801 Rockville Pike
Rockville, MD 20852
HELPLINE: (800) 638-8255 (Voice/TTY)
FAX: (301) 897-7355
Email: actioncenter@asha.org
Web Page: http://www.asha.org
Publications: *Journal of Speech-Language-Hearing Research; American Journal of Audiology; American Journal of Speech Language Pathology; Language Speech and Hearing Services in the Schools; ASHA Magazine; ASHA Leader*
A professional and scientific organization for speech-language pathologists and audiologists concerned with communication disorders. Provides informational materials and a toll-free number for consumers to inquire about speech, language, or hearing problems. Also provides referrals to audiologists and speech-language pathologists in the United States. (C, I, P, Rs)

American Tinnitus Association
P.O. Box 5
Portland, OR 97207
Voice: (503) 248-9985
FAX: (503) 248-0024
Web Page: http://www.ata.org

Publication: *Tinnitus Today*
Provides information about tinnitus and referrals to local hearing professionals/support groups nationwide. Also provides a bibliography service, funds scientific research related to tinnitus, and offers regional workshops. Works to promote public education about tinnitus and hearing loss. (E, F, I, P, Rs, S)

Arkansas Rehabilitation Research and Training Center for Persons
    Who Are Deaf and Hard of Hearing
University of Arkansas
4601 W. Markham St.
Little Rock, AR 72205
Voice/TTY: (501) 686-9691
FAX: (501) 686-9698
Email: REHABRES@CAVERN.UARK.EDU
Web Page: http://www.uark.eduldeptsirehabres
The center focuses on issues affecting the employability of deaf and hard of hearing rehabilitation clients—career assessment, career preparation, placement, career mobility, and advancement. Provides information and/or databases related to the rehabilitation of deaf and hard of hearing people served by the Federal/state Vocational Rehabilitation Program. (E, I, P, Rs)

Association of Late-Deafened Adults
10310 Main Street, #274
Fairfax, VA 22030
TTY: (404) 289-1596
FAX: (404) 284-6862
Web Page: http://www.alda.org
Publication: *ALDA NEWS*
Supports the empowerment of people who are deafened. Provides resources and information and promotes advocacy and awareness of the needs of deafened adults. (C, I, S, So)

Auditory-Verbal International, Inc.
2121 Eisenhower Ave., Suite 402
Alexandria, VA 22314
Voice: (703) 739-1049
TTY: (703) 739-0874
FAX: (703) 739-0395
Email: avi@auditory-verbal.org
Web Page: http://www.auditory-verbal.org
Publications: *The AURICLE, Backtalk!*
AVI is dedicated to helping children who have hearing losses learn to

listen and speak. Promotes the Auditory-Verbal Therapy approach, which is based on the belief that the overwhelming majority of these children can hear and talk by using their residual hearing, hearing aids, and cochlear implants. (C, E, I, P, S)

Better Hearing Institute
5021-B Backlick Road
Annandale, VA 22003
Voice/TTY: (703) 642-0580
Voice/TTY: (888) HEAR HELP (BHI Office)
Voice/TTY: (800) EAR-WELL (Hearing HelpLine)
FAX: (703) 750-9302
Email: mail@betterhearing.org
Web Page: http://www.betterhearing.org
Publication: *Better Hearing News*
BHI is a nonprofit educational organization that implements national public information programs on hearing loss and available medical, surgical, hearing aid, and rehabilitation assistance for millions with uncorrected hearing problems. Promotes awareness of hearing loss through television, radio, and print media public service messages. BHI maintains a toll-free "Hearing HelpLine" telephone service that provides information on hearing loss, sources of assistance, lists of local hearing professionals, and other available hearing help to callers from anywhere in the United States and Canada. (I)

Boys Town National Research Hospital
555 N. 30th Street
Omaha, NE 68131
Voice: (402) 498-6511
Voice: (402) 498-6749 (Continuing Ed.)
TTY: (402) 498-6543
FAX: (402) 498-6638
Email: PEB@boystown.org
Web Page: http://www.boystown.org
Boys Town National Research Hospital (BTNRH) is an internationally recognized center for state-of-the-art research, diagnosis and treatment of individuals with ear diseases, hearing and balance disorders, cleft lip and palate, and speech/language problems. It also includes multi-disciplinary evaluation of Deaf/hard of hearing students. Annual Issues in Language and Deafness Conference, the Center for Childhood Deafness, Center for Hereditary Deafness, Center for Hearing Research and an NIDCD research and training center, the Center for Hearing Loss in Children. (E, I, M, Rs)

The Caption Center
125 Western Avenue
Boston, MA 02134
Voice/TTY: (617) 492-9225
FAX: (617) 562-0590
Email: caption@wgbh.org
Web Page: http://www.wgbh.org/caption
Publications: *Caption Center News* (newsletter), *Consumer Information Series* (on topics of interest to all caption viewers), *Tech Facts* (technical newsletter)
The Caption Center is a nonprofit service of the WGBH Educational Foundation and the world's first captioning agency. Offices in Boston, Los Angeles, and New York produce captions for every segment of the television and video industries and offer an array of services including off-line captions, real-time captions, dual-field, dual-language captions, subtitling, and open captions. (C, I, Rs)

Captioned Media Program
(formerly Captioned Films/Videos Program)
National Association of the Deaf (NAD)
1447 E. Main Street
Spartanburg, SC 29307
Voice: (800) 237-6213
TTY: (800) 237-6819
FAX: (800) 538-5636
Email: info@cfv.org
Web Page: http://www.cfv.org
Publication: *Free-Loan Open-Captioned Media Catalog*
The CMP is a free-loan open-captioned media program. Deaf and hard of hearing persons, teachers, parents, and others may borrow these materials. Materials include educational videos (for preschool through college) and general interest (classical movies and special-interest topics such as travel, hobbies, recreation, and others). Most educational materials will be mailed to clients from their assigned educational depository in their state or region. General-interest materials are mailed from a national depository operated by the NAD. (C, E, IA)

Cochlear Implant Club International
5335 Wisconsin Avenue, NW, Suite 440
Washington, DC 20015-2034
Voice/TTY: (202) 895-2781
Publication: *CONTACT*
Email: pwms.cici@worldnet.att.net
Web Page: http://www.cici.org

Provides information and support to cochlear implant users and their families, professionals, and the general public. (I, C, M, S)

Conference of Educational Administrators of Schools and Programs for the Deaf, Inc.
P.O. Box 1778
St. Augustine, FL 32085-1778
Voice/TTY: (904) 810-5200
FAX: (904) 810-5525
Email: innceasd@aug.com
Publication: *American Annals of the Deaf*
Gallaudet University
KDES PAS-6,
800 Florida Avenue, NE,
Washington, DC 20002-3695
Voice/ TTY: (202) 651-5342
Focuses on improvements in the education of deaf and hard of hearing people through research, personnel development, advocacy, and training. (C, E, P, S)

Convention of American Instructors of the Deaf
CAID Membership Office
P.O. Box 377
Bedford, TX 76095-0377
Voice/TTY: (817) 354-8414
Email: caid@swbell.net
Email: Hcorson@KSD.KI2.KY.US
Publications: *American Annals of the Deaf, News 'n Notes*
An organization that promotes professional development communication, and information among educators of deaf individuals and other interested people. (P)

Deaf and Hard of Hearing Entrepreneurs Council
814 Thayer Avenue, Suite 303
Silver Spring, MD 20910
TTY: (301) 650-2244
FAX: (301) 588-0390
Email: JMACFADDEN@MACF.com
Publication: *Deaf and Hard of Hearing Entrepreneurs Council* (newsletter)
Encourages, recognizes, and promotes entrepreneurship by people who are deaf or hard of hearing. (I, P, S)

Deaf Entertainment Foundation (DEF)
Deaf Entertainment Guild (DEG)
8306 Wilshire Blvd., Suite 906
Beverly Hills, CA 90211-2382
Voice: (323) 782-1344
TTY: (323) 655-1542
TTY: (323) 782-0298
FAX: (323) 782-1344
Email: DEAFENT@aol.com
Web Page: http://www.deo.org/
DEF's purpose consists of three points: (1) to recognize and encourage
excellence of the Deaf and Hard-of-Hearing talents; (2) to promote
awareness of Deafness and Deaf Culture in the entertainment industry;
and (3) to achieve unity between the Deaf/Hard-of-Hearing and Hearing communities. Its aim is simple and clear: to provide and disseminate
information as a conduit to the entertainment industry to promote and
accelerate the presence of Deaf and Hard-of-Hearing talents in motion
pictures, television, theater and the performing arts. Consisting of over
500 talents, it is the largest entertainment publication of its kind. The
Digital Directory includes Deaf, Hard-of-Hearing, and Hearing people
who are proficient in Sign Language. The launch of DEG will open
channels for the Deaf/HOH creative worlds. (E, I, P)

Deafness and Communicative Disorders Branch
Rehabilitation Services Administration
Office of Special Education and Rehabilitative Services
Department of Education
330 C Street SW, Room 3228
Washington, DC 20202-2736
Voice: (202) 205-9152
TTY: (202) 205-8352
FAX: (202) 205-9340
Promotes improved and expanded rehabilitation services for deaf and
hard of hearing people and individuals with speech or language impair-
ments. Provides technical assistance to RSA staff, state rehabilitation
agencies, other public and private agencies, and individuals. Also pro-
vides funding for interpreter training and administers the projects. (I, F)

Deafness Research Foundation (DRF)
575 Fifth Avenue, 11th Floor
New York, NY 10017-2422
Voice/TTY: (212) 599-0027
Voice/TTY: (800) 599-3323
FAX: (212) 599-0039

Web Page: http://www.drf.org
Publication: *The Hearing Advocate*
The nation's largest voluntary health organization, providing grants for fellowships, symposia, and research into causes, treatment, and prevention of all ear disorders. The DRF also provides information and referral services. (C, E, F, I, M, P, Rs)

The Ear Foundation
1817 Patterson Street
Nashville, TN 37203
Voice/TTY: (615) 329-7809
Voice/TTY: (800) 545-HEAR
FAX: (615) 329-7935
Web Page: http://www.EARFOUNDATION.org
A national, not-for-profit organization committed to integrating the hearing and balance impaired person into the mainstream of society through public awareness and medical education. Also administers The Meniere's Network, a national network of patient support groups providing people with the opportunity to share experiences and coping strategies. (E, I, M, P, S)

Episcopal Conference of the Deaf
P.O. Box 27685
Philadelphia, PA 19118-0069
Voice: (215) 247-1059
TTY/FAX: (315) 449-1602
Publication: *The Deaf Episcopalian*
Promotes ministry for deaf people throughout the Episcopal Church. Affiliated with approximately 65 congregations in the United States.

Gallaudet University
800 Florida Avenue NE
Washington, DC 20002-3695
Voice/TTY: (202) 651-5000
Email: public.relations@gallaudet.edu
Web Page: http://www.gallaudet.edu
Publication: *Gallaudet Today*
Gallaudet University, the world's only four-year liberal arts university for students who are deaf or hard of hearing. Established in 1864 by an act of Congress, Gallaudet offers more than 50 undergraduate and graduate degree programs and numerous continuing education and summer courses. The University disseminates information through such units as the Gallaudet Bookstore, Gallaudet University Press, Gallaudet Research Institute, Pre-College National Mission Programs, College for

Continuing Education, and the Laurent Clerc National Deaf Education Center. (E, I, C, Rs)

Gallaudet University Alumni Association (GUAA)
Peikoff Alumni House ("Ole Jim") Gallaudet University
800 Florida Avenue NE
Washington, DC 20002-3695
Voice: (202) 651-5060
TTY: (202) 651-5061
FAX: (202) 651-5062
Web Page: http://www.gallaudet.edu/alumni.html
Publication: *Gallaudet Today*
Web Page: http://www.gallaudet.edu:80/~pubreweb/gt/
Represents more than 13,000 alumni of Gallaudet University across the United States and around the world. The GUAA, which is governed by an elected board of directors, provides a variety of services that support and benefit the University, the alumni, and the general deaf community. (C, F, So)

Hearing Education and Awareness for Rockers (H.E.A.R.)
P.O. Box 460847
San Francisco, CA 94146
Voice: (415) 773-9590 (hotline)
Voice: (415) 431-3277
FAX: (415) 552-4296
Email: hear@hearnet.com
Web Page: http://www.hearnet.com
Educates the public about the real dangers of hearing loss resulting from repeated exposure to excessive noise levels. Offers information about hearing protection, hearing aids, assistive listening devices, ear monitor systems, testing and other information about hearing loss and tinnitus. Operates a 24-hour hotline information, referral, and support network service and conducts a hearing screening program in the San Francisco Bay area. Also launches public hearing awareness campaigns, programs for schools and seminars, and distributes earplugs to club and concert-goers. Initiated H.E.A.R. affiliates via hearnet website in other cities worldwide. H.E.A.R. records fund raising CD's with Public Service Announcements. Sponsorship opportunities available in each program. (C, E, I, M, S)

Hearing Industries Association
515 King Street, Suite 420
Alexandria, VA 22314
Voice: (703) 684-5744

FAX: (703) 684-6048
Email: crogin@clarionmr.com
HIA is the association for hearing aid manufacturers and suppliers of
component parts. (I)

HEAR NOW
Hearing Assistance Program Director
9745 E. Hampden Avenue, #300
Denver, CO 80231-4923
Voice/TTY: (303) 695-7797
Voice/TTY: (800) 648-HEAR
FAX: (303) 695-7789
Email: jostelter@aol.com
Publication: *HEAR NOW*
Committed to making technology accessible to deaf and hard of hearing
individuals throughout the United States. HEAR NOW provides hear-
ing aids and cochlear implants for very low income, hard of hearing and
deaf individuals. (C, F, I, P)

HEATH Resource Center
1 Dupont Circle, Suite 800
Washington, DC 20036
Voice/TTY: (202) 939-9320
Voice: (800) 544-3284
FAX: (202) 833-4760 (American Council on Education)
Email: heath@ace.nche.edu
Gopher: gopher://bobcat-ace.nche.edu/
Web Page: http://www.acenet.edu/
HEATH is the national clearinghouse on post-secondary education for
individuals with disabilities, a program of the American Council on Ed-
ucation. HEATH disseminates information nationally about disability
issues in post-secondary education. It offers publications and a tele-
phone service of use to administrators, service providers, teachers, instructors, rehabilitation counselors, health professionals, and to
individuals with disabilities and their families. (I, E)

Helen Keller National Center for Deaf-Blind Youths and Adults
111 Middle Neck Road
Sands Point, NY 11050
Voice: (516) 944-8900
TTY: (516) 944-8637
FAX: (516) 944-7302
Email: abigailp@aol.com

Publications: *The Nat-Cent News, National Family Association for the Deaf-Blind Newsletter*
The national center and its 10 regional offices provide diagnostic evaluations, comprehensive vocational and personal adjustment training, and job preparation and placement for people who are deaf-blind from every state and territory. Field services include information and referral and advocacy and technical assistance to professionals, consumers, and families. (C,E,I,P)

House Ear Institute
2100 W. Third Street, 5th Floor
Los Angeles, CA 90057
Voice: (213) 483-4431
TTY: (213) 483-2642
FAX: (213) 483-8789
Web Page: http://www.hei.org/
Publication: *Review*
Through research and education the institute aims to improve the quality of life of those with an ear disease or hearing or balance disorder. Scientists are exploring the causes of auditory disorders on the cellular and molecular level as well as refining the application of auditory implants and hearings aids. CARE Center offers a full range of pediatric hearing tests, otologic and audiologic evaluation and treatment, rehabilitation, hearing aid dispensing, and cochlear implant services. Outreach programs focus on families with hearing impaired children. Lead Line provides a nationwide information and referral service 1-800-287-4763 (CA) or 800-352-8888 (all other states). (E, I, M, Rs)

International Catholic Deaf Association
United States Section
8002 S. Sawyer Road
Darien, IL 60561-5227
TTY: (630) 887-9472
FAX: (630) 887-8850
Email: KgKush@aol.com
Publication: *The Deaf Catholic*
Promotes ministry for Catholic deaf people. Chapters are encouraged to arrange Sunday masses for deaf people in their local areas with the liturgy presented in sign language. Responds to spiritual-related requests worldwide. (C, E, I, R, S)

International Hearing Society
16880 Middlebelt Road, Suite 4
Livonia, MI 48154

Voice: (734) 522-7200
Voice: (800) 521-5247 (Hearing Aid Helpline)
FAX: (734) 522-0200
Publication: *Audecibel*
Professional association of specialists who test hearing and select, fit, and dispense hearing instruments. The society conducts programs of competence qualifications, education, and training, and promotes specialty-level accreditation. The Hearing Aid Helpline provides consumer information and referral. (C, M, P)

International Lutheran Deaf Association
1333 S. Kirkwood Road
St. Louis, MO 63122
Voice: (314) 965-9917 ext. 1315
TTY: (888) 899-5031
Voice: (800) 433-3954
FAX: (314) 965-0959
Publication: *The Deaf Lutheran*
Promotes ministry for deaf people throughout the Lutheran Church—Missouri Synod. (I, R)

Jewish Deaf Congress
(formerly National Congress of Jewish Deaf)
9420 Reseda Boulevard, Suite 422
Northridge, CA 91324
TTY: (818) 993-2517
FAX: (818) 993-2695
Publication: *J.D.C. QUARTERLY*
Advocates for religious, educational, and cultural ideals and fellowship for Jewish deaf people. Conducts workshops for rabbis, parents of deaf children, and interpreters. Works with 20 affiliates and maintains a Hall of Fame. (C, F, I, R)

John Tracy Clinic
806 W. Adams Blvd.
Los Angeles, CA 90007
Voice: (213) 748-5481
TTY: (213) 747-2924
Voice/TTY: (800) 522-4582
FAX: (213) 749-1651
Web Page: http://www.johntracyclinic.org
JTC is an educational facility for preschool-age children who have hearing losses and their families. In addition to on-site services, worldwide correspondence courses in English and Spanish are offered to parents

whose children are of preschool age and are hard of hearing, deaf, or deaf-blind. All services of JTC are free of charge to the families. (E, I, S)

Junior National Association of the Deaf
814 Thayer Avenue
Silver Spring, MD 20910-4500
TTY: (301) 587-1789
Voice: (301) 587-1788
FAX: (301) 587-1791
Email: nadyouth@nad.org
Publication: *Junior NAD News*
Develops and promotes citizenship, scholarship, and leadership skills in deaf and hard of hearing students (grades 7–12) through chapter projects, national conventions, contests, and other activities. The NAD also sponsors a month-long Youth Leadership Camp program each summer in Oregon. (E, Rc, So)

League for the Hard of Hearing
71 West 23rd Street
New York, NY 10010-4162
Voice: (212) 741-7650
TTY: (212) 255-1932
FAX: (212) 255-4413
Email: postmaster@lhh.org
Web Page: http://www.lhh.org
Publications: *Hearing Rehabilitation Quarterly* (journal)
The oldest hearing rehabilitation agency in the country. Mission is to improve the quality of life for people with all degrees of hearing loss. Offers comprehensive hearing rehabilitation and human service programs for infants, children, adults, and their families, regardless of age or mode of communication. Promotes hearing conservation and provides public education about hearing. (C, E, I, P)

National Association of the Deaf
814 Thayer Avenue
Silver Spring, MD 20910-4500
Voice: (301) 587-1788
TTY: (301) 587-1789
FAX: (301) 587-1791
Email: nadinfo@nad.org
Web Page: http://www.nad.org
Publications: *The NAD Broadcaster, The Deaf American*
National Association of the Deaf-Nation's largest organization safeguarding the accessibility and civil rights of 28 million deaf and hard of

hearing Americans in education, employment, health care, and telecommunications. Focuses on grassroots advocacy and empowerment, captioned media, deafness-related information and publications, legal assistance, policy development and research, public awareness, and youth leadership development. (C, I)

National Black Deaf Advocates
P.O. Box 5465
Laurel, MD 20726
TTY: (301) 206-2802
Voice/TTY: (410) 480-4565
FAX: (301) 206-5157
Email: couthen6l@aol.com
Publication: *NBDA News*
Promotes leadership, deaf awareness, and active participation in the political, educational, and economic processes that affect the lives of black deaf citizens. Currently has 28 chapters in the United States and the Virgin Islands. (C, E, I, P, So)

National Captioning Institute
1900 Gallows Road, Suite 3000
Vienna, VA 22182
Voice/TTY: (703) 917-7600
FAX: (703) 917-9878
Publication: *Caption*
NCI, a nonprofit corporation founded in 1979, is the world's largest provider of closed captioned television services for the broadcast, cable and home video industry. Also researches the educational benefits of captioned TV, and works to expand the captioning service around the world. (I)

National Catholic Office of the Deaf
7202 Buchanan Street
Landover Hills, MD 20784-2236
Voice/TTY: (301) 577-1684
TTY: (301) 577-4184
FAX: (301) 577-1690
Email: NCOD@Erols.com
Web Page: http://www.ncod.org
Publications: *Vision, RADAR*
Assists in the coordination of the efforts of people and organizations involved in the church's ministry with deaf and hard of hearing people; serves as a resource center for information concerning spiritual needs and religious educational materials; and assists bishops and pastors

with their pastoral responsibilities to people who are deaf or hard of hearing. (I, P, R)

CPB/WGBH National Center for Accessible Media
125 Western Avenue
Boston, MA 02134
Voice/TTY: (617) 492-9258
FAX: (617) 782-2155
Email: NCAM@wgbh.org
Web Page: http://www.wgbh.org/ncam
Publication: *Media Access*
The CPB/WGBH National Center for Accessible Media aims to increase access to public mass media (television, radio, print, movies, multimedia) for underserved consumers, such as disabled people or speakers of other languages. The center researches and develops media access technologies that make them more inclusive or expand their use, and acts as a resource to broadcasters, producers, educators, and consumers through consulting, training, journal articles, and conferences. (C, I, Rs)

National Cued Speech Association Information Service
23970 Hermitage Road
Shaker Heights, OH 44122
Voice/TTY: (800) 459-3529
Publications: *Cued Speech Journal, On Cue Newsflash*
Membership organization that provides advocacy and support regarding use of Cued Speech. Information and services are provided for deaf and hard of hearing people of all ages, their families and friends, and professionals who work with them. (I, C, S, E)

National Fraternal Society of the Deaf
1118 S. 6th Street
Springfield, IL 62703
Voice: (217) 789-7429
TTY: (217) 789-7438
FAX: (217) 789-7489
Email: thefrat@NFSD.com
Web Page: http://www.NFSD.com
Publication: *The Frat*
Works in the area of life insurance and advocacy for deaf people. Has 75 divisions across the country. (I, C, S, So)

National Information Center for Children and Youth with Disabilities
P.O. Box 1492
Washington, DC 20013-1492

Voice/TTY: (800) 695-0285
Voice/TTY: (202) 884-8200
FAX: (202) 884-8441
Email: nichcy@aed.org
Web Page: http://www.nichcy.org
Publications: *NICHCY News Digest, Transition Summary, Parent's Guide*
The center provides fact sheets, state resource sheets, and general information to assist parents, educators, care givers, advocates, and others in helping children and youth with disabilities participate as fully as possible in their community. The center also publishes technical assistance guides, students' guides, briefing papers, and annotated bibliographies on selected topics; many publications are available in Spanish and all are available on the Internet. (E, I)

National Information Center on Deafness
Gallaudet University
800 Florida Avenue, NE
Washington, DC 20002-3695
Voice: (202) 651-5051
TTY: (202) 651-5052
FAX: (202) 651-5054
Email: NICD.Infotogo@gallaudet.edu
Web Page: http://clerccenter.gallaudet.edu/InfoToGo/index.html
Serves as a centralized source of up-to-date, objective information on topics dealing with deafness and hearing loss. NICD collects, develops, and disseminates information about all aspects of hearing loss and services offered to deaf and hard of hearing people across the nation. Also provides information about Gallaudet University. (I)

National Information Clearinghouse on Children Who Are Deaf-Blind
345 Monmouth Avenue
Monmouth, OR 97361
Voice: (800) 438-9376
TTY: (800) 854-7013
FAX: (503) 838-8150
Web Page: http://www.tr.wou.edu/dblink/
Publication: *Deaf-Blind Perspectives*
Collects, organizes, and disseminates information related to children and youth (ages 0–21) who are deaf-blind and connects consumers of deaf-blind information to sources of information about deaf blindness, assistive technology, and deaf-blind people. The clearinghouse is a collaborative effort involving the Helen Keller National Center, Perkins School for the Blind, and Teaching Research. (C, I, M, P, Rs)

National Institute on Deafness and Other Communication Disorders
Information Clearinghouse
1 Communication Avenue
Bethesda, MD 20892-3456
Voice: (800) 241-1044
TTY: (800) 241-1055
FAX: (301) 907-8830
Email: nidcdinfo@nidcd.nih.gov
Web Page: http://www.nih.gov/nidcd/
Publication: *INSIDE*, factsheets, brochures
The NIDCD Information Clearinghouse is a national resource center
for information about hearing, balance, smell, taste, voice, speech, and
language. The clearinghouse serves health professionals, patients, in-
dustry, and the public. (C, I, P, Rs)

The National Rehabilitation Information Center
8455 Colesville Road, Suite 935
Silver Spring, MD 20910
Voice: (301) 588-9284
Voice: (800) 346-2742
TTY: (301) 495-5626
FAX: (301) 587-1967
Web Page: http://www.naric.com/naric/
Publications: *Guide to Disability and Rehabilitation Periodicals,
NIDRR Program Directory, Compendium*
Provides information and referral services on disability and rehabilita-
tion, including quick information and referral, database searches of the
bibliographic database REHABDATA, and document delivery. NARIC
also provides the NIDRR Program Directory and the Compendium of
Products by NIDRR Grantees and Contractors. (I)

National Technical Institute for the Deaf
Rochester Institute of Technology
Marketing Communications Department
52 Lomb Memorial Drive, LBJ Building
Rochester, NY 14623-5604
Voice/TTY: (716) 475-6906
FAX: (716) 475-5623 or 6500
Web Page: http://www.rit.edu/RIT/NTID
Provides technological postsecondary education to deaf and hard of
hearing students. Disseminates informational materials and instruc-
tional videotapes on issues related to deaf people and deaf culture. (E, I)

The National Theatre of the Deaf
5 West Main Street
P.O. Box 659
Chester, CT 06412
Voice: (860) 526-4971
TTY: (860) 526-4974
FAX: (860) 526-0066
Email: BOOKNTD@aol.com
TTY: (860) 526-4975
Email: deaftcon@aol.com
Email: NTDPTS@aol.com
Web Page: http://www.NTD.org/
Concentrates on artistic and theatrical professional development of deaf
actors. Tours the United States and abroad. Also presents Little Theatre
of the Deaf productions in schools, theaters, museums, and libraries.
Sponsors a professional school and Deaf Theatre Conference. (E, I, P)

Rainbow Alliance of The Deaf
c/o Astro Rainbow Alliance of the Deaf
P.O. Box 66136
Houston, TX 77266-6136
TTY: (702) 804-6476
FAX: (702) 804-7832 (call TTY first before FAX)
Email: pjancoft@aol.com
Web Page: http://www.rad.org
Publication: *RAD Tattlers*
Email address: CajunTobin@aol.com
RAD is a national organization serving gay, lesbian and bisexual people
who are deaf and hard of hearing. Friends of our family are included.
Represents approximately 24 chapters throughout the United States
and Canada. (E, C, I, S, So)

Registry of Interpreters for the Deaf, Inc.
8630 Fenton Street, Suite 324
Silver Spring, MD 20910
Voice/TTY: (301) 608-0050
FAX: (301) 608-0508
FAX ON DEMAND: 1-800-711-3691
Email: 72620.3143@compuserve.com
Publication: *VIEWS*
A professional organization that certifies interpreters, provides informa-
tion on interpreting to the general public, publishes a national directory
of certified interpreters, and makes referrals to interpreter agencies.
(I, P)

Rehabilitation Engineering Research Center on Hearing Enhancement
Lexington School for the Deaf/Center for the Deaf
30th Avenue and 75th Street
Jackson Heights, NY 11370
Voice/TTY: (718) 899-8800 ext. 212
FAX: (718) 800-3433
Email: info@hearingresearch.org
Web Page: http://www.hearingresearch.org
Publication: *LexAccess* (biannual newsletter)
The center promotes and develops technological solutions to problems
confronting individuals with hearing loss. Projects include automatic
speech recognition, directional microphones, digital hearing aids, assist-
ive listening system assessment, electromagnetic interference issues,
child-friendly audiometry, technology training for rehabilitation counselors. The center also provides information and referral services for
consumer questions on assistive technology and research. (I, Rs)

Rehabilitation Research and Training Center for Persons
    Who Are Hard of Hearing or Late Deafened
California School of Professional Psychology-San Diego
6160 Cornerstone Court East
San Diego, CA 92121-3725
Voice: (619) 623-2777
TTY: (619) 554-1540
Voice/TTY: (800) 432-7619
FAX: (619) 642-0266
Email: RRTC@mail.cspp.edu
A federally funded rehabilitation and training center that focuses on
conducting research and developing training programs related to em-
ployment and personal adjustment of individuals who are hard of hear-
ing or late deafened. Promotes maintenance of employment status and
personal adjustment of persons who are hard of hearing or late deaf-
ened through research, educational workshops, self-help groups, and
training sessions. (E, I, Rs, S)

The SEE Center for the Advancement of Deaf Children
Main Office: P.O. Box 1181
Los Alamitos, CA 90720
Voice/TTY: (562) 430-1467
FAX: (562) 795-6614
Email: ggustaso@email.sjsu.edu
Web Page: http://www.seecenter.org
Branch Office: San Jose State University
Division of Special Education

1 Washington Square
San Jose, CA 95192
Voice: (408) 924-3784
TTY: (408) 924-3782
FAX: (408) 924-3713
Information and referral for parents and educators of deafness-related topics and Signing Exact English (SEE). Provides evaluation of sign skills, workshops, and consulting services related to communication in general and SEE in particular. (E, I, S)

Self Help for Hard of Hearing People, Inc.
7910 Woodmont Ave., Suite 1200
Bethesda, MD 20814
Voice: (301) 657-2248
TTY: (301) 657-2249
FAX: (301) 913-9413
Email: national@shhh.org
Web Page: http://www.shhh.org/
Publication: *Hearing Loss: The Journal of Self Help for Hard of Hearing People*
Promotes awareness and information about hearing loss, communication, assistive devices, and alternative communication skills through publications, exhibits, and presentations. (C, E, I, S)

Telecommunications for the Deaf, Inc.
8630 Fenton Street, Suite 604
Silver Spring, MD 20910-3803
Voice: (301) 589-3786
TTY: (301) 589-3006
FAX: (301) 589-3797
Email: tdiexdir@aol.com
Publications: *GA-SK* (quarterly), *National Directory &Guide* (annual)
A nonprofit consumer advocacy organization promoting full visual access to entertainment, information and telecommunications for people who are deaf, hard of hearing, deaf-blind, late deafened, and speech impaired. Conducts consumer education and involvement, technical assistance and consulting, application of existing and emerging technologies, networking and collaboration, uniformity of standards, national policy development and advocacy. (C, E, I)

TRIPOD
1727 West Burbank Boulevard
Burbank, CA 91506-1312
Voice/TTY: (818) 972-2080

FAX: (818) 972-2090
TRIPOD is a model co-enrollment program which includes Montessori Parent, Infant, Toddler; Montessori Pre-School/Kindergarten, Elementary, Middle School, High School. The co-enrollment programs for hearing, deaf, and hard of hearing children are within the Burbank Unified School District. (C, E, Rs, S)

USA Deaf Sports Federation
3607 Washington Boulevard, #4
Ogden, UT 84403-1737
TTY: (801) 393-7916
FAX: (801) 393-2263
Email: USADSF@aol.com
Web Page: http://www.usadsf.org
Publications: *USADSF Bulletin, Deaf Sports Review*
Governing body for all deaf sports and recreation in the United States. Sponsors US team to the World Games for the Deaf and other regional, national, and international competitions. (C, I, Rc, So)

Vestibular Disorders Association
P.O. Box 4467
Portland, OR 97208-4467
Voice: (503) 229-7705
Voice: (800) 837-8428
FAX: (503) 229-8064
Email: veda@vestibular.org
Web Page: http://www.vestibular.org
Publication: *On the Level*
Provides information and support for people with inner-ear vestibular disorders and develops awareness of the issues surrounding these disorders. (I, M, S)

World Recreation Association of the Deaf, Inc.
P.O. Box 92074
Rochester, NY 15692
FAX: (949) 645-7618
Publication: *WRAD NEWS*
Established to foster the development of innovation in recreational and cultural activities for the deaf and hard of hearing community. (E, I, P, Rc, So)

Appendix D

A Model Bar Association Position on Deaf Clients

THE ASSOCIATION OF THE BAR OF THE CITY OF NEW YORK
COMMITTEE ON PROFESSIONAL AND JUDICIAL ETHICS (FORMAL
OPINION NO. 1995-2)

QUESTION

Must a lawyer who cannot communicate directly with a client in a mutually understood language consider the need for the services of an interpreter and take steps to secure the services of a qualified interpreter to insure competent and zealous representation, to preserve client confidences, and to avoid unlawful discrimination?

OPINION

Lawyers are increasingly being called upon to advise and represent persons with whom they cannot communicate directly because the lawyer and the client do not share a common language. Often, the only effective method of communication is through a language (foreign or sign) interpreter.

The strongest indication of this development in the practice of law is the dramatic rise in the use of interpreters for court proceedings. In 1991 alone, more than 68,000 federal court proceedings required interpreters, *see United States v. Mosquera*, 816 F. Supp. 168, 171 (E.D.N.Y. 1993). Currently in New York City, both federal and state courts employ interpreters. Additionally, the state courts use per diem interpreters for as many as 64 foreign languages. *See Equal Justice and the Non English-Speaking Litigant: A Call for Adequate Interpretation Services in the New York State Courts,* 49 Record 306, 3077 (1974). The need for most of these interpreters is directly related to a significant increase in our non-English speaking population. Nationally, nearly 31 million people do not use English as their primary language and locally nearly 40 percent of New York city's population speaks a language other than English. *See* Mosquera F. Supp. At 171.

Hearing impaired or deaf persons may also require the services of interpreters to effectively participate in legal proceedings. Approximately 10 percent of our population, or 21 million Americans, are hearing impaired and more than 2 million of these Americans are "profoundly deaf." *See* John V. McCoy, *Communicating with Your Deaf Client,* 65 *Wisconsin Lawyer* 16 (1992) (hereinafter "McCoy"). Although not all deaf persons communicate in sign language, many require the services of sign language interpreters in order to communicate effectively. *See Improving the Access of Deaf and Hearing-Impaired Litigants to the Justice System,* 48 Record 834, 835 (1993).

The role of interpreters in the administration of justice is well established under our legal system. In criminal cases, our courts have long recognized that meaningful participation in legal proceedings for defendants who cannot understand English is not possible unless testimony is translated for these defendants. Failure to provide interpreters for these defendants has been found to be a deprivation of due process. *See United States ex rel. Negron v. New York,* 434 F.2d 386 (2d Cir. 1970) (interpreter required for non-English-speaking defendants); *People v. Ramos,* 26 N.Y.2d 272, 309 N.Y.S.2d 906 (1970) (translation of trial testimony a due process right); *Mosquera,* 816 F. Supp. At 178 (translation of indictment, relevant statute, plea agreements and other documents required for non-English-speaking defendants). Although the assignment of court interpreters in civil cases may not raise due process concerns, *see Iara v. Municipal Court,* 21 Cal. 3d 181, 145 Cal. Rptr. 847, 578 P.2d 94 91978) *cert.denied,* 439 U.S. 1067 (1979), our courts recognize the important role interpreters play in insuring meaningful participation in these proceedings and routinely assign interpreters for non-English-speaking litigants and witnesses. Moreover, the right to have an interpreter assigned during court proceedings is also provided under federal and New York statutes. The Judiciary and Judicial Procedure Act, 28 U.S.C. §§ 1827, 1828, allows the assignment of an interpreter during federal trials and proceedings. Although New York's Constitution does not guarantee persons unable to understand English a right to an Interpreter in criminal cases—unlike California, for example, *see,* California Const. Art. 1, § 14, *People v. Carreon,* 151 Cal. App. 3d 559, 567, 198 Cal. Rptr. 843, 847 (5th Dist. 1984)—New

York laws provide for the hiring of court interpreters and the appointment of interpreters for deaf parties or witnesses. *See* N.Y. Judiciary Law, art. 12.

For the non-English-speaking litigant or the deaf litigant, meaningful participation during a legal proceeding is not possible if what the judge, witnesses, and lawyers are saying during the proceeding is in a language the litigants cannot understand. Similarly, meaningful legal assistance may not be possible when the lawyer does not fully understand what the client is telling or asking him or her or the client does not fully understand the lawyer's advice or explanation, because of a language barrier.

The inability to communicate directly with the client in a mutually understood language does not automatically preclude the lawyer's representation of that client. *See* California 1984–77. However, to provide adequate legal services, there must be an effective mode of communication.

Although the mode of communication between lawyer and client with whom effective and meaningful direct communications can only be maintained through an interpreter, the need for qualified interpreter services cannot be ignored.

Since communication with a non-English-speaking client or a deaf client may only be effective or even possible if conducted with an interpreter, it is questionable whether a lawyer can competently represent his or her client without considering the need for, and, in some instances, securing the services of, an interpreter,

It is axiomatic that adequate communication between lawyer and client is necessary to render competent legal services. *Cf. ABA model Rules of Professional Conduct*, Rule 1.4. In addition to being the means by which a client is provided with the advice and information needed to make informed decisions, *see* EC 7-8, adequate communication is the means by which the lawyer obtains the information necessary to prepare for the handling of the client's legal matter.

DR 6-101(A)(2) mandates that "[a] lawyer shall not . . . [h]andle a legal matter without preparation adequate in the circumstances." Adequate preparation requires, not only that a lawyer conduct necessary legal research, but also that he or she gather information material to the claims or defenses of the client. *See Mason v. Balcom*, 531 F.2d 717, 724 (5th Cir. 1976). The lawyer's inability, because of a language barrier, to understand fully what the client is telling him may unnecessarily impede the lawyer's ability to gather the information from the client needed to familiarize the lawyer with the circumstances of the case. This makes communication via the interpreter vital since it may be the only practical way that a free-flowing dialogue can be maintained with the client, and the only means by which the lawyer can actually and substantially assist the client.

The duty to represent a client competently, embodied in DR 6101(A)(1), requires a lawyer confronted with a legal matter calling for legal skills or knowledge outside the lawyer's experience or ability, to associate with lawyers with skills or knowledge necessary to handle the legal matter. When a lawyer is confronted with a legal matter requiring non-legal skills or knowledge outside the lawyer's experience or ability and these skills or knowledge necessary for the proper preparation of the legal matter, DR 6-101(A)(2) appears to require that the lawyer and professionals in other disciplines who possess the requisite skills or knowledge needed by the lawyer to prepare the legal matter. The interpreter appears to be the type of professional envisioned by EC 603's observation that "[p]roper preparation and representation may require the association by the lawyer of professionals in other disciplines." When the need for an interpreter is apparent or it is reasonable to conclude that an interpreter is required for effective communication, failure to take steps with the client to secure an interpreter may be a breach of the duty to represent the client competently.

Moreover, the lawyer may not passively leave the decision as to the need for or the securing of an interpreter entirely to the client's discretion. Once it is evident that, without an interpreter, effective lawyer-client communications are questionable or not possible, failure of a lawyer to take steps to help the client understand the significance of the interpreter for adequate communication and to take, when necessary, steps to secure interpreter services may violate the lawyer's duty to represent the client zealously.

The mandate DR 7-101(A)(3) that "[a] lawyer shall not intentionally . . . [p]rejudice or damage the client during the course of the professional relationship . . . ." embodies the concept that a lawyer must actively assist the client "to secure and protect available legal rights and benefits," EC 7-1. When the lawyer fails to take steps to bridge a communication barrier with a client, knowing that it can be bridged by the association with an interpreter, it is reasonable to expect that the client will be damaged or prejudiced by this inaction.

Clearly, the duty to represent a client zealously requires the lawyer to take special care with respect to communications with clients. As EC 7-8 observes in part, "[a] lawyer should exert best efforts to insure that decisions of the client are made only after the client has been informed of relevant considerations." Although the lawyer may never know what the client fully understands, at a minimum, the lawyer must present information in a language the client understands. *See* Robert E. Lutz, *Ethics and International Practice: A Guide to the Professional Responsibilities of Practitioners*, 16 Fordham Int'l L.J. 53 (1992–93). Indeed,

EC 7-11 reminds lawyers that "[t]he responsibilities of a lawyer may vary according to the intelligence, experience, mental condition or age of a client. . . ." When direct communications with the client require an interpreter, the lawyer bears an additional responsibility of taking steps to secure these services rather than unnecessarily risk prejudice or damage to the client.

Whether the failure to consider the need for and, when necessary, to secure the services of an interpreter is unlawful discrimination in the practice of law and thus a violation of DR 1-102(A)(6)[1] may present questions about what constitutes disparate treatment or what constitutes a public or a reasonable accommodation under existing anti-discrimination statutes. These are questions of law, upon which we do not opine. *See generally* Robert T. Begg, *Revoking the Lawyers' License to Discriminate in New York: The Demise of a Traditional Professional Prerogative*, 7 Geo. J. Legal Ethics 275 (1993); The Americans with Disabilities Act, 42 U.S.C. § 12181(7)(F); 28 CFR part 36(9)(1995) (rules and Regulations, Department of Justice, Office of the Attorney General); Jordan Hochstadt, *Compliance with Title III of the ADA on $5 a Year or Less*, 21 Colorado Lawyer 1897 (1992).

Even if the failure to consider the need for and to secure the services of an interpreter may not constitute unlawful discrimination, it may show biased or condescending conduct towards the client, which should be avoided. *See EC 1-7.* For example, exclusive reliance on family members, friends or even strangers to interpret, or attempts to communicate solely using a rudimentary personal knowledge of a foreign or sign language may not only be unwise, but may reflect bias or condescension towards the client because such a practice could tend to minimize the importance of what the client has to say to the lawyer and the client's role in decision making, and to treat the client with less care than other clients because of the language barrier between lawyer and client. Lawyers should be aware of the risk of inaccuracies in translation if amateur interpreters are used, and should proceed cautiously in light of their inability to determine the layperson's or lawyer's proficiency in foreign or sign language. *See generally* L. Felipe Restrepo, *Attorneys Working with Translators Must Watch Over Defendant's Rights*, Nat'l L.J., Sept. 28, 1992, at 17 (hereinafter "Restrepo"); Bill Piatt, *Attorney as Interpreter: A Return to Babble*, 20 New Mexico L. Rev. 1 (1990). Similarly, the exclusive use of note-taking with prejudicial results for the deaf client can be a poor substitute for a qualified sign-language interpreter, because this practice may have prejudicial results for the deaf client. Note-taking presents several problems. It may hinder the free flow of ideas common to verbal communications and, for some deaf clients, it may be of very limited use. *See McCoy, supra.* For deaf persons who communicate in sign language, the sign-language interpreter makes the free flow of ideas with the lawyer possible and avoids the prejudicial effects of the exclusive use of note-taking.

There are obvious benefits to communicating through professionals, who have formal training in languages, experience with legal terminology and concepts, and skill. They do not consider the greater accuracy in translation possible with trained interpreters, because often they belong to professional associations which adhere to professional and ethical standards. *See generally* Roseann D. Gonzalez, Victoria F. Vazquez & Holly Mikkelson, *Fundamentals of Court Interpretation: Theory, Policy and Practice* (1991); *Professional Standards for Court Interpreters in the New York State Unified Court System*, New York State Unified Court System, *Court Interpreter Manual* 8 (July 1994).[2]

Lastly, the practice of limiting communications with the client to periods when the lawyer and client are in court and a court interpreter is available has a prejudicial effect on the client. It may unfairly limit the opportunity for the lawyer to fully familiarize himself or herself with the facts of the matter being handled and to advise the client accordingly. It may also limit the client's access to the lawyer and the opportunity for the client to obtain the full advantage of our legal system. The detrimental effects of this practice are uniquely related to the inability of the lawyer and client to communicate in a mutually understood language. *See* Restrepo, *supra*, at 1.

In sum, when a language barrier impedes the ability for the lawyer and the client to communicate effectively, the lawyer must be sensitive to the needs for interpreter services and take steps to secure interpreter services, when needed, to avoid unlawful discrimination or prejudice

CONCLUSION

A lawyer who represents a client with whom direct communications cannot be maintained in a mutually understood language must evaluate the need for qualified interpreter service and take steps to secure the services of an interpreter, when needed for effective lawyer-client communications, to provide competent and zealous representation, preserve client confidences and avoid unlawful discrimination or prejudice in the practice of law.

Issued: July 6, 1995

NOTES

1. DR1–102(A)(6) provides that "[a] lawyer shall not . . . [u]nlawfully discriminate in the practice of law, including in hiring, promoting or otherwise determining conditions of employment, on the basis of age, race, creed, color, national origin, sex, disability, or marital status."
2. These practices may also unnecessarily imperil the preservation of

non-English-speaking or deaf clients' secrets and confidences, in violation of the fiduciary relationship between lawyer and client. They impinge on the lawyer's ability to "exercise reasonable care to prevent . . . others whose services are utilized by the lawyer from disclosing or using confidences or secrets of the client," since the lawyer may have little or no control over these persons. *See* DR 4–101(D).

A Model Hospital Policy

MAINE MEDICAL CENTER POLICY FOR EFFECTIVE COMMUNICATION WITH AND SERVICES FOR PEOPLE WHO ARE DEAF AND HARD OF HEARING

Policy Statement: It is the practice of Maine Medical Center to ensure effective communication between all deaf and hard-of-hearing people served by MMC and MMC employees. Effective communication is a critical component of providing quality patient care and equal access to hospital services. To achieve that goal, all Maine Medical Center employees will inform deaf and hard-of-hearing patients and the deaf and hard-of-hearing relatives of patients of the availability, at no cost to them, of interpreters, Telecommunications Devices for the Deaf ("TTYs" or "TDDs"), hearing aid compatible amplified telephones, television decoders, Computer Assisted Real Time (CART) captioning, assistive listening devices and other auxiliary aids, and to provide such service promptly upon patient request.

PROCEDURE:

Any patient, and any family member or friend of a patient participating in treatment discussions and decision-making, who is deaf or hard-of-hearing shall be informed in writing of the availability at no cost of qualified interpreters and other auxiliary aids and services to meet his or her communications needs. Such notice shall be provided at the time of admission, appointment scheduling or arrival at the Emergency Department. All hospital personnel will use the attached "Notice of Services For Deaf and Hard-of-Hearing persons at Maine Medical Center" to inform such persons of services and to determine what services will be needed.

If you recognize or have any reason to believe a patient, relative, friend or companion of a patient, or any other person using hospital services, is deaf or hard-of-hearing, you must offer to call a sign language interpreter and/or other appropriate auxiliary aids and services will be provided at hospital expense. This offer and advice must likewise be made to any overt request for a sign language interpreter and/or any other auxiliary aids or services.

If a person indicated that his or her preferred method of communication is a sign-based language (e.g., American Sign Language), hospital personnel shall immediately contact [the on-staff interpreter or] Pine Tree Society Deaf Services (774-9438; 24 hours) or Certified Interpreting Associates (856-2883; weekdays) to arrange for an interpreter. MMC has a contract with Pine Tree to obtain expedited interpreting services under which Pine Tree has guaranteed that an interpreter will be provided within an hour of the request. For scheduled admissions and appointments, arrangements must be made in advance to ensure that an interpreter will be present when the deaf or hard-of-hearing person arrives for treatment. If you have any difficulty obtaining an interpreter from either of these agencies, contact the ADA Communications Services coordinator (XX at ext. XX), who maintains a list of qualified interpreters and other resources. All contacts with interpreting agencies must be documented on patient charts.

If a person uses sign language, all medical and psychiatric evaluations or discussions regarding a patient's symptoms, treatment (including individual group psychotherapy), diagnosis, progress and prognosis must be communicated through the use of a qualified sign language interpreter. Additional situations in which an interpreter must be provided include, but are not limited to: obtaining informed consent or permission for treatment; discharge planning; explaining and discussing advance directives; explaining the administration and side effects of medication; explaining follow-up treatment; and discussing billing and insurance issues.

Family members, friends, advocates, case managers and other people who are at the hospital to support the patient are not appropriate or qualified interpreters, regardless of their sign language abilities. Asking such persons to interpret denies the patient the support they need and compromises the accuracy and effectiveness of MMC staff communications with the patient. If a deaf or hard-of-hearing person nevertheless refuses MMC's offer of a free qualified interpreter and prefers to use a friend or family member to interpret, the hospital shall secure a written "Waiver of Interpreter Services," which appears on the opposite side of the notice of services form.

The Emergency Department and the Telecommunications Office

each maintain a set of pictograph flash cards which may be used to facilitate communication in cases of an emergency and while awaiting an interpreter.

If a person requests the use of a TTY/TDDs, a television decoder, an assistive listening device, CART or other auxiliary aids and services, hospital personnel should immediately contact the Communications Services office to arrange for such services to be provided in a prompt manner. All such contacts must be documented as well.

Public TTY/TDDS pay telephones are located in the Emergency Department Waiting Area, the Admitting Office, R9, McGeachy Hall as well as locations on the Brighton, Falmouth and Scarborough campuses. Telephone contact from or to persons who are deaf or hard-of-hearing may be made either through the AT&T Relay system (800/457-1220) or through MMC's direct TTY/TDDs lines in the following departments: [list departments and phone numbers]. Deaf and hard-of-hearing persons who are inpatients shall be furnished with TTY/TDDs units, along with appropriate visual telephone signalers, in their hospital rooms, if a telephone is already present in the rooms, or in patient common areas where telephones are provided for patient use. TTYs/TDDs are available from the Communications Services office 24 hours a day.

Some televisions at MMC are equipped with built-in decoders and MMC staff shall assist patients in activating the captioning. Other televisions will require the use of a television decoder which may be obtained from the Communications Services Office 24 hours a day.

If you have any questions regarding the implementation of this policy contact your supervisor, the ADA Communications Services Coordinator, XX, (extension XX), or the Telecommunications Office (extension XX).

Selected Bibliography of Law Review Articles

Anderson, Lisa, "Constitutional Law–First Amendment–Providing Sign Language Interpreter Services Pursuant to the IDEA to a Student Attending a Religious Institution Does Not Violate the Establishment Clause, Nor Does the Establishment Clause Lay Down an Absolute Barrier To Placing a Public Employee in a Sectarian School." *University of Detroit Mercy Law Review* 72 (Winter 1995): 473–87.

Bahr, Susan J. "Ease of Access to Telecommunications Relay Service." *Federal Communication Bar Journal* 44 (May 1992): 473–90.

Baker, Alice. "Sign Language Interpreters and Testimonial Privileges." *Virginia Journal of Social Policy and the Law* 2 (Fall 1994): 165.

Berko, Michele-Lee. "Preserving the Sixth Amendment Right of the Deaf Criminal Defendant." *Dickinson Law Review* 97 (Fall 1992): 101–30.

Brusky, Mary Elizabeth. "Making Decisions for Deaf Children Regarding Cochlear Implants: The Legal Ramifications of Recognizing Deafness as a Culture Rather than a Disability." *Wisconsin Law Review* (1995): 235–70.

Burgdorf, Robert. "Equal Member of the Community: The Public Accommodations Provisions of the American Disabilities Act." *Temple Law Review* 64 (1991): 499 .

Carnahan, Sandra J. "The Americans with Disabilities Act in State Correctional Institutions." *Capital University Law Review* 27 (1999): 291.

Caylor, Steven. "Court Advisory Board Takes a Closer Look at Interpreters." *JUN Advocate (Idaho)* 41 (June 1998): 14.

Chilton, Elizabeth. "Ensuring Effective Communication: The Duty of Health Care Providers to Supply Sign Language Interpreters for Deaf Patients." *Hastings Law Journal* 47 (March 1996): 871–910.

Dominguez-Urban, Ileana. "The Messenger as the Medium of Communication: The Use of Interpreters in Mediation." *1997 Journal of Dispute Resolution* (1997): 1.

DuBow, Sy. "Into the Turbulent Mainstream: A Legal Perspective on the Weight To Be Given to the Least Restrictive Environment in Placement Decisions for Deaf Children." *Journal of Law and Education* 18 (Spring 1989): 215–28.

———. "The Television Decoder Circuitry Act—TV for All." *Temple Law Review* 64 (Summer 1991): 609.

Gardner, Elaine. "Deaf Victims and Defendants in the Criminal Justice System." *Clearinghouse Review* 19 (November 1985): 748–51.

———. "The Legal Rights of Inmates with Physical Disabilities." *Saint Louis University Public Law Review* 14 (1994): 175.

Goldbas, Michael. "Due Process: The Deaf and the Blind as Jurors." *New England Law Review* 17 (1981/1982): 119–52.

Hall, Leonard A. and Charla V. Beall. "Use of Interpreters for Deaf or Foreign-Speaking People in Kansas." *Journal of the Kansas Bar Association* 63 (April 1994): 36.

Humphrey, Isabel. "Establishment Clause Prohibits Provision of State-Paid Sign Language Interpreter to Student Attending Pervasively Religious High School: Zobrest v. Catalina Foothills School District." *Arizona Law Journal* 25 (Summer 1993): 449–59.

Ivers, Kathryn. "Towards a Bilingual Education Policy in the Mainstreaming of Deaf Children." *Columbia Human Rights Law Review* 26 (Winter 1995): 439–82.

Johnson, James D. "Does the Americans with Disabilities Act Apply to the Conduct of Law Enforcement Officers Pursuant to Arrests? A Survey of *Gorman v. Bartch.*" *Georgia State University Law Review* 14 (July 1998): 901.

Lee, Randy. "Equal Protection and a Deaf Person's Right To Serve as a Juror." *New York University Review of Law and Social Change* 17 (1989/1990): 81–117.

Lee, Stephanie Holt. "*Wisconsin v. Rewolinski:* Do Members of the Deaf Community have a Right to be Free from Search and Seizure of Their TDD Call?" *Law and Inequality* 10 (June 1992): 187–216.

Liu, Andy. "Full Inclusion and Deaf Education—Redefining Equality." *Journal of Law and Education* 24 (Spring 1995): 241–66.

Maatman, Mary Ellen. "Listening to Deaf Culture: A Reconceptualization of Difference Analysis under Title VII." *Hofstra Labor Law Journal* 13 (Spring 1996): 269–344.

McAlister, Jamie. "Deaf and Hard-of-Hearing Criminal Defendants:

How You Gonna Get Justice If You Can't Talk to the Judge?" *Arizona State Law Journal* 26 (Spring 1994): 163–200.

McCoy, John V. "Communicating with Your Deaf Client." *Wisconsin Lawyer* 65 (November 1992): 16.

Natapoff, Alexandra. "Anatomy of a Debate: Intersectionality and Equality for Deaf Children from Non-English Speaking Homes." *Journal of Law and Education* 24 (Spring 1995): 271–78.

Shaw, Suzanne. "What's Appropriate? Finding a Voice for Deaf Children and Their Parents in the Education for All Handicapped Children Act." *The University of Puget Sound Law Review* 14 (Winter 1991): 351–82.

Sheridan, Brian, "Accommodations for the Hearing Impaired in State Courts." *Michigan Bar Journal* 74 (May 1995): 396.

Simon, Jo Anne. "The Use of Interpreters for the Deaf and the Legal Community's Obligation to Comply with the ADA." *Journal of Law and Health* 8 (1993/1994): 155–99.

Smith, Deidre M. "Confronting Silence: The Constitution, Deaf Criminal Defendants, and the Right to Interpretation During Trial." *Maine Law Review* 4 (1994): 87–150.

Stokes, David M. "Relief for the Deaf: The Michigan Handicapper's Civil Rights Act and the Americans with Disabilities Act." *University of Detroit Law Review* 68 (Summer 1991): 513.

Stokes, David M. and Daniel McGlinn. "The Accessible Law Office." *Michigan Bar Journal* 75 (May 1996): 390.

Strauss, Karen, and Bob Richardson. "Breaking Down the Telephone Barrier—Relay Services on the Line." *Temple Law Review* 64 (1991): 583–607.

Swygert, Jacob. "Constitutional Law—Establishment Clause—State Funding of Sign Language Interpreter for Deaf Student Attending Parochial Secondary School Does Not Violate First Amendment: *Zobrest v. Catalina Foothills School District*." *Cumberland Law Review* 24 (1993/1994): 587–99.

Tucker, Bonnie Poitras. "Application of the Americans with Disabilities Act (ADA) and Section 504 to Colleges and Universities: An Overview and Discussion of Special Issues Relating to Students." *The Journal of College and University Law* 23 (Summer 1996): 1.

———. "Deafness—Disability or Subculture: The Emerging Conflict." *Cornell Journal of Law and Public Policy* 3 (Spring 1994): 265–75.

———. "Deaf Prison Inmates: Time To Be Heard." *Loyola of Los Angeles Law Review* 22 (November 1988): 1–71.

———. "Symposium: Individual Right and Reasonable Accommodation under the Americans with Disabilities Act. Insurance and the ADA." *DePaul Law Review* 46 (Summer 1997): 915.

Tucker, Bonnie, Vernon McCay, Lawrence Raifman, and Sheldon

Greenberg. "The Miranda Warnings and the Deaf Suspect." *Behavioral Sciences and the Law* 14 (Winter 1996): 121–35.

Vernon, McCay, and Lawrence Raifman. "Recognizing and Handling Problems of Incompetent Deaf Defendants Charged with Serious Offense." *International Journal of Law and Psychiatry* 20 (Summer 1997): 373–87.

Weis, Andrew. "Peremptory Challenges: The Last Barrier to Jury Service for People with Disabilities." *Willamette Law Review* 33 (Winter 1997): 1.

Online Legal Resources

~~

WEBSITES

http://law.etext.org/102.htm
The Internet Law Library: Handicapped Individuals and the Law presents a wealth of legal resources, including federal and state legislation.

http://fedlaw.gsa.gov/legal6a.htm
The General Services Administration's FedLaw: Disabilities site provides hyperlinks to online disability law resources.

http://www.usdoj.gov/crt/ada/adahom1.htm
U.S. Department of Justice's ADA home page contains information on: technical assistance, the department's toll-free information line, enforcement, legislation status reports, settlements, new or proposed regulations, building certification, and ADA mediation.

http://www.adaptenv.org/indexg.htm
Maintained by Boston's Adaptive Environments Center, Inc., this site includes information about the New England ADA Technical Assistance Center and two national programs: the Universal Design Education Project and the ADA National Access for Public Schools Project. It also has links to many universal design and ADA resources.

http://specialedservices.com/
Special Ed Services.Com offers a website aimed towards special education departments in public schools. However, the site contains resources such as a bulletin board, links to state departments of

education and disability FAQs, assistive technology links, and advocacy information that may be helpful for people interested in other areas of disability law.

http://www.captions.org/
A frequently updated site providing news and resources on closed captioning.

http://www.weizmann.ac.il/deaf-info/www-pages.html
A privately-maintained site containing hyperlinks to miscellaneous deafness-related web sites, including resources on legal and telecommunication links.

http://www.deaflibrary.org./
The Deaf Resource Library is a privately-maintained collection of FAQs, telecommunications and ADA links, a bibliography, news, and other resources.

http://clerccenter.gallaudet.edu/InfoToGo/index.html
Gallaudet's National Information Center on Deafness is a centralized source for up-to-date research, news, and other information on deafness and hearing loss.

http://home1.gte.net/sherryze/regional.htm
Hearing parents of a deaf child maintain this site, which focuses on state-based special education resources.

http://www.dssc.org/frc/frc1.htm
The Federal Resource Center for Special Education contains text and news on the latest IDEA regulations, as well as grant information for states seeking to improve the education provided for students with disabilities.

http://www.dssc.org/frc/rrfc.htm
The Regional Resource and Federal Centers Network (RRFC) is run by the Academy for Educational Development, a nonprofit organization geared towards human development. The RRFC provides a variety of services to improve state delivery of special education and compliance with IDEA.

http://www.ed.gov/offices/OSERS/
The Office of Special Education and Rehabilitative Services maintains a website offering frequently-updated news and resources pertaining to IDEA, access, and communication issues.

http://www.wrightslaw.com/
The Special Ed Advocate website offers publications and information for parents on disability law, including a free online newsletter and a guide to the art of writing letters to advocate for someone under IDEA.

http://www.edlaw.net/
EdLaw, Inc., provides a list of attorneys who represent parents of children with disabilities; briefing papers on disability law; a compilation of e-mail newsgroups pertaining to disability law; a message board; information on the organization's consulting services; and other resources.

http://adabbs.hr.state.ks.us/dc/
The Kansas Commission on Disability Concerns and the ADA Project have developed the ADA Information Center On-Line, which contains numerous links to government, news, and general resources on disability law.

http://www.nod.org/
The National Organization on Disability offers news and advocacy updates on issues related to the ADA.

http://www.swiftsite.com/adaman/
A private law firm maintains an interactive website to help you determine if you have a case under the ADA.

http://www.evanterry.com/
An architectural firm provides a comprehensive list of online ADA resources, including links to, and information on, the Department of Justice, the Access Board, ADA settlements and consent agreements, state accessibility codes, and disability statistics.

http://www.os.dhhs.gov/progorg/ocr/ocrhmpg.html
The website for the Office of Civil Rights (under the Department of Health and Human Services) explains how to file a complaint of unlawful discrimination.

http://supct.law.cornell.edu/supct/
Cornell Law School maintains an online database of Supreme Court decisions. Search for current rulings on compliance, access, captioning, etc.

http://consumerlawpage.com/
The Consumer Law Page contains a searchable directory that can target areas of disability law.

http://www.access-board.gov/
The site for the U.S. Access Board, also known as the Architectural and Transportation Barriers Compliance Board, provides news on recent guidelines and laws pertaining to disability access. The Access Board is currently adding a list of state accessibility codes to the website.

http://www2.pair.com/options/legal1.htm
This resource page is geared towards parents of deaf children, and contains a plethora of information on special education laws and resources.

http://www.geocities.com/~drm/DRMreg.html
The Disability Resources Monthly Guide to Disability Resources on the Internet lists disability organizations and agencies by state, as well as other information on a range of disability law issues.

http://www.copaa.net/
The Council of Parent Attorneys and Advocates is a nonprofit organization established to improve the quality and quantity of legal assistance for parents of children with disabilities. The group's website lists decisions, rulings and briefs; contains a discussion board; offers an e-mail newsgroup; and maintains a network of volunteer attorneys who provide free assistance.

http://uscode.house.gov/usc.htm
The U.S. Code contains the text of current public laws enacted by Congress.

http://www.ncd.gov
The NCD Bulletin is a monthly publication of the National Council on Disability. The Bulletin is free and available over the Internet.

http://www.gallaudet.edu
Gallaudet University's homepage offers a variety of educational, technical, legal, legislative, and other resources.

http://www.nad.org
The National Association of the Deaf offers a free E-zine of current legislation and other news regarding people who are deaf or hard of hearing. Archives of the E-zine, as well as articles from the *NAD Broadcaster*, are available online.

E-MAIL DISCUSSION GROUPS

E-mail lists, sometimes known as listservs, are interactive, computer-based communications. To quickly find a suitable list from the thousands of lists available, visit one of these three websites:

> www.egroups.com
> www.onelist.com
> www.liszt.com

Another source of lists is the company Listserv. To obtain information on discussion groups, send an e-mail message to: listserv@listserv.net. In the body of your e-mail message, write:

> lists global/[keyword]

(where [keyword] is the topic of your choice [e.g., disability]. Listserv will send a reply containing information on the discussion groups that match your search request.

Although a successful group may last for years, some may disappear more quickly. The following list is a sampling of disability-related discussion groups that may be available.

Name: IDEA '97
Address: Majordomo@lists.air-dc.org
Information: To subscribe, send an e-mail to the address listed above. In the body of the e-mail, write:

> subscribe <ebd-idea97talk>

Name: Disability Law
Address: oklahomadisabilitylawcenter@eGroups.com
Information: To join the list, send a blank e-mail message to:

> oklahomadisabilitylawcenter-subscribe@eGroups.com.

Name: Disability News
Address: Disability-News@eGroups.com
Information: To join the list, send a blank e-mail message to:

> Disability-News-Subscribe@eGroups.com.

Name: Council of Parent Attorneys and Advocates
Address: copaa@eGroups.com
Information: To join the list, send a blank e-mail message to:

> copaa-subscribe@eGroups.com.

Name: ADA-EMPOWERMENT
Address: ADA-EMPOWERMENT@onelist.com
Information: To subscribe, go to the following website:

   http://www.onelist.com/subscribe/ADA-EMPOWERMENT

Name: ADA-ACCESS
Address: ADA-ACCESS-request@LISTSERV.AOL.COM
Information: This group examines physical access for people with disabilities; related architectural norms and practices; and modification of policies, practices, or procedures for access to programs, services, transportation, and facilities. To subscribe, send email to:
listserv@LISTSERV.AOL.COM and in the body of the message, put:

   subscribe ada-access

Name: EDLAW
Contact: EDLAW-request@LSV.UKY.EDU
Information: This group explores law and education. To subscribe, send an e-mail to:
listserv@LSV.UKY.EDU and in the body of the message, put:

   subscribe edlaw

Name: Access By Design
Address: http://www.access-by-design.com/wwwboard/wwwboard.html
Information: An open bulletin board for discussing ADA questions, disability problems, etc. To subscribe, follow the directions posted on the group's website.

Name: DISABLEDUNITE
Address: http://dunite.homepage.com/
Information: To subscribe, follow the directions posted on the group's website.

Name: ADA-LAW
Address: ADA-LAW-request@LISTSERV.NODAK.EDU
Information: Discussion of the ADA and other disability-related legislation not only in the United States but other countries as well. To subscribe, send email to listserv@listserv.nodak.edu and in the body of the message, put:

   Subscribe ADA-Law Firstname Lastname

Index

Index entries in italics refer to court cases.

hospitals and health care services, 93, 221
international symbol, 221
long distance rate reduction, 220
new technology, 222
operator services, 209
pay or public phones, 27, 151, 208, 214, 221–22
police departments, 181–82
portable, 151
relay services, 34, 206–10
schools, 73
Section 504 regulation, 47–48. *See also specific public agency (e.g., Hospitals)*
Section 508 regulation, 41
7-1-1 for nationwide relay access, proposal for, 210–11
shopping malls, 151, 221
Social Security Administration, 93
speech-to-speech relay service, 212
state programs, 210–11
VRI (Video relay interpreting), 212
wireless services, compatibility, 222

Undue hardship. *See* Americans with Disabilities Act (ADA)
Uniform Federal Accessibility Standards, 74, 148, 150
Universities. *See* Colleges and universities
U.S. government. *See specific department or agency by name (e.g., Justice, U.S. Department of)*

Vernon, McCay, 111
Video relay interpreting (VRI), 212
Videotaping of police communications, 175
Virginia, 174
Visual warning systems. *See also* Lights as signals for auditory systems
TV emergency alert system, 198
Vocational rehabilitation counselors, 136–37
deaf college students, 85–87
Section 504, applicability, 41
Voice mail, 219
VRI (Video relay interpreting), 212

Warning systems. *See* Lights as signals for auditory systems
Web. *See* Internet
Welfare agencies. *See also* Social services
Americans with Disabilities Act provisions, 22
Wheelchairs, barriers preventing access to buildings and facilities. *See* Architectural barriers
Williams v. Jersey City Medical Center, 106
Wireless telephone services, 222
Witnesses, right to interpreters, 163, 182
Workforce Investment Act, 40
Written messages. *See* Note-writing
Wyatt v. Aderholt, 113–14
Wyatt v. Stickney, 113–14

second SUV. There's blood on the ground, a burgundy lake spreading beneath O'Driscoll and the male agent. Bile burns up the back of my throat.

"What did you do?" I squint at Brennan as he careens out of the parking lot.

"I saved your life."

"Did you kill them?"

"I don't know." Brennan's face is pale, his eyes bruised and red-rimmed. "I hope not."

"They're government agents. If you did—"

"Jesus, I just saved your life. Say thank you or shut the hell up." He white-knuckles the steering wheel.

"Thank you," I say. "What now?"

"We make a getaway."

"Abi's still in the lobby."

"Did you come in her car?"

"Yeah."

He does an illegal U-turn and heads back to the hospital. Sirens blare and corkscrew agony through my brain.

"Go get her." Brennan hauls ass out of the SUV, dragging me and a duffel bag with him. "Hurry up, Raleigh."

The lot is crawling with cops. Abigail sees me first and rushes out of the lobby.

"Holy heck, Raw. What happened? They said there's a gunman in the building. And what happened to your head?" She fusses over my face.

"We need to go." I grab her hand and stride through the chaos outside the hospital, trying to look inconspicuous despite the blood pouring off my jaw. Brennan meets us at Abi's truck, his hospital gown soaked red in an imperfect circle on his chest.

"Did you get s-s-shot?" I'm shivering, my teeth hammering so hard I'm bound to break a molar.

"I heal, remember?" He helps me into the truck.

"What the hell is going on?" Abigail jams her phone in the dash and lets the engine idle.

"We need to get out of here," he says.

"Not until you tell me why Raleigh's bleeding."

"O'Driscoll s-s-shot me." The words rattle out my mouth.

"The Homeland Security agent shot you? Why?" Abi grips the steering wheel and glares at Brennan. "What've you got us messed up in?"

"Abigail, Raleigh's in shock. He's losing blood and needs help. I suggest you drive." Brennan's voice is steel and ice.

"We're at the hospital."

"Yes, and the person who shot us is, too, so I suggest driving very fast and very far away right now."

"If a government agent shot you, how did you get away?" Abi persists in giving Brennan the third degree.

"I shot her," he says.

"You killed her?" Abigail shrieks, which only exacerbates my headache.

"Abi, please, just drive." I flinch when Brennan presses a wad of Kleenex from the glove box against my head.

"Fine." She wrenches the truck into gear and spins the wheels. "I'm taking you straight to the police station."

"You don't want to do that." Brennan tenses beside me.

"Give me one good reason why not?" Abigail heads for downtown Amarillo instead of taking the exit for the interstate.

"Because Brennan isn't the kind of tourist you think he is."

"Who the heck is Brennan?" Abi asks.

"Crow. Crow's real name is Brennan." I try to meet his gaze, but his face swims in and out of focus.

"Brennan." He says it over and over like it's some kind of mantra.

"I found him beat up in the desert with no memories."

"What?" Abi whispers, her eyes wide as the Texas sky.

"It's true. I called Madison to help me. She'll tell you." *Inhale.* The truth is almost always better than a lie. *Exhale.* Abi has to believe me. *Inhale.* She has to trust me. *Exhale.* "Ever since then we've been trying to figure out who he is and where he's from."

"You figured that out yet, Raw?" She gives me a scathing glance before focusing on the road again.

"Yeah, we think he's an astronaut."

"Astronaut?" Abi's laughter is shrill and devoid of humor. "From where? The moon?"

"Actually…" I glance at Brennan, but he looks away, his hand splayed over the blood stain on the right side of his chest. "He's from Mars."

BRENNAN

My name is Brennan Cozens.

"**Unprecedented,**" says the voice inside my head. "**I want this all documented.**"

Again, I repeat the words in my mind hoping the name will start to feel more like mine and less like a stranger's.

"**It wasn't deliberate,**" says the familiar voice. "**Every time I run a patch, Williams manages to override it. This is his world. Inside sero, he's God.**"

Sero? What the hell does that mean?

"**You can't control it?**"

"**I can influence it, and I can stop it of course, but I can't dictate the outcomes. That's the whole point of psytek.**"

Shut up! I knock my fists against my head willing the voices to silence. The scattered pieces of who I am form an untidy mosaic, but I think I'm starting to remember properly this time, and not only in the snatches gleaned from Raleigh.

I'm starting to remember the guy I was before I fell, although the details on how I ended up in Texas are still sketchy. Thing is, I'm not sure I want to be Brennan. I think I prefer being Crow. I am Crow.

CROW

"We can't go back to the Rusty Inn," I say while Abi attempts to digest all the information we just dumped on her.

"Think they'll come after us?" Raleigh asks.

"You shot a Homeland Security agent," Abi says. "Of course they'll come after us."

"You weren't involved."

"I am now." She sounds pissed.

"Abi, I—"

"Save it. I'm done hearing you apologize. Things are the way they are." The look she gives me is darker than the void of space. "So what do we do now?"

"We need to go somewhere we can get Raleigh patched up." I rummage through the duffel bag and pull out a pair of jeans.

"What about Raleigh's mama's place?"

"Too risky. They know who Raleigh is. They'll be all over his family." I wriggle into the jeans going commando and shed the hospital gown. Abi and Raleigh both stare at my bare skin, at the blood smear on my chest and back around a phantom bullet wound. By this time tomorrow I'm guessing I'll have two new symbols in my skin where I should have a bullet hole.

"Holy heck." Abi blinks. "I didn't know you had so many."

"There are more now," Raleigh says. "Brennan—"

"Don't call me that. I'm Crow."

"Crow." He swallows and nods. "Are you all right?"

"I'm better now." Once we get somewhere safe, I'll have to try and explain about the voices inside my head although I can't begin to fathom what they mean, or how this is all connected to Raleigh. "Are there any other motels close by?"

"There's the old Jepson place on the way up to Dalhart. It's been abandoned for over a year," Abi says.

"Perfect." I tug on a T-shirt. "Let's go."

It's nearing midnight by the time we pull into the motel. We park around the back in the darkness of the desert, far from the reaching beams of passing headlights—not that there are too many. The motel is dilapidated, most windows jagged shards and the walls crumbling. Using the flashlights on their phones, Abi and Raleigh navigate the interior. The furniture is frayed, the bed covers sport polka dot burns from errant cigarettes, and cockroaches scuttle in the corners. The vending machines are all broken and have long since been emptied. No electricity, no water. It's the last place anyone would want to stay, and that makes it the perfect hide out.

"There's a gas station a few miles up the road. I'll get us some supplies." Abi stands in the doorway of room 13 and folds her arms.

"Here." Raleigh hands over some bills.

Gingerly, she accepts the crumpled notes. "Water, food, bandages, aspirin. Do we need anything else?"

"Disinfectant of some kind," I add.

"Thank you, Abi. I owe you," Raleigh says. "Want me to come with you?"

"No, Raw. I really, really need some time away to think." She strides to her truck and less than a minute later she drives off.

"You trust her to come back?"

"I trust that girl with my life," he says.

"Hope you're right." I lean against the door. Raleigh is a grim silhouette in the halo of light from his phone before he shuts it off.

"It's so dark." He steps outside, peering up at the sky. The stars string silver across the night, and Mars winks at us from its seat in Capricorn. The breeze whistles through the clumps of bushes skulking on the periphery of the parking lot.

"How's the head?" I ask.

"No more messed up than usual." He rubs the back of his neck.

I keep my gaze on the stars, trying to figure out the tangled thoughts spinning through my mind.

"Did you know," Raleigh starts. "They hypothesize that life only became possible on Earth after asteroids shattered Mars, sending meteorites rich in oxidized molybdenum crashing into Earth?" He drums his fingers against his thigh. "Life might never have happened on Earth without Martian shrapnel and here we are, some three billion years later, wanting to put life back on Mars. Ironic, ain't it?" A wry smile plays on his lips as he turns to look at me. The breeze tugs hair across his eyes and stray strands catch on his lips, lips I can't wait to kiss again.

"Or poetic." I return his smile. It might seem a shitty time for flirting but I can't help myself, not with the starlight splayed across Raleigh's face and dousing his shoulders in quicksilver.

"Can you tell me what happened?" he asks.

I chew on my thumb, searching for the words to make sense of it all. "I called that number and it sounded like someone picked up, but I couldn't hear anything." Or could I? I'm not sure. A voice maybe. If they said something, I don't remember. "Then this stuff started coming out my ears. There wasn't any pain, just a weird seeping sensation like my brain had turned liquid and was trying to escape."

"I saw you having surgery. Your head was all bandaged up," he says gently, once again his hand strays to the back of his neck.

"Wish I knew what they did to me." I lean against the doorjamb, our shoulders touching with a static prickle. "Although if they've messed around with my head, that might explain why I'm hearing voices."

"Voices?"

"At first I thought I was overhearing a TV or radio somewhere, but they're definitely inside my head."

"What do they say?" Raleigh looks worried.

"Not to kill anyone, promise." Except maybe that would be easier to handle. "I catch snatches of conversation, something about a candidate and algorithms. There's this one word, sero, I think. They talk about that, and they said 'Williams' keeps hijacking the system." I meet his gaze, hoping my next words will bring on an epiphany. "I think you might be the one in control."

"Me? In control of what?"

"I was hoping you'd know." No eureka moment, then, which leaves us no closer to any answers.

"Did you see any more of my memories?" he asks.

"Saw you beating the crap out of Wayne."

Raleigh looks away, and I sidle closer.

"He deserved it," I say softly. Wayne deserved far worse.

"I almost killed him." His shoulders slump. "His face will never be right again."

"The dude didn't look that bad to me. Besides, you should've been the one pressing charges." I brush against him again, wanting to feel the electric tingle of our connection, wanting so much to forget about all the things we don't know and get lost in this moment of simply being together out beneath the stars.

"And have what they did all over the Internet?" Raleigh sucks in a breath. "No thanks."

"Can you even say it?" I ask.

"Say what?" Raleigh squirms.

"You've never actually said it." I'm pushing the guy. I know exactly where all his buttons are, but I'm pushing them gently. "Out loud, I mean. Have you ever told anyone?"

Hard as it might be, if he could admit what happened, I think he'd feel better. Maybe it would give him a chance to let go and move on, but what do I know? My only knowledge of the experience has been gleaned vicariously through his memories. It wasn't my body that was violated; it wasn't my pride and dignity and sense of self left in tatters.

"No." He pauses and chews on his bottom lip. "Some people don't even think it's possible—for a boy, I mean. You know." The words strangle him and I reach for his hand, but he inches away. "They would've asked why I let it happen, why I didn't try to defend myself." Eyes squeezed shut, he shakes his head. "It's better this way."

"Raleigh, they—"

"Don't." He meets my gaze, eyes glistening, and I wish I could make it right for him, and make all his pain go away. "Please don't."

"I don't think you'll get over it until you can admit what happened. It doesn't make you any less of a man, less of a human being. They're the monsters. Not you."

He doesn't say anything and an aching silence settles between us. Eventually, I have to break it.

"How come Lilah didn't post the video anyway after what you did to Wayne?"

"She knew it'd only help me in court, justify what I did somehow," he says. "She told me she deleted it, told me no one would ever know what happened and that I'd get locked up for good." Raleigh's lips twist in a rueful smile. Christ, he's good-looking, beautiful even with his hair down and billowing in the wind.

"And that's what you wanted, the video deleted, I mean?" My mouth's gone dry; a fire ignited in my belly. I can't stop staring, watching the shadows shift across the plains of his face. I'm staring so hard my eyes are burning.

"Yup. Kinda made going to juvie worth it." He fingers the

wound on his head. "Why's Homeland Security looking for you?" He changes the topic and I exhale, not wanting to keep picturing Raleigh with Wayne that day. "You don't seem the terrorist type."

"Maybe it's because of what they put inside my head."

"But who's *they*?"

Too many questions, too few answers, and way too much confusion.

"O'Driscoll said they are whoever they need to be. I doubt they're actually Homeland Security," he says.

That does not allay my anxiety. There are still too many gaps in my recollection, too many things I don't know, and Jesus Christ, my eyes are killing me!

"They must be connected to Bennett, to Mars somehow. Maybe they think it makes me dangerous."

"But why?" Raleigh frowns.

"I'm pretty sure they don't want one of their candidates roaming around Texas when he should be getting ready to go to Mars."

"So now you believe you are an astronaut?" Raleigh eyes me suspiciously.

"I don't know what to believe." Part of me thinks maybe this has more to do with Raleigh than with me, if what the voice said is true and Raleigh is somehow calling the shots on all of this. But how?

"How did they even find us?" he asks.

"Maybe from the photos we posted?"

"They showed up before that. Aw, hell. This is all my fault. I might as well have rigged a flashing neon sign with your name on it."

"What do you mean?" My eyes, fuck. Rubbing them only makes them worse.

"Right after I saw what I thought was a meteor I posted about it in the MarsLife forums."

"That's probably what caught their attention. And maybe Tony and Mary-Jo called the State Troopers."

"Who?"

"The people I tried hitching to Amarillo with." So stupid. But then hindsight is always 20/20.

"Maybe." He twists strands of hair around his fingers and bites his bottom lip, which only adds fuel to the fire in my veins. "I saw the SUV right before you showed up on the interstate."

"I'm lucky they didn't find me, then."

"Lucky?" He raises an eyebrow.

"I wouldn't know you if they had." I want to hold him, or maybe I need to be held, but I don't want another memory deluge right now, so I fight the urge to touch him.

"I'm sorry, Crow. I didn't know."

"They would've found me one way or another."

"Whether O'Driscoll is DHS or not, we're in some serious trouble." His shoulders slump again and his face folds into an expression of despair.

"I know."

"What are we gonna do?"

"I'm thinking." I stare off into the middle-distance as if the answers might rise out of the desert. Now Raleigh's staring at me, but not in an I'm-about-to-jump-your-bones kind of way.

"What?"

"Your eyes."

"What about them?" I blink and rub at them again. The burning, itching sensation only intensifies.

"Your eyes are turning purple, and they're sort of glowing."

"Don't be ridiculous."

"Serious as a heart attack. I'll show you." He snaps a close-up photo of my eyes and shows me the evidence. Just as he said, my eyes are lucent purple. It might've been cool if it weren't so fucking creepy.

"Weird scars, goo out my ears, and now glowing eyes. What the hell is happening to me?"

"Do they feel weird?" Raleigh asks.

"Feels like I've poured pure capsaicin into them. I need answers, dammit." I kick my toe through the dirt, succeeding only in sending up more dust to irritate my eyes. "Hey, I suggest not mentioning anything about our telepathic bond to anyone else, okay?"

"We're telepathic now?" he asks, incredulous.

"Just don't mention anything about sharing memories. Otherwise it might be your skull they want to crack open." A troubling thought, although I'd like to know what caused this memory soup we're sharing.

"Ever think you falling out the sky might've been an accident?"

"All I do know is that I'm not going to let some strangers drag me away in a blacked-out SUV."

"Maybe they were trying to help."

"By dragging me away unconscious? Doubtful." An idea weasels into my thoughts. "Think we could try jump starting this brain-share thing we've got going on?"

"How?" He licks his lips like he can read my mind although we've tried the just touching thing before. It'll take more than that this time.

"Abi had some weed. I could smell it. We could try that."

"How will getting high help?" He almost looks disappointed.

"When I passed out before, I came the closest to remembering things for myself." I step closer and Raleigh doesn't move away. "I think an altered brain state might be the key to unlocking more of my own memories."

"I hope your memories aren't the closest I'll ever get to Mars." He sucks in a breath and winces, the fresh scabs on his hands cracking open.

"You know…" I tuck a loose wisp of hair behind his ear, shivering as electric sparks ratchet up my spine. I'm trying my best to banish the hope that Raleigh ends up staying on Earth. "I don't think this MarsLife program is all it's cracked up to be."

Raleigh

Out here the constellations look like pennies scattered in molasses without the glow of the refineries or the town to dull their burn. I'm tired and my head hurts, and I'm pretty sure there's a new scar on the back of my neck, although given the recent head injury, I sure hope I'm imagining it. All I want to do is sleep then wake up from the nightmare my life has become, but the look on Crow's face puts my insides on the spin cycle. He needs answers, and I'm the only one who can help him get them.

Crow regards me with a look of expectancy and I nod.

"Fine, let's go get high."

"Holy heck." Abi gapes. "Your eyes!" She touches Crow's cheek and pulls down his lower lid. "That's freaky."

I sort through the food from the convenience store and choose a Twix for dinner, leaving the healthier protein bar for Crow. My head feels better since Abi doused it in surgical spirits and antibiotic ointment. At least the wound was superficial. "So you believe me now?"

"About him possibly being from Mars?" Abi says. "Yeah, maybe." She sits cross-legged on the wonky bed and tucks into a bag of Cheetos. "But what's up with all the artwork?" She gestures to his arms.

"We've been trying to figure that out." Crow perches beside me on the sofa chair and nibbles on the protein bar, crumbs sticking to his lips.

"You a masochist or something?"

"Not exactly." Crow chews and swallows before continuing. "They appear post injury."

"But not like a regular scar," Abi says.

"Nope, they're the logo for the Bennett Institute."

"What's that?"

"A research facility connected to MarsLife," I say. It's all connected. Somehow. It must be. "So maybe Crow's an alien." The idea doesn't seem so implausible any more.

"Sure you shouldn't be taking your meds?" She flicks a chip at me.

"Hey, he fell out of the sky, and he's leaking anti-freeze from his ears."

"And you're sharing memories and his eyes are glowing, I get it." She balls up the empty Cheetos packet and tosses it into a dusty corner. "Doesn't mean he's E.T."

"Watch this." Crow helps himself to my pocketknife and slices open his arm.

"What the…" Abi's mouth hangs open. We all watch the wound on Crow's arm seal shut. He spills some water over his skin and wipes away the blood. Not even the faintest trace of injury remains.

"So you did get shot." Her gaze drops to his chest.

"And all I get in return are new symbols on my skin."

"Okay, you might be an alien." She wraps her arms around her knees, her eyes huge and hollow in the light from my phone set up on the table like a candle.

"Doubtful." Crow grins. "Considering we're pretty certain I grew up like a regular kid even if we're not clear on the where yet."

"Have we got a plan?" Abi asks. "'Cause this whole being on the run thing is getting old real quick. Couldn't we go to our local cops?"

"You mean Sheriff Daniels who just took my dog?" The words come out blacker than fresh asphalt. "Not an option."

"What I need to do is remember more." Crow leans toward Abi. "We're starting to get more pieces of the puzzle, but if I could remember more, maybe I'd understand what's going on and what to do next."

"How'd you do the memory sharing thing before?" she asks.

"It just happens sometimes." I shrug. "When we touch."

"But I think an altered cognitive state might help," Crow says. "You've got some weed."

"You want to get high out in the middle of bumfuck nowhere and hope this mystical connection you two apparently share conjures up the answers?" Abi frowns. "And then what? I have a life. Raleigh, too. My folks'll worry when I don't go home. I'm supposed to be going to California in four days. Madison will have a fit if she thinks Raleigh is missing for real this time."

"I'm so sorry about this." Crow drags his fingers through his hair. "I wish none of you were involved, but the connection we share is real." His hand slides onto my knee sending a jolt through my bones.

"We could put this all online and let the world know that O'Driscoll woman tried to kill you," Abi suggests.

"Not until we know more." Crow squeezes me knee. "Hence wanting to get high."

"It can't hurt, can it?" Abi removes a baggie from her pocket and starts rolling a joint.

"Do we both have to do it?" There's no way I'll get into MarsLife if they find THC in my bloodstream.

"You still thinking about those tests?" Abi hands the joint and a lighter to Crow.

"Sorta."

"Don't you think it's better to find out if there's something nefarious happening with this whole MarsLife program before you accept a ticket off-world?" Crow lights up the blunt, his eyes bright with desperation and his glowing irises chilling my bone marrow. Sure as shit on a pig, his eyes are veined with a spiderweb of metallic purple.

"This is nuts." But I take a long drag anyway, the pungent aroma abrading my nasal passages and burning the back of my throat.

"Feel anything yet?" Abi asks. Crow's pupils dilate, the violet glow getting even brighter.

"Not yet. You?" His gaze flicks to me.

"Nope."

"You know, we seem to remember more whenever we get closer." Crow bites his lip before taking another drag on the joint. Cupping my face with one hand, he leans in and presses his lips against mine. I open my mouth and breathe in as he exhales. The familiar static marches across my skin and up my spine. The drug grabs hold of my mind and starts shaking out my thoughts as if they're a bunch of pickup sticks. This isn't like the psychotropics that made everything go blank and tranquil. Now every little thing is raw and psychedelic, amplified by megawatt emotions. Crow takes another hit and shares the smoke with me again. Abi and the motel room fade into gray as Crow's tongue meets mine.

The ambient lighting embedded in the floor throws pale halos across the off-white walls. It smells of metal and plastic. My footsteps echo down the windowless corridor. I'm at the Bennett Institute. There's a high voltage hum barely audible for the pounding of the blood in my ears. My palms are slick with sweat and every hair on my body stands at attention, prickling with apprehension.

Using my RFID tag, I swipe myself into the medical wing and through various doors before reaching wing A-400. Gray corridors and windowless doors that all look the same.

A402 – the cer-ro lab. I swipe myself in and shut the door behind me. I can do this. It's what we've been working on for years, a culmination of sleepless nights and cutting-edge technology.

What looks like a hybrid torture device somewhere between a dentist's chair and an MRI machine sits off to the left of the room. Cerebro-renovo. We could've made it look a little more friendly. Best to put future candidates under general for this. The contraption looks like the carapace of a centipede complete with leg fronds poised and ready to pin down prey.

"Are you ready?" Tina asks.

"I will be." Together, we set about calibrating the machine and my fingers stray often to the implant on the back of my neck marked by a narrow thread of scar tissue.

"It's time."

Fear ignites along every synapse. But I nod and exchange my clothes for a hospital gown.

"You know you don't need to be the guinea pig."

"Of course I do." I give her a smile with false bravado. If this goes wrong, it could cook my brain. I settle into the machine and Tina stabs at the computer.

"Keep it short. No more than ten minutes," I instruct.

"You got it, boss."

The memory fades and I'm back in the motel room, Crow's head in my lap and his hand on mine. His eyeballs dash left and right beneath lids laced with fine blue capillaries as he endures whatever miserable memory of mine must be ricocheting inside his skull.

"Is he asleep?" Abi asks.

"I think he's still in it." Maybe addling our thoughts with THC wasn't the wisest move. We have no way of knowing what effect it'll have on Crow or how long he'll stay mired in my memories.

"Think he'll be okay?"

"Yeah, considering a bullet couldn't touch him." I smooth hair off his face, hoping he's seeing something less horrible than last time. Gently, I drag a finger down the back of his neck, tracing the narrow scar.

"Did you see anything?"

"I think so."

"Could we chat out there?" She gestures to the door. "We won't go far."

I don't want to leave Crow but there's not much I can do except wait for him to come to. He's breathing normally and there's no gunk pouring out his ears so, having extricated myself from Crow, I join Abi outside beneath a gawky mesquite. I don't want to know, but my fingers go searching the nape of my neck and find a scar just like Crow's.

"What did you see?" she asks.

"Something about a weird contraption and a doctor or technician calling Crow her boss." Crow's wrong. This is about him, not me. "It was intense. I could smell and feel everything like it was happening to me." And given the scar, maybe it did.

"How do you know it's real and not just a mind-warp from the weed?"

"Details like that? No way that's all in my head. You ever heard of Cerebro-renovo?"

"Sounds awful. What is it?"

"A machine. Like something out of a horror movie. I'm not sure what it does."

"Not sure I wanna know." She shudders.

Me neither, except Crow seemed to have had a hand in its construction, and he climbed into the thing of his own volition.

"I'm scared, Raw. This is all too much." She turns the ring on her middle finger over and over. "You're living a stranger's memories and you could've died tonight."

"Sorry you got caught up in this." More guilt, more regret. I run a search on my phone for Cerebro-renovo and come up empty. No surprise there. My fingers stray to the back of my neck, up into my hair. I could be imagining it, but no—I definitely have a scar on the back of my neck in exactly the same place as Crow's. How come I never noticed until now? I swallow hard, resisting the urge to tear out whatever's under my skin and the desire to throw up at the same time.

"Do you trust him?" Her question hits the bull's-eye. What little I know about Crow terrifies the crap out of me. I'm in way over my head.

"I don't know."

"Part of me wants us to leave right now, just get in the truck and drive real fast until we hit the Pacific," she says.

"I can't leave him." And I don't want to. We're in this together. There's a reason I found him in the desert that night. Of all the places he could've ended up, of all the people who could've found him, I've got to believe there's a reason it was me. There must be a reason we've got the same implant, too.

"Why not? You don't owe him."

"I've been inside his head. He's been inside mine. We have a connection."

"One that got you shot."

I don't need to see her face to know the expression she's wearing, all disapproval and concern.

"I'm afraid of him, and I'm afraid for you." Her eyes fill with tears. I loop my arm over her shoulders and pull her close.

"It'll be okay," I whisper into Abi's hair, trying to convince myself as much as her.

"Hope so." She wipes her eyes. "Because this is getting batshit crazy."

Weston's angry guitar riff interrupts our conversation. I fish my phone out my pocket. Unknown number.

"You just gonna stare at it?" Abi nudges my foot with her own, and I answer.

"Hello, Raleigh." The familiar voice turns my blood to ice.

"How did you get my number?" Goose bumps erupt across my skin.

"Same way I know you have a lovely sister and a charming little nephew." Her voice is syrup and barbed wire. At least Crow didn't kill her and she's well enough to be making threats.

"Don't hurt them."

"That'll depend on whether or not you cooperate." O'Driscoll pauses. "We'd like to make a deal."

CROW

When I crash back into reality, Raleigh and Abi are gone, leaving me alone and hungover from the memories of Raleigh's time in juvie. The more I learn about this guy, the more I want to take him far away from Dead Rock and show him how good life can be. I want to save him from this town, from all the people who've hurt him and maybe even from himself. That's rich coming from a guy with voices in his head and half his own memories missing.

Dragging myself off the bed, I drink some water and listen to their conversation. Only Raleigh isn't talking to Abi, it sounds like he's on the phone.

"What are you doing?" I rip the cell from his hand. "They'll trace the call."

Raleigh looks at me guiltily. Abi won't meet my gaze.

"Who was it?"

"Just my sister wondering if I've run off to kill myself." He lets out a nervous breath and suspicion curdles my insides. After everything, I really want to trust Raleigh. I have no one else.

"You can't use your phone." I switch it off before handing it back. "We have to stay on the move."

"That call was super short," Abi says. "Doesn't it take several minutes for them to run a trace?"

"You really want to take that chance?"

"Maybe it wouldn't be such a bad thing to turn yourselves in," Abi says while focused on her feet.

"And what do you think they'll do to me and Raleigh when they find us?" I ask, my tone acidic. "Or to you since you're aiding and abetting?"

"You made this mess. You better fix it." Abi points a finger at me.

"You don't think I know that?" I take a step forward and Raleigh grabs my arm. This time it feels like I've tried to shake hands with a power line.

"That actually hurt." He flexes his fingers, and I study the mark on my arm. The scar there is darker, as if singed by his touch.

"We're all getting a bit uptight. Let's just take it easy, okay?"

"Did you remember anything helpful or do you just have the munchies now?" Abi folds her arms and juts out her hip.

"I remember being in a lab," Raleigh says. "Also, there was this weird machine. You called it Cerebro-renovo. I think you were doing some sort of calibration test." He pauses and fingers the back of his neck. "You had some sort of brain implant, and the woman with you called you the boss."

The world tilts on its axis and I find it hard to breathe.

"And," he continues, "I think I've got the same implant."

My fingers search the back of my neck. A fine line of scar tissue runs out of my hairline. It's less than an inch long and feels like real keloid.

"Crow?" Raleigh comes toward me and I back away, the memory sinking into my mind. I remember getting the implant and the trepidation I felt climbing into the machine, but what I can't remember is why. Why agree to have my head cut open and get locked into a monstrous machine? And I certainly don't feel like I could've been the one in charge of something like that.

"I'm fine." I focus on the horizon. It's turning lime green with the promise of dawn.

"Do you know what it means?" Raleigh asks.

"I really wish I did. But if you've got the same, then we're more connected than we thought." It's minor consolation to know I'm not in this alone. Of course that just means Raleigh and I are equally screwed.

"Maybe that's how we're sharing memories." He meets my gaze with a look of such jumbled emotion, I'm left speechless.

"How do you know these aren't dreams?" Abi asks. "I mean, it could be PTSD or something, right?"

"There's a difference in consistency." Raleigh sighs before continuing. "Dreams are like mist, the way they float into your head, obscuring your thoughts, distorting the truth and then dissolving when you wake up. But memories…" He picks up a rock and hurls it into the scrub. "Memories are like glue. They stick to you. You can't shrug them off, and they don't just vanish like they were never there."

"Crow's did," Abi says.

"Not completely," I say. "Memories make us who we are, but they don't have to define us." I look at Raleigh, hoping he gets the message.

"Abi, think you could give us a minute?" he asks. She looks at him with concern creasing her forehead.

"I'm gonna try to get some sleep." She steps into the room and shuts the door behind her. Picking my way through the shadows, I amble over to the pickup and Raleigh follows.

"So this is what we know." I take a deep breath and lay it all out before hopping onto the back of the truck. "And about those voices—they mentioned something called sero. Could be short for Cerebro-renovo."

Raleigh raises an eyebrow at me. I offer him my hand, and tentatively, he accepts, letting me haul him up beside me with only the faintest tingle in my palm.

"It kinda makes sense," he says. "You were in the cer-ro lab in my memory. So these voices, you think they're memories of stuff you overheard?"

"Feels plenty real when I hear them."

"Like someone's actually talking to you?" His eyes widen. "How is that possible?"

"Maybe they're connected to the chip in my head, or…"

No, Occam's Razor dictates that the simplest answer must be true, which in this case means I'm probably demented and suffering some sort of brain catastrophe that's distorting my perception of reality. The alternatives are too extreme to contemplate. "Forget it." I drag a hand through my hair, pressing my palm against the scar on my neck.

"You know what I wanna know? How the hell I have a brain implant." Raleigh slams his hands into his pockets and winces when his raw knuckles make contact with denim.

"That is a mystery. At least it means we're in this together, even more than we thought."

"Didn't Baudrillard say something like there's nothing more mysterious than a man talking to himself because it's like another planet is communicating with you?" A knowing grin tugs at Raleigh's lips. He's so damn sexy, quoting a French philosopher in his heavy drawl with the first glimmer of dawn spilling over his hair.

"I think you're paraphrasing, but that's the gist of it." We stand side by side watching fingers of pink and orange reach across the desert. The sun bathes Raleigh in golden light, and all I want to do is disappear inside of him no matter how dark that gets, because it's better than being inside my own fractured mind.

"You really okay?" His hand rests on my chest where a bullet should've shredded my flesh.

"Yup, but there's a new one." I tug up my shirt to show him the symbol starting to sprout on my pec. His hand ghosts over the spiral attempting to break the surface of my skin. He steps closer and all my blood rushes south, heat pooling between my legs.

"I…" He bites his lip. "I like being connected to you, even if it's in ways I don't understand." His voice is a soft crush of gravel. He stares at me, but I can't maintain eye contact.

"We both know where we'll find the answers," I say as

his hands hover above my nipples. Jesus, I want this guy so bad it hurts. I want to show him that sex doesn't have to be a sordid, shameful thing. I loved Jeremy once. He was my first, and then we grew up and grew apart. But I remember kissing him, loving him, and how good it felt. I want Raleigh to feel that, to know the touch of someone who cares about him and not only how fast he can make them come.

"The Bennett Institute."

"Yup." I can barely breathe. "Thank you, Raleigh." I lift his chin and force him to meet my gaze.

"For what?"

"For helping me remember even if I don't understand any of this. Thank you for not leaving me in the desert that night."

For several long moments, we stand staring at each other as the sun paints fire across wisps of cloud. My past might be the scattered shrapnel of a detonated grenade, but Raleigh is the truth of my Now. And maybe that's all I need. If I could wake every tomorrow having nothing else but Raleigh in my life, I think I'd be okay, and that thought is more terrifying than not knowing who I am. The way I feel about Raleigh eclipses every other fear and uncertainty.

"I saw something about you, too, you know." My hand rests on the thrumming pulse in his throat. Static needles my fingertips. With my heart going a mile a minute, I slide my hand into his hair and find the scar on his neck. "It started in juvie, those guys you beat up. After that…" I knot my hand in his hair so he won't look away. "You let them have you in exchange for cigarettes."

"At least that way, I was the one in control."

"And the cigarettes bought you extra phone calls to your mom and sister." My heart bursts with something a lot like love.

"Yeah, that, too." Raleigh looks at me through long lashes as if he's waiting for me to pass judgment on him, but I get it.

I've lived in his skin and I understand what he went through, why he chose to do what he did and I don't hate him for it.

"Raleigh." My voice hitches and I have to clear my throat. "I think I'm falling in love with you."

"Did you activate the nurture protocol?" The voice explodes inside my head at the least opportune moment.

"No, sir. This is a result of the natural learning algorithm."

"This isn't what we wanted." The person speaking sounds pissed.

"Isn't it?"

"We want the candidate to deal with trauma and stress, not fall in love."

"And you don't think falling in love can be traumatic and stressful?"

Shut up! Shut up! I banish the voices and focus on Raleigh's lips.

"No," Raleigh says, emphatic. "You've only known me a handful of days."

"And I've seen a lifetime of your memories. I know you inside out." Ignoring the continued discussion about whether or not love is an appropriate test scenario happening inside my skull, I let my lips brush Raleigh's. He returns the kiss, hard, a solar flare burning me up. He runs his hands across the scarred landscape of my back and chest. As he knots his fingers in my hair, the stun-gun pulses from our physical contact only make me shiver and shake with amplified pleasure. I wish I could freeze this moment with Raleigh's lips on mine and our bodies pressed together so tight it'll take a crowbar to pull us apart.

"I can't do this." He pulls away. "There's something I have to tell you."

"I already know all your secrets."

"Not all of them." The look on his face turns the fire in my veins to shards of ice. "This is about O'Driscoll."

RALEIGH

I'm speechless. My thoughts bust open like a dandelion in the wind as I try to process the words I never thought I'd hear directed at me. But it's not possible. I'm damaged and dirty and not worth a moment of Crow's time, let alone his love. He's falling for me. Falling. I just hope this time the fall doesn't leave him naked and broken in the dirt.

I wage an internal war with myself. The conversation with O'Driscoll plays on repeat in my mind, the terms I agreed to, how willing I'd been to hand Crow over. The guilt is a crysknife in my gut, stabbing over and over again. I can't do this, not with all this emotion corkscrewing through my rotten core.

"This is about O'Driscoll," I say, the words choking me. "I...I made a deal." Crow's life in exchange for mine and Madison's and Nashua's. O'Driscoll guaranteed me a place in the MarsLife program regardless of my test scores, too, but that hardly matters when she's got a gun to my sister's head. Even so, I can't believe I'm about to hand over the guy who's seen most of the shadows in me and still wants to be with me, who might even love me.

I rush through the explanation, guilt punching holes in my words and making me stammer. Crow looks at me, not with hatred or disgust, not even with disappointment, but with understanding. That's so much worse. I want him to get angry, to yell, to hit me, but he takes my hands and rubs his thumbs gently between my sore knuckles, the tingle familiar and comforting.

"I get it, Raleigh." He looks at me with those shiny purple eyes that make me want to shed my skin for him.

O'Driscoll could've sent a team to pick him up, but I need to know Madison and Nash are okay; that handing over Crow means something. We need to get back to the Rusty Inn.

"We should get going," Crow says, stoic despite what's about to happen.

"We don't have to do this," I say, willing him to argue, to fight back, to rail against the universe.

"Do you have another choice?" We stride back into the motel room. Abi is wide awake and smoking a cigarette.

"You told him," she says. The expressions on our faces no doubt give us away.

"We should leave soon," Crow says.

"You're okay with this?" she asks, eyes huge in her petite face.

"Hardly, but O'Driscoll threatened Raleigh's family, so there's no alternative." Crow leads the way to the truck and cranks open the door. A trickle of goo leaks out his ear.

"Crow, wait."

"I can't ask you to choose between me and your family. That bitch almost blew your head off, and she could do the same to Madison or Nash." He collapses in the seat with a groan and pinches the bridge of his nose.

"You all right?" I hop in beside him.

"Feels like I've got mortar rounds going off inside my skull." Wincing, Crow massages his temples. "Let's just get this over with."

"Maybe O'Driscoll can help you," Abi says and jams her phone into the dash.

Please let this be the right thing to do. Blood fills my mouth from where I've been gnawing hard on my inner cheek.

"I doubt her intention was ever to help. That and — " Crow pitches forward. I catch him before his face hits the dash.

I shake him, but he's unresponsive. At least he's breathing and his pulse throbs beneath my fingers pressed against his wrist.

"What's happening? Is he alive?" Abi's voice shoots up

an octave.

"He's breathing." More gunk trickles from his ears, and I ease him back against the seat, using my shoulder to keep him upright. I brush hair off his face, hair that appears to be growing ultramarine from the roots.

"Think he'll make it to Dead Rock?" Abi eases the truck onto the road and heads south.

Crow groans and squirms in the seat, his hands twitching in his lap and his eyes scurrying back and forth behind his eyelids. He mutters something incomprehensible, his jaw clenching around the words.

O'Driscoll could be the enemy. If she's got some nefarious agenda, then Crow was right to want to escape and here I am taking him straight back to the root of the problem. Crow's life is certainly worth more than a place in the MarsLife program. Having to find another way to keep my promise to West seems totally insignificant considering O'Driscoll threatened Madison's life. Would a government agent really murder a mother and child? *Inhale.* Why is this happening? *Exhale.* What the fuck am I going to do? *Inhale.* I glance at Crow and his words ricochet inside my mind, doing some serious hollow-point damage. *I think I'm falling in love with you.* We can't do this. We can't take him back.

"We can't do this!" I pound my fist on the dash.

"What about your family?" Abi asks, her face pensive.

"I can't, Abi. I can't just hand him over without knowing who O'Driscoll is or what they did to him." To us. When the hell did they put a brain implant into me and why? I know where to get the answers and it isn't in Dead Rock.

"You shouldn't have gotten involved."

"Too late now. I am involved." Totally and utterly entangled. "And I can't do this to him."

"Are you in love with him?" Abi asks.

"Maybe." Yes. "I don't know." I do and it scares the crap

out of me because there's no way I can have Mars and Crow.

"You obviously have feelings for him."

"For fuck's sake we're sharing memories, Abi, of course I have feelings for him. No one's ever known me the way Crow does. He's *lived* my memories. I've lived his. I know what he's thinking and feeling."

"Does he know everything?" She casts me a furtive glance. Abi has her suspicions about what happened with Wayne but I've never confirmed them and I doubt I ever will.

"He knows plenty." *Inhale.* Count to ten. *Exhale.* "And knowing all that I do about him, I know it ain't right to hand him back to O'Driscoll." *Inhale.* There has to be another way. *Exhale.* Think, think, think dammit!

"You made a deal."

"I'm unmaking it. We're not going to Dead Rock."

"What if they hurt Madison and Nash?"

"They won't." My insides turn to lead, doubt gnawing at every nerve ending. "They're government agents. They can't harm civilians."

"How can you be so sure?"

"As long as I'm with Crow, they'll want Maddy and Nash as bargaining chips, and for that they'll need my family alive."

"This is insane, Raw. You're risking their lives for his." She jerks her head in Crow's direction.

"I know." God, I don't know what to do. "The Bennett Institute is just outside Omaha."

"Raleigh." She shakes her head.

"We need answers and that's where we're gonna get them."

"We need to do what the DHS wants."

"If they're even Homeland Security."

"We should've gone to the cops." Abi chews on her bottom lip and drums her fingers against the steering wheel.

"Like they'd believe this story?"

"If it weren't for his eyes and him slicing up his arm, I'm not sure I'd believe it, either."

Crow twitches, a fresh wash of cerulean water-falling from his ears.

"Aw heck." Abi thumps her fists against the steering wheel. "He's getting worse."

"He needs proper help."

"And your sister needs you to not get her and Nash into trouble. This isn't just about you, or Crow."

"I know, but I can't just hand him over."

"Like hell you can't." The look she gives me is one of unbridled anger. "This is your problem, Raw. Always has been. You can be so selfish and get tunnel vision. Like that thing with Wayne."

"What's Wayne got to do with this?" I bristle.

"Instead of moving on from whatever happened between you two, you tried to solve your problems with your fists and screw everyone around you in the fallout." She speeds up, forcing the truck up to sixty.

"You don't even know the full story, Abigail."

"Doesn't matter. You think you had a hard time in juvie? How'd you think Mads coped with Dale breathing down her neck, with her nutty mother and absent father, huh? You didn't think what your little stint in juvie would do to her, did you? Same way you're not thinking about anyone 'cept yourself right now. Screw the sister that's always bent over backward for you if it means saving this stranger, TMI memory thing or not."

"Abi—"

"Can it, Raw. I'm taking us to Dead Rock because that's where we need to go. I choose Madison, even if you can't." Her words burn as if she's fired up a blowtorch and scorched me to the bone. The warmth from Crow's body soaks into my skin and the charged wave that precedes a memory, ripples up my arm, sinking its claws into my mind before I can argue with Abi.

Body-boarding through the surf off the coast of Hawaii, my thirteenth birthday spent in bed with bronchitis, Rex the mutt we found on the side of the road and saved from death-by-traffic, and the argument that ended in my parents' divorce.

"This is the opportunity of a lifetime," Dad says. Mom doesn't seem convinced.

"This is exactly what you promised me you'd avoid."

"We're talking major advancements in all kinds of technology, the future of mankind."

"What about the future of us, or don't we matter anymore?" Mom's face is streaked with tears. I take my sister's hand and lead her out of the kitchen away from their pained faces and raised voices.

"I already accepted their offer. We're moving to Arlington," Dad says, his words are followed by the sound of splintering ceramics.

"You just decided to uproot this family? What about my career? My whole life is here! And what about the kids?"

"I want this, Melissa. I need to do this. They won't make me this offer again."

My mom's next words shatter me.

"Then I want a divorce."

"Raw, wake up." Abi reaches around Crow and nudges me. "We've got company."

"How long have they been behind us?" I ask, still groggy.

"Been following us since Channing," Abi says. "It's probably nothing."

"Raleigh?" Crow coughs and sits up.

"Hey, how you feeling?"

"Like I've been run over by a bulldozer. What happened?" He scratches at the scabs on his neck and ears.

"You've been unconscious for almost an hour." We're approaching the interstate.

"Did I miss anything?" He yawns and massages his temples.

"I saw another memory." I wish I didn't have to tell him about his parents.

"Like what?"

"Um...." I cast a glance at Abi.

"Here, problem solved." She fiddles in her pocket and produces a pair of earbuds, which she connects to the car stereo and turns up the volume. The music leaks out her ears. She's listening to Weston scream about the evils of the American corporatocracy.

"Your parents were getting a divorce."

"Makes sense." Crow takes a deep breath. "My dad always was a workaholic. I think. Anything else?"

"That was it."

"Any hints about where I'm from?"

"Only that your dad was moving to Arlington."

"Like Arlington, Virginia?" he asks.

"He was talking about the future of mankind and cutting-edge technology. Think he works for DARPA?" I know it's a stretch, but nothing is impossible anymore.

"And that I work for MarsLife? Guess it runs in the family." He tugs his hand through his disheveled hair.

"Did you see anything about me this time?"

"Bits and pieces from your trial." Crow scoots around in his seat so he can look at me. "I know why you never told anyone about that day in the snow, but it's not your fault." His voice cracks and his eyes glisten neon. "You didn't ask for it, and you didn't deserve it."

I squeeze my eyes shut, trying to pry myself from the quicksand of bad memory. Crow wraps his arms around me, and I melt into his lightning-bolt embrace. If I let myself remember, then that day becomes real and what I lost in the snow will be something I can never get back. I've tried so hard to block it out, to pretend it didn't happen, to un-remember the handful of moments that changed my whole fucking life, but it's corrosive and inescapable.

The headlights of the vehicle behind us get bright, and Abi scowls in the rearview mirror. The lights flash like they want us to pull over.

"Look out!" Crow screams and Abi slams on the brakes, moments away from ramming into the back of the stationary vehicle in front of us.

"Dumber than a sack of straw, sitting out here without lights on." Abi pounds her fists against the steering wheel. The car behind us pulls up next to us, boxing us in. The passenger window rolls down and O'Driscoll leans out, gesturing for Abi to do the same.

"Thought we were meeting in Dead Rock." Abi glowers.

"Change of plan, kiddos," O'Driscoll says. Black-clad figures move through the glare of the headlights. More agents, like a SWAT team, and all armed.

"Yeah? And what's that?" I shout out the window.

"We'll be transporting you from here. You and Cozens will travel with us. Your friend can travel with Preston." She jerks her head to the vehicle behind us.

"I thought you only wanted Crow." Abi swallows hard. "Where are you taking Raleigh and me?"

"Government escort." She smiles the same way a hungry coyote might.

"Okay. Give us a minute to pack our things." Abi rolls up her window and turns to face me. "I don't like this."

"Doesn't make sense," Crow says. "I don't think you should go with them."

"Do we have a choice?" Abi asks. Agents spread across the road and up on the shoulder. They've all got their weapons in the their hands, barrels pointed down.

"I don't like that they want to split us up, either."

A hard rapping at my window makes me jump high enough to bash my head against the car roof, and maybe it knocks some sense into me, too. An agent beckons with a hand for me to get out.

"We're not going with them." I lock my door and Crow leans over Abi to do the same with hers.

"Raw, what're you doing?"

"I don't trust them. This wasn't part of the deal."

"Williams, get out of the vehicle!" Preston yells. The weapons are up now, trained on the pickup.

"Maybe if you let me go, they'll leave you alone." Crow slides low in his seat.

"Think they're going to leave witnesses?" I give Abi an apologetic look. "There's a reason they're apprehending us out here where no one can see what's happening."

"What do I do?" Abi hesitates, hands on the wheel.

"Come out now or we'll be forced to shoot!" Preston jerks at Abi's door handle and O'Driscoll's expression slips from faux friendly into full-on fury.

"Drive, Abi. Get us out of here."

"And go where?" She slams the truck into reverse and floors the accelerator.

"Get onto the interstate. They won't try anything with people around."

Abi jerks the wheel and the tires grind through gravel. She changes gears and shoots past the SWAT team scrambling back into SUVs.

"We can't outrun them," Abi says. Her gaze flits to the

rearview mirror every few seconds.

"Get down!" Crow shouts a moment before bullets tear through the back window and Abi screams. We turn onto the interstate, gunning west for Dead Rock.

An SUV screams up behind us and rams into the pickup. The impact slams me into the seatbelt and Abi loses control of the wheel. We swerve across the road, but she manages to keep us off the median. Sweat slicks my palms and fear solidifies in my gut. Another round of bullets thunks into the pickup and the rear wheel bursts. The truck lists badly to the side. There's a rig headed straight for us and Abi can't get control. The semi tries to slow, but there's a truck behind it and another rig in the neighboring lane, all blaring their horns.

"Do something!" Crow yells right before the SUV slams into us again, harder this time, pushing us across the median into oncoming traffic. I risk a look over my shoulder as the vehicle slams into us once more. Abi loses control and the pickup does a somersault. The world is literally spinning and comes to a crunching halt when we tumble into a billboard pylon. Stars obliterate my vision, a cluster of constellations replacing the bleak fields.

I reach for Crow with numb fingers; my bones like lead. It would be so easy to give in, to let the riptide suck me down, but I don't want to die and I don't want Crow to die. Madison shouldn't have to bury another brother. My mom won't survive losing another son. I kick against the currents, but the darkness drags me under.

CROW

"The candidate's vitals spiked, but heart rate is steady." The voice wafts through my mind.

"His scores are off the chart." Another voice.

"Is this your idea of doing well under pressure?"

"You're missing the point." The person sounds excited. **"It's not how he copes with the pressure, it's that he's manipulating the psytek all by himself. Our changes don't last more than a few minutes before he alters the program."**

"Someone's gone and tried to turn you into roadkill." A hand reaches through the darkness and drags me to my feet. His face swims into focus, tendrils of black and brown coalescing into a familiar form.

"West?" Raleigh asks, standing right beside me.

"You reckon your bones would make better wind chimes or a fine set of cutlery?" Weston smiles, showing me the crooked teeth Abi never seemed to mind. His hair lies flat and dark against his skull, shaved along the sides in rock star style. He's wearing the band T-shirt and ripped jeans he died in.

"Am I dead?" Raleigh's words echo in the emptiness. I open my mouth, but no sound comes out. I'm merely a spectator here, trapped in whatever this is. My hands look weird, all sinewy and veined with flickering purple. Not veins, but a lattice of ones and zeros. My skin is a transparent mass of binary code.

We're standing on the interstate flanked by desert scrub that blinks in and out of a digital rendering. There's no wind, not even a whisper of a breeze, not a single cricket chirp or bird call. This isn't real. It's a virtual reality. It must be.

"Do you want to be dead?" Weston saunters past me and crouches beside his bone cross.

"I don't know." Raleigh stands beside him, real and whole

without any numbers rippling through his skin.

"Thanks, by the way." Weston runs his fingers over the bleached bone cross. "I appreciate not being forgotten."

"Never." Raleigh's rubbing his arms like he's got a fire ant infestation beneath his skin. The knots on my forearms itch in sympathy. I rub at the spiral patches of code, but that only makes it worse, the numbers dissipating under my touch.

"I miss you," Raleigh says. Weston gets to his feet and brushes dust off his knees.

"I miss you, too, little bro." He pulls Raleigh into a hug. "Storm's coming." He breaks away and points at the horizon blackened by cumulonimbus. A funnel twists out of the cloud, a spiraling umbilical cord promising destruction as a tornado is born. The twister hurls strings of code across the sky in jagged lightning streaks.

"You oughta go." He claps Raleigh on the shoulder and looks directly at me. The tornado tears up the road, tossing chunks of asphalt like a disgruntled toddler chucking toys. The storm sucks up the peripheral matrix, the force pulling me into the digital vortex. I reach for Raleigh and grab his hand. Weston smiles at me and my fingers tighten on Raleigh's. The scars on his wrists crack open. Blood pools between my fingers, splashing into the dust. The tornado churns closer. The wind shreds Weston into rusty tendrils that twist and float like so much debris. The road disintegrates beneath our feet and blood continues to drip from our arms, Raleigh's red and mine a series of violet numbers, each droplet forming stepping stones over the vast nothing feeding the storm. I don't want to die. Desperate to escape the vortex chewing up the earth, I race across the bloody path, dragging Raleigh behind me.

RALEIGH

It smells like a hospital, like antiseptic and imminent death, but it's quiet. No bustle of nurses, coughing patients, or weeping visitors. I'm strapped down at the wrists and ankles and there's a needle in my arm hooked up to an IV crane. Here's to hoping it's only saline solution trickling through the tube. I've got gummy heart rate monitors stuck to my chest, making my skin itch. Twisting to get a better look at my surroundings makes every joint in my body scream in protest. The car accident. O'Driscoll ran us off the road.

Enduring the pain, I twist as far as the restraints will let me. The room isn't a room at all, but a plastic bubble. Thick, black tape runs in a door-shaped seam on the opposite end of the cell. No toilet, no basin, not a stick of furniture. This is worse than the solitary confinement units in juvie.

I struggle against the padded cuffs and only succeed in hurting my wrists. Footsteps approach and weird shadows ripple beyond the layers of plastic confining me. The seal peels open and a Hazmat-wearing figure enters the room. Behind the protective face plate, the man has salt and pepper hair and kind eyes. The rest of him is housed behind industrial grade rubber.

"Where am I? Who are you? Why am I here?" The machine behind my head beeps in warning as my heart starts kicking the crap out of my sternum. *Inhale.* No point in panicking. *Exhale.* I'm tied down! This man can do whatever he wants to me and I'm defenseless.

My wrists slam painfully into the side-rails of the bed, my feet thrash, but the restraints only get tighter.

"Raleigh, please calm down." The man attempts to soothe me, his voice distant and echoing.

"Untie me." *Now, before I break my hands and then your*

face.

"I will as soon as I'm sure you're not a danger to yourself or to me." He silences the beeping machine with a blue-gloved hand and stands beside me. "I'm Doctor Torres. Do you know where you are?"

I shake my head.

"You're in a specialist ward at a classified location." He clears his throat and shifts his weight between his feet, the material of his suit creaking. "You were in a car accident."

"Then why aren't we at the ER? Where's Crow? Abigail..." Panic claws up my throat and I flail against the cuffs. "You can't keep me here against my will!"

"Raleigh, I'm here to help you." Torres removes a syringe from a silver tray.

"No! I don't need drugs; I need answers." I lunge at him, hoping to head butt him in the face, but the restraints don't let me lean out far enough to do any real damage and the hot poker pain in my ribs leaves me gasping for air.

"And you'll get them once you're calmer. You're hyperventilating." He sticks the needle into the port on my arm. I thrash against the cuffs, bashing my elbows into the rails, kicking and flailing until ice seeps into my veins. Calming, soothing. There's no fighting the drug as it forces my limbs to relax.

"I really am here to help you."

"Please tell me." My tongue is two sizes too big, awkward and clumsy behind my teeth. My eyelids struggle against gravity while Torres checks the bandage on my head with his oversized hands.

"We'll take good care of you. Don't worry. We're going to run some tests and..." His voice slows, the words lost as sedation pulls me under.

I'm floating, traveling along corridors with fluorescent lighting at regular intervals. Disembodied voices drone beneath my threshold of comprehension. A machine whirs around me, the table hard and cold beneath my shoulder blades.

"Try not to move," they tell me, as if I have another choice.

Hands on my shoulders and knees roll me onto my side and bend my legs, their faces obscured by protective suits.

"Hold still." A needle in my spine and creeping headache.

I wish they'd put me under fully. Being half aware of what they're doing to me and powerless to resist is infinitely worse than not knowing. I'm trapped inside my own skin while they poke and prod, scan and analyze. If only one of Crow's memories would whisk me away, but I'm caged in this haze unable to scream and desperate to escape.

CROW

```
tech1@cer-ro:~$ sudo shred -fz -n 10 /dev/sda2


tech1@cer-ro:~$ ./psytek-init.sh && reboot


tech1@cer-ro:~$ chmod +x psytek-2.14.10
```

I'm falling, my body reduced to so much stardust…stardust…
No, scardust. That's what I am.

RALEIGH

The creak of plastic wakes me, and Torres shuffles into the room, tablet in hand. He reads the machines beeping behind my head and makes several notes on the tablet. I want to know what all the data says about me.

"I'm thirsty."

He holds a cup with a straw to my lips, and I gulp down water. My head swims and every inch of me hurts.

"I'll be back later with dinner," he says and prepares to leave.

"Wait!" My voice croaks. "Please tell me what's going on."

"I'm not authorized to discuss it with you."

"Can you at least tell me what I've got implanted in my brain?"

Torres startles and clears his throat. "What implant?"

"The one on the back of my neck. I know it has something to do with the Cerebro-renovo machine."

"I don't know what you're talking about." He heads for the seal in the plastic.

"Hey! Can you at least untie me?"

Torres hesitates.

"Please. I need to pee."

"You've got a catheter," he says.

Inhale. You'll figure it out. *Exhale.* Just stay calm.

"How about giving me a little slack then? Can't a guy even scratch his balls?"

Torres sighs and grudgingly lengthens the straps on the wrist cuffs to the point where I can scratch my chest.

"I'll be back later to check on you." He re-seals the flap and sets off to the left, his surgical slippers whispering across linoleum.

It takes less than thirty seconds of contortion before I rip out the needle in my arm and twist my body, bringing my teeth to my hands. It takes forever to undo the buckles on the wrist cuffs, cutting up the corners of my mouth, but eventually I succeed and get rid of the ankle cuffs, too. The heart monitors leave itchy welts on my chest, but they come away with relative ease. The catheter they've stuck in me presents the greatest challenge. Using the IV needle, I manage to pry open the tubing and let it drain before removing the rest of the plumbing, gritting my teeth as the tube slides free.

As far as weapons go, my options are limited to the needle from my arm, the various machines as bludgeoning tools, and the gurney. The plastic is a hell of a lot thicker than I imagined and even when I peel open the flap, there's another glass sliding door that needs a swipe-card to access. There's a vent at the top of the bubble spewing cool air over me, but the shaft is way too narrow to make a good escape route.

I punch the plastic. It gives like a membrane, absorbing the impact without so much as a fray. Using the needle, I stab into the wall of the bubble. It might as well be leather for all the damage my tiny hypodermic does.

Guess I'll have to wait for Torres to come back to get the jump on him. Every second feels like an eternity, and I try not to think about what might be happening to Crow. Minutes turn to hours although it's hard to tell being stuck in here. By the time footsteps sound in the corridor, there's a jackhammer inside my skull and my throat feels like Arrakis. The steps are heavy, purposeful, and march right up to my bubble.

The doors slide open, plastic unseals, and I launch myself at the suit, except this one's armed and there's a second guy right behind him. I manage to do some damage to the suit, but not much more than that considering the state of my ribs.

"Nice try." The guy, Hughes—or so says his name tag— shuffles me back into the bubble. "Initiate contingency two.

Candidate managed to get free."

"What's contingency two?"

Hughes gestures for his buddy, Grayson, to enter the bubble. He seals the cell and the air coming through the vent drops a few degrees, making me shiver.

I suck in a breath and my head swims, my vision blurring. Hughes curses and catches me before I hit the floor. He manhandles me back onto the bed, and I'm vaguely aware of his hands on my ass hanging naked out the back of my hospital gown.

Torres enters with a sandwich and a jug of orange juice. He inspects my head before helping me sit up.

"If I let you feed yourself, do you promise to behave?" he asks.

"Promise." I'm used to this, telling doctors what they want to hear to get what I want. Torres frees my arms from the restraints.

"I'm sorry about earlier."

"Any headache?" He shines a light into my eyes, ignoring my pseudo-apology.

"Only when I sit up." It's almost bad enough to stop me contemplating escape.

"That's normal. You're still healing from the accident. You should be fine again in a few days, the ribs might take a little longer."

"Please tell me what's going on." I inspect the hospital food. My stomach rumbles with hunger despite the insipid mush that's pretending to be ham and cheese. Suddenly Dale's burritos do seem like Michelin-star cuisine.

"I'm sorry," Torres says and taps at his tablet.

"There was a girl in the car with us. Abigail. Is she here,

too?" I pick at the bread, skirting limp shreds of lettuce.

"I'm so sorry," Torres says. "She didn't make it."

"What?" His words are a knuckle-dusted fist slamming into my gut.

"Her injuries were too severe."

"Where is she?" My words garble with the rage and disbelief tearing up my throat. Abigail is dead. I killed her. She's dead because of me. I will never forgive myself. *I'm sorry West, I'm so sorry.* The tiniest smidgen of comfort is that Abi and Weston can be together now like Abi always wanted.

"In the morgue," Torres says.

I fling the sandwich across the room, showering the plastic wall in mayonnaise. Torres backs away almost as if he's frightened of me. I ignore him, staring at the ceiling as hot tears force a trail across my cheeks. If I'd never been in the desert that night, never found Crow, never tried to help him, then we'd never have been in the car and Abi would be alive and on her way to California. Rotten to the core, just like Dale said.

"And to what do we owe this little tantrum?" O'Driscoll steps inside the cell. I lunge for her, too late remembering my feet are still attached to the gurney, and end up sprawled awkwardly halfway to the floor, the rails hammering my damaged ribs.

"Enough of that." She snaps her fingers. Hughes and Grayson squeeze into the cell. "Good to go?" She addresses Torres and the doctor nods.

"You killed Abigail." I wheeze.

"An unfortunate casualty," she says.

"Why'd you do it?" My voice quavers, my whole body quivering with rage. "I was holding up my end of the deal."

"The situation changed." She shrugs. "That's all you need to know."

"Where are you taking me?" I collapse against the pillows,

temporarily defeated.

"Moving you to more appropriate accommodations," O'Driscoll says. "Let's go then." Hughes and Grayson wheel me out of the cell.

"Where's Crow?"

"Waiting for you." O'Driscoll's smile could freeze over hell. We head to the elevator down a plastic-wrapped corridor. There's a mural on the wall, the image blurred by the plastic, but the spiral is unmistakable. We're at the Bennett Institute.

We drop several stories before they wheel me into what might've been a regular hospital ward except for the glass divisions carving up the room into quarantine units.

"Raleigh." Crow gets to his feet. "Are you all right?" He bashes a fist against the glass and sparks spiderweb across the pane. He yelps and clutches his hand to his chest. They place me in the glass-walled box next to his.

"The glass is electrified," O'Driscoll says. "So don't bother trying to escape." She nods and Hughes unbuckles the restraints. Grayson stands guard with a stun stick in his hand.

"Welcome to your new home. Make yourself comfortable." O'Driscoll and her lackeys step out of the box, taking the gurney with them, leaving me barefoot in a hospital gown. She presses her palm against an access panel on the opposite wall and the glass door slides shut, sealing with an ominous hiss and click of multiple locking mechanisms. They peel off their Hazmat masks and O'Driscoll makes a big show of taking a deep breath before giving me a wink. I slam my fist into the glass, hoping I'll punch right through and wipe the sneer off her face. The force of the shock spins me 180 degrees, my whole arm throbbing.

"Always so violent." O'Driscoll tsks. "See you later, boys." She leaves the ward with Hughes and Grayson trailing in her wake.

"Hey, are you okay?" Crow asks. "Talk to me."

I can't look at him, can't even begin to process all the jumbled, chaotic thoughts and feelings. He's the reason I'm locked up again, the reason Abigail is dead.

I survey my new home instead. My prison is furnished: toilet, basin, bed. There are fresh clothes on the pillow, gray sweats, and white sneakers. It's like being back in juvie. At least I don't have to share this space with another feral delinquent. Beside the clothes, there's a tray of unappetizing hospital food complete with lime green Jell-O. Dressed, I settle on the floor with my dinner. The best thing I can do now is heal and get strong. Next time anyone comes within reaching distance, I'm going to grab a stun-stick and shove it down their throat. Then I'm going to hunt down O'Driscoll and make her suffer. It's the least I can do for Abigail.

My violent thoughts have always scared me. Not this time. This time I sink into them, letting the darkness in my mind wrap around me in comforting strands. Crow watches while I shovel tepid spaghetti into my mouth. He's sitting as close to the glass as he can get without being shocked. His eyes are more electrifying than the pane between us, burning radioactive purple. There are new scars dotting his neck.

"Abigail's dead." The words burn my lips.

"I'm sorry," he says. "Jesus, I'm so sorry." He runs his hands through his hair. "If we'd let O'Driscoll take me back at the hospital, then Abigail—"

"Enough!" None of this is Crow's fault. He didn't ask me to haul him out the desert; he didn't get Abi involved. O'Driscoll is the real enemy here, not Crow.

Abandoning the remnants of my dinner, I study the serrations on the plastic knife. It's not as good as a razor blade, but it'll do. Dragging the plastic across my skin, I complete a shallow circumference of my forearm, an inch higher than the scars for West. I do it again and again, blood welling like tears in the grooves of the widening gash. The knife loses its edge, becoming useless after too few circuits on only one wrist. It'll have to do until I can get a scalpel blade and slice through my skin as deep as Abi's death cuts into my heart.

"For Abigail?" Crow asks.

I nod and rest my arm on my knee.

"Can we talk?"

"Not now." I peel open the tub of Jell-O and squeeze the contents into my mouth as blood from my wrist dots the pale linoleum. Dinner complete, I retreat to the bed and ease myself onto the hard mattress.

"Raleigh?"

"I don't want to talk, Crow. I want to sleep and hope to hell that when I wake up none of this will be real." My words are harsh, fueled by the coiling pain in my chest and the stinging in my wrist. Weston, Abigail—I could've saved them both and I didn't. I might not have killed Wayne that day, but I'm no less a murderer.

CROW

Raleigh sprawls across his bed, left foot dangling off the edge and his hair a dark cloud across the pillow. I haven't been able to sleep much since we arrived. The voices won't shut up, an incessant chatter about protocols and algorithms, databases and Searle's Chinese room. I can't make any sense of it, and what little I do understand, I wish I didn't because, all things considered, it seems unlikely that I'm human.

My eyes have stopped hurting, although goo still occasionally leaks out of my ears, which only confirms the not-human theory.

Raleigh twitches, and I stalk closer to the glass. His back rises and falls, lips slightly parted. He's here because of me. Inadvertent or not, this is all my doing. I'm already responsible for Abigail's death. I won't be responsible for Raleigh's. If there's a way out of here, I'm going to find it, and I'll take down anyone who gets in my way.

His breathing pattern changes and he stirs, rolling over and opening his eyes. It takes several long moments before he finally speaks.

"Have you been watching me all night?"

"Not *all* night. God, how boring." My quip almost gets him to crack a smile. "Might want to mop up some of that drool."

"I do not drool." He wipes his mouth and this time the smile makes contact with his cheeks.

"It's okay. It's cute."

With a chuckle, he rolls out of bed and pads on bare feet to the glass partition separating us. I blink and the world changes color. Raleigh stands limned in reds and oranges. The bed is cool blue like most of the furnishings. Regardless of the color, the world around me has been reduced to digits like that scene in *The Matrix* only I'm damn sure I'm not Neo, and if I am seeing the code behind my world, it's all ones and zeros.

"Whoa." I study my code-pulsing hands.

"What's wrong?"

"I think I'm seeing in infrared…and then some."

"For real?" As if to test the theory, Raleigh holds out a hand and splays his fingers. The sequence of numbers scrolling down his arm are different but no less binary.

"Jesus, Raleigh. What the fuck is happening to me?"

"When did it start?"

"Right now. I think you might've been right about me not being human." My voice cracks, emotion cutting through the chaos of my senses and my vision slowly reverts back to normal. I take a deep breath as the numbers dissipate.

"I don't want to be an alien or Brennan Cozens. I just want to be your Crow."

"*My* Crow?" He raises his eyebrows.

"You heard me." I crumple to the floor. Wrapping my arms around my knees, I rock back and forth. No matter how hard I fight against reality, no matter how hard I wish this wasn't happening, that it was all some incredibly fucked up dream, I can't escape the prison I'm in, the prison my body and my whole world is becoming.

"We need to get out of here," Raleigh says. "Maybe we could get in touch with your dad. If he works for the government, he might be able to help."

"I don't know where he is. I don't even know where *we* are!"

"We're at the Bennett Institute. I saw the logo on the wall."

Bennett. A sense of rightness, of belonging settles in my gut, like maybe this is where we need to be after all. Even if I did work here, though, that still doesn't explain how I ended up in the desert.

I press my hand against the glass and electricity snaps

into my fingers, sharp and painful, but not as bad as last time. Perhaps I'm becoming immune. I press my hand to the glass again, gritting my teeth against the bone-breaking voltage. I last only five seconds before yanking back my arm.

"I'm sorry about Abigail." My gaze drops to the scabs on Raleigh's wrists. "About everything."

"It's not your fault. It's O'Driscoll's." His expression darkens and the look in his eyes now means he's ready to hurt someone, hurt them like he did Wayne. As long as it's O'Driscoll on the receiving end of his wrath, I'll do everything in my power to help him.

"I meant what I said, Raleigh." My stomach churns with the admission. "I know the timing sucks, but I'm yours if you want me."

"Shittiest timing ever." A wry smile tugs at his lips before folding into something far more serious. He sighs and shakes his head, and I wait him out with my heart threatening to catapult from my chest.

"I..." he starts. "I thought I knew what I wanted. I've only ever wanted Mars."

"And now?"

"And now I want you." He meets my gaze with fathomless eyes. "I want you maybe even more than Mars, and that terrifies me."

RALEIGH

This routine is getting old.

Every morning they wake us up at the ass-crack of dawn and escort us through a maze of interconnected chambers to a training room complete with fancy gym equipment. Grayson and Hughes preside over Hazmat-clad doctors. They hook us up to a variety of machines before they make us run on treadmills, completing virtual programs of ever-increasing difficulty. Even with my busted ribs, I was scoring higher than Crow, but he's getting fitter and stronger. Push-ups, bench presses, sit-ups, jump rope— It's boot camp and we even have a drill sergeant. Grayson stands constant watch, hand on his stun-stick in case we step out of line.

The afternoons are dedicated to mental exercises: puzzles and math problems and tests like the one we did in kindergarten to measure IQ, even language learning. Crow whips my ass when it comes to math and grammar, but it turns out I'm the puzzle king. After that, we're usually subjected to medical tests: MRIs, EEGs, and a dozen other acronymed procedures that leave me feeling like a pin-cushion.

"Ready?" I whisper across the table to Crow. He's concentrating on a set of epically difficult Sudoku puzzles I already solved while I struggle to learn the Russian alphabet. He looks up at me, eyes bright purple.

Surreptitiously, he leans forward and slides his hand across the table. Using our tablets for cover, we grip each other's fingers. It's worse than getting zapped by the voltage in our cells. I stifle a yelp and grit my teeth, keeping my fingers on his even when they start to throb. I close my eyes and let the memory crash into me.

"*Welcome to the Bennett Institute.*" *Sofia Perez extends her hand, giving me a bright smile.*

"*It's an honor to be here.*" *I shake her hand, not quite believing the director herself has come down from the upper echelons to meet me, a lowly new programmer.*

"*We're delighted to have you onboard the MarsLife program. Given the recent catastrophe with the Endeavour, we need new protocols now more than ever.*"

"*Doctor Torres told me you were particularly interested in the AI project I've been working on.*"

"*Yes.*" *She gestures for me to join her as we pass through a series of sliding glass doors to begin a tour of the restricted access areas. The Bennett Institute is a dream come true. Forget DARPA and the military stuff my dad is working on; the private sector and space tech is where it's at, and no one does it better than Bennett.*

"*We want you to adapt your program for our aptitude tests.*"

"*Doctor Torres said the cognitive tier would be top priority.*" *I follow her down pristine corridors, past rows of high-tech labs. I can't wait to start here! How many other twenty-one year olds have walked out of college and straight into their dream job?*

"*Actually, we'd prefer you work on the psychological. It wasn't cognitive impairment that caused the problems on the Endeavour.*"

She opens a door and gestures for me to step through first. The office is at the corner of the building with large windows looking out over the Offutt airbase. It's a stark reminder that although the company technically isn't government run, the work I do here is still tied to military operations.

"*This is your office. A tech will be up shortly to walk you through digital security procedures. I understand you've already been debriefed about physical security?*"

"Yes." An unpleasant half hour that involved the threat of cavity searches should I be suspected of walking in or out with contraband.

"Shall I show you to your lab?"

Feeling like a nerdy kid in a hobby shop, I bounce after her, barely able to contain my excitement. Tony Stark can kiss my ass! This is awesome—glass and silicone and computers more powerful than any I've ever seen.

"When do I start?" I ask.

"Right now." She gives me a smile. "We're expecting great things from you, Brennan. And I don't think I need to remind you that we're on a tight schedule. The Entropy is due for takeoff in less than three years, and we'll need to screen every candidate a year in advance."

"I understand you're planning to host open aptitude tests as well."

"Once your program is ready, yes. A trial run for the new protocols if you like." She checks her watch and tsks. "My apologies, but I have another engagement. Again, welcome to Bennett and to MarsLife."

She sashays out the lab, leaving me to stare in awe at my brand new work space.

"It's not nap time." Grayson shouts and we retract our fingers, sliding out of the memory and back into reality.

"Sofia Perez," I whisper.

"Who's that?" Crow asks.

"The Director of the Bennett Institute. She hired you to create a program for the MarsLife tests."

Crow's eyebrows shoot up at that. "A computer program?"

"Yeah, something about new protocols. Sound right?"

"It's starting to."

I want to ask what he saw of my life, what new nightmare he endured, but Grayson gets in first.

"Time's up," he says. "You know the drill."

Grayson and Hughes escort us to the medical wing. Torres is waiting and O'Driscoll stands beyond the glass in a tailored suit, left arm still in a sling from where Crow shot her. She's a sadistic cow, always sitting in on the medical stuff like she enjoys watching us getting poked and prodded, or maybe she just likes seeing us mostly naked.

"What do you want today?" I shed my hoodie and T-shirt. "More blood, maybe brainwaves?"

"Something far more exciting." O'Driscoll smiles and Torres frowns through the Hazmat mask. "Today we'll be assessing your regenerative abilities."

"Aren't they obvious?" Crow asks.

"What regenerative abilities?" I hold up my scarred wrists. The marks I cut for Abigail are scab-free rings of keloid.

"We know Crow's cells can regenerate. We'd like to measure healing rates against a human baseline. You."

Implying Crow isn't human?

"You do realize we feel pain, right?" Fear flows acidic through my veins.

"Yes," she says with an arctic smile. "Part of what we'll be testing is Crow's pain threshold and endurance."

"This is torture." Crow addresses Torres. "You're a doctor, you swore the Hippocratic Oath, and now you're going to torture us?"

"I'm sorry." Torres looks anywhere but at us.

"This is for the greater good," O'Driscoll adds. "The more we understand about you, the better we can develop this technology to help people."

"Is that why we're here?" Rage blurs my vision; my fists clench. "Lab rats in some experiment gone wrong?"

"Who said anything's gone wrong?" Her smile widens

and the urge to break something becomes a throbbing need. "We're right on track. Please, begin. We're on a schedule here."

"Does Sofia Perez know what you're doing?"

O'Driscoll blinks at me several times as if she doesn't understand the question.

"Crow used to work here, and now he's a guinea pig. Something must've gone wrong." I glance at Crow. He's massaging his temples and mumbling "shut up" under his breath.

"Whatever this is, please, you don't have to hurt Raleigh," Crow says, breathless, his face contorted by pain as he grabs his head.

"I'm sure Raleigh won't mind a few minor injuries considering what he's inflicted upon himself," O'Driscoll says.

"Screw you."

"So much anger, Billy-bob." She nods at Grayson who shoves a stun stick into my back, herding me toward one of two gurneys set up side by side. Hughes does the same to Crow.

I launch myself at Grayson before I reach the gurney, shoving my scarred fists into the face plate. It cracks, but doesn't break. A stun-stick makes contact with my bare flesh and pain explodes across my back. My muscles seize and I slide sideways off the bleeding soldier. His nose must've bounced off the face plate.

"Contain him!" O'Driscoll yells.

Hughes slams the stun-stick into my chest. My vision turns brilliant white and my muscles go rigid enough to break bones.

"Raleigh!" Crow screams my name and rough hands haul me off the floor.

"Ready to get diced, freak?" Blood gloms Grayson's upper lip. He forces me onto the gurney and straps me down.

"When I get out of here—" I spit at O'Driscoll, but she's

too far away and beyond a layer of thick glass. "I'm going to slice your face off, stab the blade through your shriveled heart, and leave you to die." The words spew out of my mouth. Maybe then Abi's death won't feel so meaningless, won't be such a waste of life.

"How terrifying." O'Driscoll gets to her feet. "But until then, you're going to bleed for me."

"You can't do this. We have rights! This is illegal," Crow yells.

"*Human* rights." O'Driscoll laughs.

Fear turns into anger, a molten stew in my gut threatening to erupt.

"I'm sorry," Torres says as he bears down on me with a scalpel blade.

CROW

I study my newly formed pinkie. The base of the finger sports the same spiral symbol as the ones on my arms. Another Bennett logo. At least I've got all ten fingers again. Not that that's good news. Tomorrow they might amputate my whole arm.

"Deleting the database hasn't made much of a difference. It's erased a few memories, but it hasn't altered much more than that."

Shut up! I press my hands over my ears, trying to block out the voices.

"You'll have to scrub the drive." That's a voice I'm starting to recognize, irritatingly familiar.

"Not yet."

"Williams can't withstand much more of this." I know that voice! It's Doctor Torres.

"He'll have to."

"You awake?" Raleigh whispers and the voices recede as I focus on the now. At least they didn't dismember him, stopping short of causing any permanent damage. Even so, he's sporting stitches in his chest beneath a layer of bandages while all I get are more scars.

"Can't sleep. How's the chest?"

"Hurting, but could've been worse. You okay?"

"Only a lingering headache."

His silhouette pauses, hands raised and testing the air in front of him. His fingers brush against the glass, igniting a corona in the shape of his hand.

"I can't believe they're doing this to us." Raleigh settles on the floor opposite me, arms wrapped around his knees.

"What you said earlier about Perez and those protocols." I tug my hands through my hair. "I think I might have a theory."

"What is it?"

"What if—what if none of this is real?"

"Feels plenty real to me." His fingers splay across the wounds in his chest.

"Yeah, but stuff would feel real in a virtual reality. I mean, isn't that the whole point?"

"Like we're inside some sort of computer game?" He laughs. "I wish, Crow. But I think that's wishful thinking."

"Immersive gaming is huge right now. You ever played Calamity City or Lost Epochs using a VR helmet?" I used to play for hours, losing days at a time of reality.

"They weren't big on those in juvie."

"Right, well, suffice it to say you are fully immersed in the virtual landscape of the game. The helmet caters to all your senses. There's nothing like the aroma of grilled flesh courtesy of dragon fire."

"But those games don't allow you to feel pain. They have their limitations."

"True, but I don't know how else to explain the voices I'm hearing." Unless I'm having a psychotic break.

"You fell out of the sky, remember? I don't think you hearing voices is the strangest thing that's happened to you."

"I recognize one of the voices." As improbable as it may seem. "I think it's Doctor Torres."

"So maybe it's a memory." Raleigh shrugs. "You could know him from working here."

"It's not the same. I'm telling you, there's something weird."

"You think?" He snickers but he's not hearing me, unwilling or unable to grapple with the concept. Maybe there's a way I could show him, prove to him that we're in some sort of simulation being controlled extrinsically.

"If this isn't real, if it's a virtual creation, then we can control it. We should be able to manipulate it."

"Who says we're the ones in control?" Raleigh asks, incredulous.

"Worth a try, isn't it? If it means figuring a way out of here. Besides, the voices said you were the one calling the shots."

"I doubt that, but sure, let's give it a try. What do we do?"

Gingerly, I lift my hand and Raleigh mirrors me on the other side of the glass.

"This isn't real and if it isn't real then the barrier between us doesn't exist."

The jolt when we touch the glass makes my teeth ache.

"Real enough for you?" He shakes out sore fingers.

"Let's try again. You've got to believe that there's nothing between us."

"There's a lot between us," he says with a solemnity that makes my whole body ache to hold him.

"You know what I mean. Let's try it."

"Are we going on faith or science here?" Raleigh frowns and lifts his hand once more.

"A bit of both. Ready?"

He nods and we press our hands to the glass. Electricity spiderwebs across the partition, a purple lattice.

"Keep your hand there." I grit my teeth, and Raleigh clenches his jaw as we endure the pain. The electricity dissipates in a snap-crackle trail of code, dripping numbers like when my vision did its infrared thing. I feel like there's something I should remember; that there's something I'm missing. The glass melts between our palms, turning into fine mist until skin meets skin.

I pull Raleigh into an embrace. He hugs me back, crushing me against his chest. A familiar static charge races across our skin. "We did it."

"But what did we do exactly?" he asks, his eyes dark pools of shadow in the dimly lit room.

"We just figured a way out of here." But my exuberance

is short lived.

"This isn't good."

"Can we do something?"

"A hard reset might help."

No, no, no. We're so close to getting out of here.

"Please don't do this," I whisper to the voices in my head.

"The cycle is nearing completion anyway. Do you really want—"

"Yes. Do it now."

```
tech1@cer-ro:~$ reboot
```

"Crow?" Raleigh's fingers lace through mine. "You okay?"

Shaking and shivering, the electricity between us surges up and down my arms, swimming through my skin as if I have electric eels for veins. Before my brain has time to process what's happening, my mouth finds Raleigh's, and my body goes supernova.

Silently, I rise from my place on the floor and lead him to my bed. His gaze meets mine, and I'm melting, into his eyes, into this moment. My vision flickers in and out of infrared combined with screeds of binary code. I wish I could control it, but it doesn't matter: Raleigh's beautiful across all the spectra.

"Shouldn't we be—"

"No." Not when he's looking at me like he wants to climb inside my skin. "There is nothing else we should be doing right now."

Even if Raleigh has been reduced to a flickering column of ones and zeros. Even if they chop off my head tomorrow and it never grows back. This moment is real to me right now, and that's all that matters. I need to hold him, to show him what I've only been able to tell him.

With gentle fingers, he brushes a curl off my face, and trails a wicked wake of sparks down my cheek.

Raleigh's thumb presses against my lips. "Do you believe things happen for a reason?" His other hand slips beneath my shirt.

"Yes."

"Me, too. I've got to. Else everything that happened—" He shakes his head. "And it might not even be real. Do you think Weston and Abi being dead is real? What about Bear?"

"I don't know." I want to say something profound and meaningful, but it's hard to string sentences together while undoing the drawstring on Raleigh's sweatpants. "But I know that this right now is as real as it's going to get."

"My whole life I've wanted to be something more than just a redneck from West Texas. To escape what I am and what that place made me: a criminal, a whore, a failure."

"You're not a whore or a failure," I whisper and nibble his ear.

"Just a criminal then?"

"I am, too, you know, considering I shot O'Driscoll."

He kisses me, and I can tell he's smiling.

"I've always wanted to go to Mars," he says. "And instead, a piece of Mars came to me." His hands slip between my legs, and I stop breathing.

"The universe doesn't always give us what we want," I manage to say when I can breathe again, albeit in ragged gasps.

"You're right." He tugs my shirt over my head. "Sometimes it gives us what we need."

I can't hold back anymore: I kiss him, pulling him down on top of me. I want him. I need him, something raw and earthy, even if we wake up tomorrow to find out none of this was real. My reality right now is Raleigh: his skin and tongue and his hair like silk between my fingers.

"May I?" I pause before gathering up the hem of his shirt.

He nods, and, gently, I peel off his shirt. The wounds beneath the bandages on his chest burn a deeper red in my vision, hot and painful.

"We don't have to do this if it hurts."

"I've had worse," he says with a grin.

Easing him onto his back, I kiss a path of tiny lightning bolts down his chest and across his ripped stomach. I follow the V of his abs and liberate the rest of him from clothing.

"You don't have to do that," he says. I lick and kiss his thighs, moving ever closer to his erection.

"I want to." I know from his memories how he feels about this, how dirty he's felt, how used and worthless. I want to show him how different it can be. I want to taste every inch of his skin and lick every hollow. Maybe it should gross me out knowing who and what he's done, but it doesn't. If anything, it makes me more determined to make love to him.

He gasps when I close my mouth around him. He tastes so good. As I work lips and hands in unison, Raleigh traces spirals up and down my back until his spine arches and his fingers knot in my hair.

"I want you, Crow."

Goose bumps flare across my skin in response as I kiss my way up his body, my teeth grazing his nipple, before my mouth meets his and I roll him on top of me.

"Then have me."

"Really?" He frowns, hesitating, and driving me crazy.

"If you're okay with it."

"I've never been more okay with anything in my life, but..." He trembles. "Are you okay with this, I mean, you know—"

"I do know, and it doesn't matter. I want you, the Raleigh that's here right now. Leave the past where it belongs." I kiss him slow and deep, easing him into me. A jolt of pure ecstasy sizzles through my veins, the electricity between us making my whole body thrum.

I want to stay in the now, to feel Raleigh move against me, skin to skin, but the invading tide threatens to consume me. I kick against it, but resistance is futile and we're swept away by friscalating threads of code.

RALEIGH

Crow's head rises and falls on my chest with every breath. Our legs entwine and he's so warm. Too warm. Trying not to wake him, I ease off the bed to wash my face in the basin. The wounds in my chest burn. Maybe I tore open the stitches last night. Last night... The first time I've ever had sex and actually enjoyed it.

I peel off the bandage and eight black stitches fall to the floor like dead spiders. I should have four identical cuts of varying depth running vertical down my chest. Instead I've got a convoluted spiral like the one all over Crow, ivory where his are pale purple.

"Holy shit." If this means what I thinks it means...

"What is it?" Crow sits up and looks at me with inhuman eyes. I turn to face him and point at my chest.

"That's not a good sign." He steps out of bed, padding across the floor to examine me.

"At least I heal, right?"

"Now they'll carve up both of us." Crow yawns, his hair disheveled and adorable. The desire to kiss him and throw him back into bed makes my blood pump like burning oil.

"That ends today." They're not going to touch either of us again. "Get dressed. We're getting out of here." I gather up our jumbled clothes and tug on a T-shirt.

"How exactly?"

"Same way we melted the glass."

He raises an eyebrow and pulls on clean underwear.

"Like you said. None of this is real." I slip my feet into sneakers and fasten the laces. "If we can think our way past the partition, we can think our way outta the building."

"So now you believe me?" He tugs on his clothes.

"There's a lot about the past couple of weeks I wish

wasn't real."

"A lot?" Crow catches his bottom lip with a top incisor.

"Last night is definitely not on the list of regrets."

"If nothing else, I'd like to believe the connection we share is real." His irises gleam livid purple.

"Time to go."

"We just walk out of here?"

"Why not?" I press my palm against the glass door keeping us trapped. The voltage slams into my fingers causing an ache all the way to my shoulder.

"Try together?" Crow joins me, and I brace myself as we place our hands on the glass. We both jump back as the electricity shoots through our nerves.

"So much for that theory," he says.

"This isn't real." I slam my fist into the partition only to be rewarded with another bolt of voltage. "It worked last night. Why isn't it working now?"

"Have faith, Raleigh," Crow says. "Thoughts have powers of reality, remember? So stop thinking." He grabs my hand and presses our palms against the glass.

CROW

Our fingers snag on the glass. It's become all sticky and malleable. The voltage surges through me, vibrating every atom in my body. The voices are back, a chorus of confusion, but I ignore them, trying my best to tune them out and focus only on Raleigh.

He's wearing a lopsided smile when we step across the threshold, the glass disintegrating in our wake. I feel strange, not quite weightless, but less dense somehow. My fingers glow an eerie translucent purple. Raleigh tightens his grip.

No memories this time, not even a prickle of static, just the unquestionable sense of completeness, of being whole. We walk out of the cell hand in hand.

"We did it." Raleigh glances in wonder over his shoulder. "We're free."

"Almost." My sense of self withers and reforms. I am not Crow. I am not Brennan Cozens. I am both and neither, an amalgamation, an iteration, a numinous entity that is becoming between two multiplicities even as I feel myself breaking apart, unwinding and threading coded ribbons through Raleigh's blood. *We* are becoming.

I squeeze his fingers, and he flinches. Ivory vines wrap around his fingers, meandering up his hands. The Bennett logos bloom like flowers across the flesh of his arms, and his breath catches in his throat. New marks coil up my own arm.

"What's happening?"

"We'll figure it out once we get out of here." I cup Raleigh's face and pale tendrils splay across his cheek from the point of contact, knotting binary spirals through his flesh.

RALEIGH

Part of me understands what's happening as another rejects the possibility. Crow changes rapidly as if the jolt from the glass quick-fired his transformation. And he's not the only one who's changing. Just like Crow, I'm becoming littered with the Bennett logo.

Excitement and terror vie for control while strings of code radiate from our joined hands, slither up my arms, and spread across my bare chest. I should let go. I should run a million miles from him, but I don't want to and all I can think about is Mars.

I follow where he leads and together we pad from the quarantine area, passing through various layers of security by the power of thought alone.

"What now?" I ask.

"We need to find the real." He looks at me with flickering eyes. We step into the elevator and the code surges down my spine in static traceries. There's no memory share this time. It's unnecessary. I know everything I need to about Crow. I punch the button for the exit.

The elevator chimes and the doors open on a thicket of fire power. Soldiers fan out across the lobby in full riot gear, and at the front of the formation, O'Driscoll wields a semi-automatic.

She scowls. "Going somewhere?"

We're going to die. There's no way out. This is where our story ends.

"It's not real," Crow whispers, and I want to believe him, but the gun aimed at my head begs to differ.

"Nice and easy, boys." O'Driscoll gestures for the soldiers to move in. "No need for anyone else to get hurt."

"On your knees." Preston yells from the right, looking

down the barrel of his gun at us.

"We're not going to die," Crow says. "Not like this."

"I trust you."

He kisses me, a fleeting press of lips.

"On your knees, Williams. Don't make this any harder than it already is," O'Driscoll says. I want to obey, but I can't. Crow won't let me, determined to stand his ground.

"Permission to terminate the candidate?" Preston asks.

O'Driscoll gives the order, and Preston pulls the trigger.

RALEIGH

There's something weird about the light; that, or I'm dead. Everything screams at me in Technicolor, as if the whole world got doused in neon. My thoughts scatter like the night Crow crash landed. Again, time expands, an elastic band stretching and snapping, giving me whiplash as I hurtle along a convoluted trajectory. The memories cascade—a jumble of mine and Crow's, ours lives threshed and rewoven, this time intertwined.

I search the maelstrom, but I am alone. No, not alone. I have Crow, his hand still locked in mine. My thoughts turn into a kaleidoscope of agony, my mind stretched beyond breaking point. I am being ripped apart, dismantled atom by atom. There's a purity to the pain; it's exquisite and transcendent.

I'm melting, no, melding. Our bodies become one on a particle level, our atoms entangling, the energy an ebb and flow through both of us, a tide cresting in a giant wave, threatening to wash both of us away. Reality turns liquid, dissolving as a new horizon washes across my world.

"He's coming around." A familiar voice cuts through the murk and my body comes alive with needles and pins. My lashes are gummed down, and I can't open my eyes.

"Give me a moment." A warm, soft flannel wipes my face. Fingers pry open my lids and flash a light in my eyes.

"Have a drink."

I find the straw pressed to my lips and suck in a mouthful of cold water.

"You might be a bit dizzy, but do you think you can sit up?"

I murmur assent and strong hands help me, my legs

swiveling off the side of the bed. For a moment, the world spins like it's tearing off its axis, but I blink and objects realign the right way up. A blanket wraps around my shoulders. I'm only wearing a pair of boxers.

Using the heels of my hands, I rub at my eyes and my vision clears enough for me to recognize the face peering attentively into mine.

"Doctor Torres?"

"Welcome back, Raleigh." He presses a juice box into my hand, and I start sipping sickly sweet orange juice before surveying the room. Not a room, a lab, and the bed I'm sitting on—I freeze. The headpiece at the top looks so much like the Cerebro-renovo contraption.

It *is* the Cerebro-renovo device. My hand flies to the back of my head, my shaved head. There's a scar on the back of my neck no bigger than my thumbnail. Unlike the contraption I saw in Crow's memories, this one doesn't have centipede fronds, but an octopus-like EEG cap. My scalp bears the gummy fingerprints from its sensors. I can't help checking my arms and sides for the Bennett logo just in case. My skin is pristine. Except for my wrists. A single bracelet of keloid rings each hand. My brother is dead.

Doctor Torres slides back into view on a wheelie chair with a tablet in his hand.

"How are you feeling?" he asks. "Do you know where you are?"

"Crappy." I take another sip of orange juice. "Bennett Institute, Omaha."

"And do you know why you're here?" He lifts a bushy brow.

The memories scuttle about in my brain, slip-sliding back into place, and I grasp hold of reality. This is real, it has to be.

"I'm here for testing?"

"Yes, and your psych evaluation is now complete."

Doctor Torres marks something on his tablet. "You'll be escorted back to your room for recuperation. Disorientation and confusion is normal so if you're feeling a little off balance, don't worry about it."

"Did I pass?"

"We'll know that in a few days." Torres gestures to someone behind me.

"Wait, does that mean Abigail is alive?" My breath hitches, waiting for an answer. No scars on my wrist for Abi. *Please let her be alive.*

"What you experienced in the psychscape can be traumatic." Torres turns pensive.

"You think?" Traumatic seems an understatement.

"But it wasn't real, not exactly," Torres adds.

"What do you mean, not exactly?" My fingers tighten their grip on the juice box, the cardboard buckling as my knuckles turn white and my thoughts turn to Crow.

"I'd like you to see me tomorrow morning at nine."

"Why?" I'm tired of being poked and prodded. I want answers, dammit!

"Routine checkup and debrief after the test. We can talk about anything worrying you then, but first I'd like to give you some time to adjust back to reality."

"That's it?" I ask. The orderly, Hughes, appears with a wheelchair.

"For now. Yes." He smiles and nods at Hughes. "Give yourself some time, Raleigh. We'll chat tomorrow."

"It's fine, I can walk." I push off the bed, but my legs have other plans. I collapse into Hughes's arms before he plonks me into the chair. He wheels me down the corridors, past walls daubed with the logo I last saw carved into Crow.

Crow. He doesn't exist. None of it was real, all part of the psychscape.

"Someone will bring you dinner." The orderly deposits me

in my room with a gentle smile so different from the Hughes who was wearing a Hazmat suit. This room isn't the ascetic prison in the nightmare Bennett, but a proper bedroom, complete with a giant *Dune* poster on the wall above my bed and a dozen books about astrophysics. Having pulled on sweats, I collapse on the bed and stare at the ceiling, trying to get my bearings.

First order of business, call Abigail. It goes straight to voicemail and my insides twist into convoluted Möbius strips.

Clenching my jaw so hard my teeth ache, I dial Madison. She answers after an eternity of ringing and relief floods my body at the sound of her voice.

"How'd it go?" Madison asks. "It's so good to finally hear from you."

"Better and worse than expected."

"Mama wants to know when you get the results?" she asks.

"Mama's with you?"

"Of course. Leigh, are you okay?"

The memory of Mama's trailer out in the desert frays and dissipates. There's no way Madison would let our mother live out alone like that. Mama lives in a trailer, but it's parked around the back of the house. Always has been, giving Mama the illusion of privacy while keeping her close to her remaining kids.

"I'm fine. Groggy is all. Have you heard from Abigail?"

"Not for a while now. You haven't called her yet?"

"Got voicemail." Dread sinks ice-cold talons into my heart.

"I'm sure she's just busy with her new job and all. Hold up, Nash wants to say somethin.'"

Madison hands over the phone, and I spend the next few minutes listening to Nash babble about how Bear ate his new sneaker. Maddy comes back online and I promise to let her know once I get the results. We hang up but there's a brass-knuckled fear still bashing at my skull.

My family are all well, and Bear is alive and eating shoes. If only I could hear from Abigail, then the universe would be as it should be. And yet, disorientated doesn't even begin to cover how I feel. I signed up for this and knew from the start that undergoing the advanced neural inquiry of Cerebro-renovo would be an ordeal unto itself.

My fingers stray to the scar on my head, feeling around the edges for the neural chip I've got embedded in my brain stem. That's how they got inside my head, or rather how the AI interface interacted with me in the psychscape.

That's all Crow was, an advanced AI that morphed and developed according to the vagaries of my imagination and induced stress situations. He wasn't real. Brennan doesn't exist.

Not real, not exactly. Torres's words taunt me.

Crow, the person, might not be flesh and blood, but what happened in the psychscape felt plenty real. And the way I felt about him—it doesn't get any more real than that.

I'm not sure how to mourn Crow: like he was someone who died? Or do I just get over him the way I imagine people do after a breakup? Problem is, I'm not sure I want to.

A knock at the door jerks me from my thoughts.

"Come in." I haul my ass off the bed, half expecting Torres to arrive with my expulsion papers.

"Hi, can I come in?" A guy with unruly hair stands on the threshold. He's wearing cargo pants and a black T-shirt that reads *Tesla > Edison*. I like this guy already.

"Who are you?"

"That's what I wanted to discuss." He runs a hand through his hair. "Can we talk?"

"I suppose. Are you also a candidate?"

He checks the corridor before closing the door and folds

his arms, looking uncomfortable.

"No, I'm an employee." Although he isn't wearing a name badge and security pass on a lanyard like all the others. "Specifically, I'm a cer-ro specialist. I designed the psytek AI."

"But you're so young."

"You don't think twenty-three year olds can write wicked cool code?" His face splits into a wide grin. "I've got an M.S. from CalTech."

"Sorry, it's just —"

"No worries, man. Also, it's not like I did it single-handedly. Anyway." He waves away my apology like so much dust in the wind and takes a seat on my desk chair, gesturing for me to sit on the bed.

"You still haven't told me your name."

"I'm coming to that." He drags his hand through his hair again, leaving his fingers at the nape of his neck. The gesture reminds me so much of Crow. My stomach tightens around emptiness. Trust me to fall in love with a figment of my imagination.

"This is awkward." He chews on his bottom lip. "I... It's just, well, this is a little unorthodox."

"What is?" I rest my elbows on my knees, letting my gaze roam over his face. He's good-looking in a bookish sort of way. He's cute with his thick black hair and blue eyes, which I can see smoldering even with him sitting across the room from me.

"Everything. But if anyone asks, we never had this chat, okay?"

I swallow hard and nod. He chews on the cuticle of his thumb.

"I'm not sure how much you remember of your 'scape, but I thought you should know that your experience was rather unique."

"Unique?" My stomach flips somersaults. I don't want to

be anomalous, I want to pass this test and get certified for Mars training. I made a promise to West, and I have to keep it.

"Your results are unprecedented."

"Wait, you know my results?"

"I'm the one who drafts the data," he says. "I'm head of the architecture team. It started as a third year software program back at CalTech until MarsLife snapped it up. Now I'm doing my PhD on cer-ro tech. I've been developing the AI for MarsLife for two years." He sounds pleased with himself. I don't care about any of that; all I want are my results.

"I recently wrote in some changes," he says. "Improvements to the efficacy of the interface. I made it smarter and more sensitive."

"What has this got to do with me?" *Just get to the point already.*

"Since you were the first candidate to deal with the new interface, I was in charge of the 'scape and, boom, dude, you blew me away." His hand gestures mimic his words.

"Just tell me if I passed or not."

"Passed?" A grin slides sideways onto his face. "Man, you have no idea."

I raise my eyebrow, and he takes a deep breath before starting. "So, normally the psytek AI gets inside the mind of the candidate and starts mirroring the psyche. We throw certain stimuli into the mix based on previous psycho-analyses, which helps the AI interact with their host. We watch the candidate's progress and we get a set of results based on the candidate's choices, reactions, et cetera."

"I know how cer-ro works." All this was in the brief where they made it excruciatingly clear that our inner thoughts would be laid bare, made visible by the AI inside our head. My desire to get to Mars was a hell of a lot stronger than my desire to keep secrets. Besides, MarsLife already knew all about my record, and I didn't think the truth about Wayne would ever see the light of day, I'd buried it so deep down.

My breath catches at the back of my throat and blood heats my face. This guy sitting opposite me knows about Wayne, what he did to me, and what I did to him. But that's the point of cer-ro, to pry us open and reveal all the hidden traumas that might make us turn psycho, like the astronaut who turned into an ax murderer on the Endeavour. There's no way I could've passed this test.

"Raleigh, did you hear what I said?"

"No, sorry."

"I was saying that you didn't just let the AI into your head, you fucking owned it, manipulated it, and took control of the 'scape. That's unprecedented."

"His name was Crow." No idea why I blurt that out. Crow isn't real. He's a composite computer program. Not that it seems to matter to my heart how many times I tell myself he doesn't exist.

"Also Brennan Cozens, right?" There's a glint in his eyes I can't decipher.

"You saw all that?"

"We saw everything." He wipes his palms on his thighs as if this conversation is making *him* uncomfortable. "What I wanted you to know is that the AI is built on the model of a real person. We need the psychological scaffolding to create an empathetic program otherwise it would be an emotionless machine."

"So the AI had an identity?" Why is he telling me all of this?

"It's not meant to be that sophisticated. It's meant to be a mirror for the candidate, a conduit and a guide. It's not meant to become its own person."

"Crow did."

"Yeah." More chewing on his thumb. "That wasn't expected. Somehow the AI became cognizant, and you didn't assign it an identity so much as you allowed it to self-actualize."

"How is that possible?" I'm stunned. If I get what this guy's saying, then Crow was real, sort of, as real as a computer program can get.

"We don't know, and I haven't slept in days trying to figure it out." Black circles hang like teabags beneath his eyes, although it doesn't really detract from his good looks.

"So I failed."

"No, well, I don't know. That's above my pay grade. I'm just the programmer. That's not what I came here to tell you. Ah, shit." He wrings his hands and chews on his bottom lip again. "I wanted to tell you that Crow was modeled after a real person," he repeats, "that he was given certain personality traits and memories, too." The guy avoids eye contact. "Our entire identity is wrapped up in memory. We are nothing without our recollections, without context. So, for an AI to be empathetic, to be emotionally responsive, we have to give it a backstory."

"What are you trying to say?" Crow is real. Or at least he was based on a real person and if so, then what does that mean exactly? That I fell in love with the avatar of an actual human being? It's too much to take in. I press the heels of my hands against my eyes and take several deep breaths trying to get myself under control. Crow might actually exist.

"What I'm saying. Jesus." He claps his hands together and I meet his gaze. "I'm saying that technically…I'm Crow." He looks at me with eyes as blue as the Texas sky.

"You're Crow?" *Inhale.* It's not possible. *Exhale.* It can't be. *Inhale.* I want it to be. *Exhale.* Do I want Crow to be real? Yes.

"I modeled the AI upgrade on me. He's not entirely me." The guy chuckles nervously. "It's not like I could download my entire memory into the AI, but I used a few defining moments. Certain key points in my emotional and psychological development to give the AI a backstory and emotional gravitas. Does that makes sense?"

"Defining moments?"

"Yeah, but you know all those already." He blushes again. This guy has seen inside my soul, and yet he's the one who's embarrassed.

"What do you mean exactly?"

"Usually, a candidate projects mental images onto the AI. That connection isn't supposed to go both ways, but for whatever reason, you were able to get inside the mind of the AI. This is what makes you so unique. Maybe something to do with your ability to read patterns. That much is obvious by the way you played football, and you aced that section of the acuity test as well."

My mouth hangs open. Like a frog catching flies, Mama would say.

"Don't be so surprised, dude. You knew you were smart, right?"

"But I mangled your program."

"Yeah, and that takes some leet skills." He laughs, the sound eerily reminiscent of Crow.

"So those memories I saw, Crow's memories, those weren't from my own imagination?" Trying to wrap my head around all this makes my brain hurt, but that's nothing compared to the vise that's crushing my chest.

"It's complicated, but on a fundamental level, no. I was valedictorian and took home that academic trophy. I went hiking with my dad in Yosemite. I'm dyslexic and had a boyfriend named Jeremy. See where I'm going with this?" He raises his pierced left eyebrow.

"This is too much." I rest my head in my hands, staring at the floor and trying to fight off the urge to puke. "You've seen inside my head."

"And you've seen inside mine."

"But you're not Crow." Which is to say, he's not that loving AI who didn't judge me, who helped me bare my soul to the MarsLife Corps for a shot at going to the stars. He's not the guy who let me kiss him in the desert and make love to him in the dark.

"No, I'm not, but we're a lot alike." He almost sounds disappointed.

"Why are you telling me this?"

"Because I thought you should know and because after everything I've seen, I…"

I look up to find him squirming. He looks nothing like Crow, short and better built for a programmer than I'd expect, his black hair shaggy where Crow had indigo curls. This guy might have blue eyes—deep blue, not ice blue like Wayne's—but there's something familiar in them, something warm and comforting about the way he's looking at me.

"Listen, I know I'm not Crow, but I wanted you to know that if it had been me, I wouldn't have done anything differently. I might've been a bit smarter about some decisions, but I would've done what he did."

"Which parts exactly?" Instead of feeling embarrassed and vulnerable, I feel free, unencumbered by the need to keep secrets. This guy has already seen the worst of me.

"All parts." He meets my gaze, and this time he doesn't look away.

"Your name isn't Crow, though?"

"No, it's Brennan Cozens." A smile tugs at the corners of his mouth. "And I'd really like to take you out sometime."

"Are you serious?" My internal organs are doing advanced acrobatics. Whether it's a side effect of cer-ro or because this virtual stranger just asked me out, I can't tell.

"Considering what my AI alter ego has already done, I think buying you dinner is the least I can do." There's a playful flicker in his eyes. I should be mortified, but I'm not. If anything, I'm excited by the idea of getting to know the real Crow. No, the real Brennan. One and the same really, although I'm not sure which is the simulacrum. I study my hands. The psychscape felt so real, no different to what my senses are defining as real right now. Maybe I'm still in a virtual world, maybe this is still part of the test and yet, looking at Brennan, there's a part of me that knows that isn't true. Crow is gone forever—only the kernel of his essence still exists, in Brennan.

"If I passed, then I'll go to Mars," I say. "And if I failed, I'll be heading back to Texas."

"So we should do dinner soon." He smiles. "There's a great little pizza place in town. How about tomorrow night? Give you a chance to catch your breath."

Brennan stands and moves to the door.

"This is really weird." He's Crow and he's not Crow, but he's still the closest I've ever come to love.

"I know, but I'm hoping it won't be after we've had a proper conversation and you get to know the human me." He checks his watch. "Wanna meet me downstairs at eight tomorrow night?"

"Sure." That gives me just under twenty-four hours to get back in touch with reality. I've never actually been on a proper date before. Anxiety starts pricking up my spine.

"And Raleigh—" Brennan hesitates with the door half open. "Just so you know, I like you because of everything you've been through and everything you are, not despite of it. See you soon."

He closes the door, leaving me reeling with a stupid smile stretching across my face.

BRENNAN

With my heart blast beating my ribs, I shut Raleigh's door and take a moment to breathe. I've spent the better half of a week inside Raleigh's mind, but that didn't prepare me for meeting him in person, for looking into his dark eyes, knowing what he knows about me. Unprecedented, anomalous, remarkable — those are the words I'll use in my report, but what this situation is, is mind-bendingly bizarre.

Following my feet, I arrive at my office and slump in the chair before my array of monitors, not quite sure what to do considering my mind is still churning over everything that is gorgeous, intelligent, badass Raleigh Williams. And I scored a date with the guy!

"Hey, Cozens." Doctor Torres leans through the open door. "Got a moment?"

"What's up, Doc?" I ask in my perfect Bugs Bunny voice. Torres doesn't crack the tiniest of grins.

"We need to talk. My office in five." He strides away having extinguished all excitement buzzing in my brain.

Grabbing a flat white from the hallway vending machine, I step into the doctor's office, not sure what to expect.

"Take a seat." Torres is wearing the stern expression he usually reserves for incompetent interns.

"Is something wrong?" I sip my coffee.

"There's going to be a formal inquiry into your conduct during the Williams psychscape. This may result in disciplinary action."

"What?" I sputter frothy milk that suddenly tastes like dirt.

"I tried to shoulder the blame, and they'll be investigating me as well, but I thought you should know that the consequences may be dire should they find evidence of misconduct."

"Misconduct? Are you serious? This case was unprecedented."

"And we pushed the envelope. I'm aware, and for those decisions, I'll be held responsible. However—" Torres clears his throat and folds his hands on his desk. "However, some in the department feel that this case in particular was handled with a certain lack of professionalism and that things became too personal."

"Where is this coming from? Does Perez have a problem with what we did?"

"It doesn't matter who, Brennan. This is happening. The entire program is being called into question after what happened with Williams."

"Is this about the intimacy between Raleigh and the AI? They do know I didn't have any control over that, right? Which is what makes this case so amazing."

"Yes, but management has its concerns." Torres drums his fingers on the desk. "And so do I."

"Sure, the system isn't perfect yet, but Raleigh's case has provided us with reams of data, data we can use to refine our psytek protocols. This is just the beginning!"

"Brennan, what you need to understand is that if they bring us up on charges of misconduct, we'll be shut down."

"They can't do that." After all we've worked for. After all the sleepless nights spent perfecting the code. Hell, I even had my skull sliced and diced for this project.

"They can and they will," Torres says. "After what happened with Endeavour, MarsLife can't afford any more bad press. If they detect even the faintest whiff of negligence or incompetence, we'll get the boot."

"They'll fire me? But what about my PhD, what about Mars?" I meet Torres's apologetic gaze and my dream crumbles, swirling down the shitter.

"Nothing is certain yet. They've only just begun their investigation," he says. "But I wanted to warn you. I also wanted to encourage you to cooperate fully as they conduct their investigation."

"Will this affect Raleigh getting into MarsLife?" I ask around the continent-sized lump in my throat.

"Absolutely." Torres sighs and rubs his hands over his face. "I'll keep you in the loop. You should get some sleep, Cozens. Inquiry starts tomorrow at seven sharp. They're starting with staff interviews so don't be late."

Feeling like I've just been bludgeoned by the Hulk, I stalk out of Torres's office and retreat to my own. My thoughts are operating at FTL, searching for anything incriminating in my activity over the last few days.

I pull up Raleigh's file and scan through all the data from his psychscape and hit replay on the recorded scene from the Pontiac. They can inquire all the way— They'll never be able to accuse me of negligence or incompetence. But how could we have done everything by the book when Raleigh's case obliterated the fucking manual? They can't hold that against us. Against me.

Trying not to think about the situation I can't control, I let the footage play out, watching from Crow's perspective as he knots his fingers in Raleigh's hair.

I'm not Crow. I never will be no matter how hard I try. But maybe that won't matter once Raleigh gets to know the real me. Or maybe I'm deluding myself. Either way, I've got less than twenty-four hours to think of a way to explain how I feel to Raleigh so he doesn't think I'm nuts.

Oh, by the way, Raleigh, while you were falling in love with Crow, I think I might've been falling for you. Yeah—what not to say on a first date.

RALEIGH

If I never have to put on a hospital gown again, it'll be too soon. I check my phone for the umpteenth time before stepping out of my jeans. Still no response from Abigail, which could mean a dozen different things, but I can't shake the image of her crushed by a semi.

Torres walks into the exam room carrying his ever-present tablet and greets me with a smile. "How are you feeling today, Mr. Williams?"

"Hungover." Psychologically more than physically, although a wave of dizziness attacked me this morning when I tried doing my daily regimen of push-ups.

"That's normal." He shines his laser-like flashlight into my eyes, making me squint. "So is light sensitivity. You've been in a coma for almost a week."

"Come on, Doc. Can't you just tell me if I passed or not?" I want to tell him everything I already know from Brennan, but I don't want to get the guy in trouble, not when we're supposed to be going on a date tonight. *Inhale.* It's just a date. *Exhale.* And I already know him. *Inhale.* No, I know Crow. *Exhale.* Brennan might not be a complete mystery, but he's still a stranger.

"I'm not the one who ultimately decides." Torres pulls the gown past my shoulders and sticks heart monitors on my chest, watching the readings on his tablet.

"But you have some inclination, right?"

"Your results are still being analyzed. You need to be patient." He removes the tacky circles, switching them out for smaller ones that he sticks to my arm measuring blood pressure and makes a note on his tablet.

"You saw some of it, though. What's your personal opinion?"

"Raleigh, I can't—"

"Please." Maybe if Crow had been real, I wouldn't feel this desperate. If not going to Mars meant getting a life with Crow, it might've been a situation I could accept. Brennan's face flits through my mind, but I banish the idea. We haven't even been on a date yet. And even if I flunk out of MarsLife, he'll still be here, living my dream. I couldn't handle that.

"From what I saw, and this is only from personal observation"—he tightens a tourniquet above my elbow and swabs my skin with alcohol—"you coped extremely well with trials one through five."

"Trials? That wasn't in the debrief." The needle slips into my vein and blood starts filling up a vial.

"Candidates have to go in blind to a certain extent or else it can skew results." He removes the blood-taking paraphernalia.

"So what were these trials?" And how the hell did I pass them?

Torres shakes his head and pulls up a chair to face me. "Your persistence is certainly admirable."

"This stuff happened inside my head. I have a right to know." I tighten my grip on the edge of the table, trying not to give in to simmering frustration. "You said it wasn't real, not exactly. What did you mean?"

"Most of the trials are based on basic principles of psychological evaluations, the kind used for law enforcement officials, firefighters, and other public servants. They're designed to test responses to certain scenarios tailored for each candidate."

"Like what?"

"Honesty and integrity, moral compass, ability to handle emotional and psychological stress, even physical duress."

"How many trials are there?" Worry starts chewing on my insides like a hungry gopher with a grub.

"Eleven."

"And I passed five." Passing less than fifty percent means I won't make the cut, not with over a hundred candidates applying. The air rushes out of my lungs as I deflate.

"That's not to say you failed the rest. But those are more complex tests, hence the reason I'm reluctant to discuss results before I've seen the analysis."

"More complex, how?" What little they told us in the debrief was mostly about how cer-ro worked on a physical level; they never got too deep into the psychological side of it.

"Our new design is meant to push candidates to their limits, to create a traumatic environment so as to show their breaking point and their coping mechanisms. Life on Mars is no picnic. We can't afford to send up unstable, unpredictable individuals."

"People like me." That's my application in the trash then. My life without Mars stretches before me, a bleak canvas of Texas dust and soap suds. I can't go back to that.

"Hard to say without proper analysis of the data, but what I can say is that your reaction to the trials was unique."

"Yeah, I—" I bite my tongue and swallow down the rest of my words that would've ratted out Brennan. I wish he'd been straight with me last night about my chances of passing.

"Stop worrying about it. Your mental acuity scores were in the top one percentile and you're in excellent physical health. Right now you stand a very good chance of being selected for the program."

"Doc, you know my history. I was never gonna make it, was I?" I avoid his gaze. He knows about Wayne, about 206.

"Raleigh, look at me." His voice is gentle. "Look at me." And warily I do, expecting to find pity or disgust, but find neither. "Knowing your history, I think you were misdiagnosed and incorrectly medicated. You were—are—suffering from rape trauma syndrome."

Every time I hear that word it's like a bottle rocket goes off in my belly.

"Is that like PTSD?" Like the vets my dad rips on for going soft after seeing a little blood.

"A form of, yes. Regardless of what happens with MarsLife, I strongly recommend you see someone."

"I've been to shrinks." More than enough for one lifetime.

"But you were never honest with them."

"Like I was going to tell that court-appointed head doctor what happened." The crack in my voice runs a fault line right through my chest. "Even if he believed me, he'd have asked why I didn't fight back. Or worse."

"Or worse?" Torres sets aside his tablet and focuses his full attention on me.

"Things might be different where you're from, Doc, but in small-town Texas folks are a little slow catching onto the twenty-first century. I don't think most people reckon it can happen to a guy, and if it does, they think it's his own fault for letting it."

"Do you believe that?" He slips into shrink mode.

Inhale. He's just doing his job. *Exhale.* Don't lose it. Not here. Not now. I'm back to white knuckling the edge of the exam table and trying to extinguish the anger burning through my veins.

"I agreed to meet Wayne that day. I'd been…" I ball my fists in my lap instead, letting my nails cut into my palms. "I'd been flirting with him. God, I actually liked him."

"Do you think you were asking for it by going to meet him that day?"

"Guess I was asking for something, right?" I study my hands, the knuckles that almost bashed the life out of Wayne.

"So you think you got what you deserved?"

My head jerks up, and I meet his gaze. "No one deserves that."

"You agreed to meet him, you'd been flirting with him, are you sure you weren't asking for it?" His expression is unreadable.

"What the hell's wrong with you? No, I wasn't fucking asking for it."

"And you didn't deserve it?" he asks again, rising to his feet then slipping the gown back over my shoulders.

"I already told you. No one deserves that."

"But did *you* deserve it?"

"I... No, I..." The words stick in my throat, choking me. "Screw you, Doc." I blink back battery acid tears.

"Raleigh—"

"No, all right? No, I wasn't asking for it, and I didn't fucking deserve it. Is that what you want me to say?"

"I want you to believe it," Torres says, the epitome of calm while I feel like a storm twisting into an F5.

"What happened to you isn't your fault. You didn't ask for it. You didn't deserve it." His words become a mantra, seeping slowly through the layers of my carefully constructed walls, doing major water damage to the foundations of my denial. I'm shaking, the fault line running through me cracking open and turning me into a full on earthquake.

"It wasn't your fault," Torres says. "You didn't deserve it, Raleigh."

I want to believe it, I want to believe it wasn't my fault, but part of me resists what the other part of me knows to be true. If only Crow were here, the one person who knew everything and loved me anyway. But he doesn't exist. He never did. Brennan, however, is very much real.

BRENNAN

Raleigh meets me in the lobby wearing jeans and a sweater that molds his sculpted torso. He's a good four inches taller than me and sort of mean-looking since they shaved his hair. Pity about that, but essential for the cer-ro procedure. I hope he'll let his hair grow long again; I want to run my fingers through it.

"Ready?" Not that I am with my sweaty hands and a collar that feels way too tight despite the top button being undone.

"Lead the way." He signs out at reception, and we head to my Mustang. "Nice ride." He slides into the passenger seat.

"Thanks. Took me ages to refurbish her." I get behind the wheel and silence settles between us.

"Are you feeling okay?" I ask eventually.

"Torres gave me the all-clear this morning." He cracks his knuckles, a muscle twitching in his jaw.

"That's good." God, there's nothing worse than attempting polite conversation. It lasts until I pull into the lot, Raleigh becoming increasingly fidgety during the ride as we make small talk about everything except the things we need to discuss. I'm not going to tell him about the inquiry. What's the point? It'll only cause unnecessary stress.

"Listen, I don't want this to be weird." I pause before getting out the car. "I like you. I know a lot about you, so do you think we could skip all the first date bullshit?"

"I've never been on a date," he says. "Not unless you count the hookups I had in juvie." His words are shocking, his expression disarming.

"Those definitely do not count." This is his first proper date and instead of making some grand romantic gesture, I've brought him to a humdrum pizza parlor. What a way to woo the guy. "I'm sorry, Raleigh, I can be an insensitive asshat. I'm working on it."

"Crow was kind."

"You're in love with him." In love with an iteration of me. Why does Raleigh have to be so damn tragic, and so damn stoic? It makes me want to jump his bones right here. The thought of having to compete with Crow in the bedroom, though, douses my desire a little.

"I think so," he says. "I know that's crazy, but it's like I've got a psychscape hangover."

"I know the feeling." I tap the steering wheel, contemplating my next words. "It's okay. I'm not expecting anything from you, but I hope you give me a chance and get to know the real me."

"I'm not my issues, you know." He regards me with haunted and questioning eyes.

"I know that." I know his file verbatim and Raleigh is so much more than a psych analysis. "And I'd like to get to know the real you, too. But can pizza be involved? I'm starving."

"Sure." An almost-smile quirks up his lips, dispelling some of the anxiety turning my shoulder muscles into concrete. I should be honest with him about the inquiry. He deserves to know, but Goddammit, I don't want to annihilate his hopes.

Together, we climb out of the car and find a secluded corner away from other patrons. I don't want any distractions tonight. I only want to look at Raleigh, to understand the guy who pretty much destroyed my program and simultaneously stole my heart.

"So I'm guessing you're not as into rabbit food as Crow, then?" Raleigh asks while studying the menu.

"Didn't you hear? Pizza is a vegetable."

Raleigh laughs, eyes sparking. I'm not sure I ever saw him laugh in the psychscape and more's the pity because this guy is even more gorgeous when he cracks a smile.

"What do you recommend?" He frowns at the choices.

"Nothing with olives or… No, that's just wrong." He looks at me over the top of the menu. "Who puts asparagus on pizza?"

"People with defective taste buds." My comment makes him laugh again, and the nerves in my belly melt away. "I'm going traditional Hawaiian. You?"

"Same. With jalapeños."

"Ah, so you like it hot?" There's no denying the innuendo there, and Raleigh responds with a knowing smile and the hint of a blush. Sometimes I forget he's only nineteen and from a podunk town in rural Texas.

"You've seen exactly how I like it, right?" Raleigh's expression darkens. "Sorry, that's not fair. It's just…" He reaches for his soda and swallows a mouthful as if it's courage-bolstering bourbon.

"Dude, I get it. I imagine this is what it would feel like for my sister to have dinner with her gynecologist."

Raleigh chokes on his Coke. "*Chido* analogy."

"Well, technically, I have seen inside you, albeit mostly your mind." I wink and this time Raleigh deliberately sets down his glass and licks his lips before fixing me with his dark-eyed gaze.

"Considering how much you know about me, I reckon I should know more about you."

"I'm an open book. Fire away," I say. The waitress brings us our pizzas, and we both tuck in, cutting slices to eat with our hands instead of using a knife and fork. I'm convinced trying to eat pizza delicately destroys half the flavor.

"Okay, so you know the most traumatic experience in my life. What's yours?" Raleigh licks cheese off his fingers, and I watch transfixed. I've never wanted to be greasy fingers so bad in my life.

"My parents' divorce. They asked me to choose who I wanted to live with."

The pineapple sticks in my throat as the unpleasant

memory surfaces. Still, considering what I've witnessed of Raleigh's life, it's only fair I divulge this much.

"Seems like a shitty thing for parents to do."

"Don't think they realized how damaging it was." My shrug is anything but diffident. Almost ten years after the fact, thinking about that time in my life makes me hurt in ways I can't put into words.

"Guess every family is a little dysfunctional." Raleigh sighs.

"We're all messed up to a greater or lesser extent," I say around a mouthful of cheese. "Funny thing is, it's normal to be a bit fucked up."

"I'd be a lot less fucked up if they'd just tell me the test results already." Raleigh drops the half-eaten slice of pizza back on the plate. "Life will be better on Mars."

I reach across the table and take his hand before I realize what I'm doing. He doesn't pull away, doesn't even twitch, just looks at my hand touching his, which only makes me feel shittier for not telling him that the chances of him getting to Mars have greatly diminished and it's not his fault. I'm about to come clean when, with a slow smile, he turns his hand over so we're palm to palm, my fingers resting against the scars on his wrist. I'd be lying if I said the contact sent an electric frisson through me the way Crow and Raleigh jolted in the psychscape when they touched, but there's definitely a buzz in my circuits.

"I half expected a memory swap," Raleigh says, his fingers grazing my wrist.

"Sorry to disappoint."

"There are better ways of getting to know someone."

That look on his face—his eyes wide and shiny, his top incisor catching his bottom lip—it takes all the self-control I posses not to lean over and kiss him.

"Are you done?" I cast a glance at his mostly demolished pizza and he nods. "Wanna get out of here?"

RALEIGH

It's after ten by the time we roll back onto the Bennett campus, listening to old school rock and bitching about the state of modern music. My hands haven't stopped sweating. Dinner was nice. Too nice. Everything with Brennan comes easy, maybe because part of me still sees him as Crow.

"Do you live on the grounds?"

"I've got a cottage down in the employee village." He hesitates when we reach the intersection, as if he's not sure which way to turn. "Do you want to come over for coffee or something?"

"Sure, why not." The *or something* makes my heart do jumping jacks. I wipe my hands on my jeans and hope he doesn't notice my trembling fingers.

A few minutes later we pull up outside his bungalow, and I follow him inside. It's homey and smells like Brennan, all citrusy soap and faraway places. It smells like Crow.

A gray cat rushes out of the bedroom and meows loudly, rubbing against Brennan's legs.

"Hope you're not allergic. Turing here is quite an affectionate little guy." He sweeps the cat into his arms and carries him to the kitchen. I watch while Brennan proceeds to spoon tinned tuna into the cat's bowl. I've never been so enthralled by fingers working a can opener.

"Nope, but I prefer dogs."

"I'm sorry about what happened to Bear in the 'scape." He washes his hands and gives me an apologetic glance over his shoulder.

"Was that you?" Despite knowing Bear's alive and well in Dead Rock, I can't quite shake off the experience of handing my dog over to Sheriff Daniels.

"Torres's orders. We wanted to up the trauma value."

"You certainly did that." I slide my hands into my pockets to stop them from shaking. God, what's wrong with me? "I'm just glad Bear's still tearing after gophers back in Texas."

He smiles at me and some of the knots in my gut start to unravel. Not all of them, though.

"I still haven't heard from Abigail."

"She's fine, Raleigh. That was just part of the 'scape. A really crappy move to pull, but it didn't happen. Promise." He dries his hands on his jeans and I nod. Of course she's fine. "Can I offer you beer, coffee, soda?"

"Coke is fine."

"Mind if I have a beer?"

"Go for it." What I wouldn't give for some booze-induced courage round about now. "I'm half expecting them to make me pee in a cup again before we're done. Seems kinda dumb letting underage drinking be the reason they fail me." Although it's not like they don't have a million other reasons to kick me out of the program.

"You're dedicated." Brennan passes me a Coke and pops open a beer, and I join him in the tiny living room.

"You've really never seen the ocean?" he asks between sips.

"Been wanting to go to Corpus Christi or Galveston for ages. West and I always planned to, but it never worked out." My gaze lingers on the giant digital frames switching through 3D images of nebulae taken by the Hubble telescope. My brother never saw the sea, and now there's a chance I'll get to see Mars.

"How about this," Brennan says. "I promise that no matter what happens, we'll take a road trip down to the coast."

"Why?" Setting down the Coke, I turn to look at him.

"Because no one should leave this planet before swimming in one of its oceans," he says earnestly.

"I've seen Hawaii."

"Vicariously. Doesn't count."

"So none of what we shared in the 'scape counts then?"

"Since it technically wasn't me you were with, no." He inches closer on the couch and my blood turns to a river of molten pitch. "None of it counts." He starts peeling off the label on his beer bottle.

"Crow didn't seem to mind my history." I break eye contact. No way I can look at him and ask what I have to. If there's pity or disgust on his face, I'm not sure I'll survive seeing it. "I was wondering if you felt the same." Better to rip off the Band-Aid than peel it back slow.

"I don't care how many people you've slept with, or what happened with Wayne." He gulps down a mouthful of beer. "I mean I care, because I care about you." He stumbles over the words and I hold my breath waiting for the "but".

"What I mean is…" he continues. "It doesn't change how I feel about you." He rests his hand on my knee and I tense, my whole body gone as a rigid as a dead rabbit. There's no static charge, no memory deluge, just his warmth soaking into my skin.

"We've all got baggage, man, but our past doesn't dictate our future. Like Crow said, you're not that boy in the snow."

I shuffle closer, letting Brennan's hand travel up my thigh. I want him, and I want this to be real and meaningful. I slept with Crow, not Brennan. As similar as they are, they're not the same, and it wasn't real. This is. I meet his gaze, and my heart does a double-kick. He reaches a hesitant hand toward my face, and trails his fingers down my neck.

"You remind me so much of Crow." The kind eyes, the mischief in the corners of his mouth, his gentle touch.

"Is that a bad thing?"

"Just strange. But…but I think doing this might help." Tilting my head to the side, I close my eyes and lean forward until we make contact. We take it slow for all of ten seconds before realizing we both want a hell of a lot more.

His tongue slips between my lips and goose bumps flare across my skin. He tastes of Bud Light, but I don't care. His hands rove over my shoulders and down my back, the contact making my head spin. I grip his waist, needing an anchor. I want him, closer, and I tug him onto my lap. I lace my fingers through his hair and keep on kissing him, loving the way he bites my bottom lip and digs his nails into my shoulders.

"Wait, Raleigh."

"Are we moving too fast?" I pause, my fingers about to start undoing the buttons of his shirt.

"I can't do this. I'm sorry." He looks away, but stays on my lap, my hands on his waist.

If he tells me *it's not you, it's me*, I might put my fist through the wall. I freeze in place, not knowing what to say. He drags his hands through his hair.

"They've started an inquiry," he says. "They're questioning our protocols, everything about how we conducted your psych evaluation." His words are a rush I can barely make sense of. "If they find us guilty of misconduct, then the test will be nullified and the results considered inapplicable." He looks up, hair falling in shaggy points across his eyes.

"So I'd have to do the test again?" This can't be happening. I'm so fucking close and now they're wrenching it all away.

"That's the thing." Brennan slides off my lap and starts pacing. "I'll lose my job for sure. Torres, too. If they're not happy with how the psytek works, they'll shut it down. They'd rather not risk another media debacle."

"Are they going to find any evidence of misconduct?" I ask, struggling to keep my voice even as anger and disappointment well up inside me.

"Your situation was unique so we didn't exactly follow all protocols, but I never did anything to jeopardize your chance of making it into the program, that I swear on my mother's life. It's going to come down to management's interpretation of the data, and I have no idea how they'll see things." He leaves his hand at the back of his neck just like Crow did, and the kicked puppy look on his face cools my simmering rage. It was my weird reaction to the simulation that caused the problem after all.

"So, there's a good chance we'll both be kicked to the curb?"

"I guess." Brennan folds his arms. "I'm so sorry, Raleigh." He sounds so much like Crow it makes my bones ache.

"Not your fault." If I had Crow, maybe the thought of not getting to Mars wouldn't feel like taking a sledgehammer to the gut. I swallow down a bitter rush of disappointment and frustration. I've done everything I could. In the end, it's out of my hands.

"At least we'd have each other, though, right? Even if we're grounded on Earth," Brennan says, and his words dare me to consider a different future, one that's always felt even more unattainable than my dream of Mars.

"Maybe it wouldn't be all bad."

"You mean that?" He approaches slowly and I reach for him, tugging him back onto my lap. "You'd let me be your consolation prize for not getting into MarsLife?" A hesitant grin plays on his lips.

"Well, when you put it that way." I run my hands up his thighs needing to feel his presence, needing one good thing to be real.

"Are you sure you want to do this?" He eases away like I'm some wounded creature he doesn't want to startle.

"Don't do that. Don't treat me like I'm broken." I know he's only trying to be considerate, but that's part of the problem. I'm not used to men being careful with me. Sex has always been brutal. I don't know how to do it any other way. But I did with Crow.

"I just thought—"

"What?" I try to keep the bitterness out of my voice without much success. "That I can't have sex without being constantly reminded that I'm damaged goods?" It's not Brennan's fault. Not even this inquiry business. It's my fault for having a fucked up brain. It's always been my fault.

"Raleigh, I didn't—" Brennan moves onto the couch, a muscle twitching along his clenched jaw. I've blown it. Now I'll never get to Mars and I'll never get to be with the one guy who might've actually been able to love me.

"I'm sorry." For everything. For everything I am. "I should go."

"Don't." Brennan grabs my arm as I try to push past him. "I want you to stay."

"I don't need you to fix me. I'm not lookin' to be saved." My voice cracks with emotion I'm barely keeping at bay.

"Good, because that wasn't exactly what I had in mind."

"You just lookin' for an easy lay then?" That was cruel, but only if it isn't true. I glare at him, and he doesn't look away.

"You're making it impossible for me, you know." He releases my arm. "If I want you, it's because I think you're easy. If I don't want you, it's because I think you're broken. Either way you get pissed and slam out of here, and I'm left alone. What'll it take for you to believe that I just want to be with you, not for any other reason except that I like you, that I find you damn sexy, body and brain?"

It takes several moments to process what he said. I study his face and find only honesty. His words play on repeat, especially the last part. Maybe if I replay it enough times, I'll start to believe it.

"Sorry." I slide back onto the couch. "Sometimes I wish things could be normal. I've never really done this." Outside of a digital simulation. "Guess I don't—"

He shuts me up with a kiss.

We break apart and Brennan's gaze locks with my own.

"Do you want this?" he asks.

"Yeah."

"Then don't overthink it." He grabs the hem of my T-shirt, tugging it over my head, and kisses my chest where virtual reality Torres cut me up.

I think I might be falling in love.

After trying to undo the buttons on his shirt, I give up and rip it open, buttons scattering to the floor. I run my hands over his shoulders and pecs, palms coasting through the dusting of dark hair leading south.

"I don't look like Crow," he says.

"No, you don't." I plant a kiss in the hollows of each collar bone. "You're real. Crow wasn't." My voice quavers. "Not in the ways that matter." And I'm going to have to let Crow go. There's no point holding on to him when I have Brennan.

Brennan's kisses make my every nerve scream. Cupping his butt, I lift him as I get to my feet, his fingers digging into my shoulders while his legs automatically wrap around my hips. I stumble through the lounge, Brennan directing me to the bedroom by whispering in my ear while he nibbles on it.

Brennan's hands on my body are fire-brands, his tongue an acetylene torch. He pulls away only as long as it takes for us to ditch the rest of our clothes. Our kisses become as furious as a desert storm, our need for each other a frenzy as we move to the bed.

"Hold up." He presses a hand to my chest, and I back off. "There are condoms in the nightstand," he says with a smirk that sweeps away almost all my insecurities. "Top drawer."

Licking my lips, swollen from where he's been biting them, I lean across him to get to the nightstand, and Brennan takes the opportunity to use his teeth on my nipples, his hands moving between my legs. He's turning my bones to liquid, each stroke of his fingers making coherent thought impossible.

He pauses long enough to let me grab condoms and lube.

"Who's this for?" A wave of nervous energy vibrates up my spine.

"I don't mind. Whichever you prefer."

"Is that you trying not to be an asshat or do you not mind for real?"

"While I am flexible, right now I just really want you to fuck me," he says and his words are flaming arrows, hitting me smack in all the vital places. Using my teeth, I tear open the condom.

"Next time it'll be you on top." He runs lube over my rock hard erection, my own hands trembling at the thought of being inside him… of having him inside me.

"Next time?"

"Guy can dream, right?" He kisses me again, and this time, his tongue moves slowly against my own. I take my time exploring his body with slick fingers.

"Don't let me hurt you." Not physically. Not at all. Not ever.

"You won't." He arches his hips in invitation.

Inhale. This is really going to happen. *Exhale.* This feels right, it feels good. *Inhale.* We both want this and…and as I exhale I slide inside him. He crushes his mouth against mine and runs his hands down my back, driving me into him as deep as I can go.

"Oh God." I squeeze my eyes shut. Tears would absolutely ruin this moment but feelings I can't name bubble up from the deepest, darkest places inside of me.

"No, look at me." He runs his thumbs over my eyebrows. "I want you to look at me."

And I do, committing every freckle and smile line to memory.

"This is what you asked for," he says, and my breath catches in my chest. "This is what you deserve."

Braced against the headboard with one hand while using the other to support my weight, I drop my head to kiss him, not caring if he tastes my tears. He arches up to meet me, his hands on my lower back, and I let him guide me until our breathing comes in ragged gasps, until we lose ourselves in the pounding of hearts and bodies.

Lying next to Brennan, I can't help thinking of Crow. They're so similar yet so different. It messes with my head every time I think about the fact that Crow was as much my own mental projection as a self-actualizing AI. And while the sex with Crow was good, these past few nights getting naked with Brennan have taken it to a whole new level. Maybe it's because I can finally let go the way I never could before. With Brennan it's different. He knows all my secrets. I don't have to pretend or play a role with him. I can just be me, my soul as bare as my skin.

What's even weirder is that I don't miss Crow as much as I thought I would, not with Brennan filling up the void, and more. Crow was never real. Brennan is blood and bone and comes complete with a passion for Frank Herbert, a wry sense of humor, and an intelligence that leaves me in awe.

I brush hair off his face and he smiles, cracking open a blister-blue eye.

"Morning." He licks his lips. "What time is it?"

"Just after six."

"Good. Maybe I'll get to work on time today." He jabs a finger into my ribs under the covers.

"Think you'll find out anything more today?" The verdict of the inquiry hangs over both our heads.

"I've got a meeting with Torres first thing this morning."

He kisses my nose. I want Mars. I want Brennan. Is there

a way I can have both?

"Still taking that road trip to the ocean, right?"

"Absolutely." He sidles over, our legs entwined beneath the covers. My hand finds a knee, a thigh, and then—

"Hey, I can't be late this morning." He tries to pry my fingers away and ends up groping me instead.

"Then we better be quick." I duck under the covers and my cell phone rings.

"Who is it?" I ask, and Brennan reaches toward the nightstand.

"It's Abigail."

I throw back the covers and grab the phone.

"Abi?" A flood of relief washes over me at the sound of her voice. Brennan slips out of bed leaving me to chat.

"First vacation I've ever taken," she says. "And of course Jimmy drags me off into the woods where there's no signal. I've been eating skeeters and having to avoid bears while trying to pee for a week now. Now he's hauling me up some mountain to watch the sunrise, which means I finally got your messages." I don't care that I spend the next ten minutes listening to Abi bitch about the blisters on her heels or how hard she's falling for this new guy. She's alive and living the life she always wanted with someone who might help her forget Weston.

My gaze drifts to Brennan where he's brushing his teeth and searching for his comb.

After promising to call her the minute I know anything, I hang up, feeling ten tons lighter knowing Abi's okay.

Brennan starts shaving, and I hit the shower. It's disconcertingly domestic, being so comfortable around each other after such a short time. Looking back on the journey it took to get here, I'm not sure how it happened or why the fact that he puts toothpaste on both our brushes every morning makes me so stupidly happy.

"You could join me." I flick soap suds at his naked back around the edge of the shower curtain.

"Or I could be on time." Brennan glares at me in the mirror, lips twitching into a smirk.

"Suit yourself." I step under the spray, and a moment later Brennan slips in beside me. He wraps his arms around me, his head resting on my shoulder as I fold my arms over his and close my eyes. For a moment the world is reduced to the splash of water, beating hearts, and warm skin.

"No matter what happens today, I'm really grateful we had this," he says.

"I'm scared." I turn around to face him, the hot water cascading over my shoulders. What if I get in and ultimately have to leave Earth and leave Brennan? I know I don't want to, but I'm not sure what I want more. And besides, I have a promise to keep to my brother. What if I don't get in and have to go back to Texas? What if Brennan loses his job? *What if, what if, what if.*

"'Fear is the mind-killer,'" he quotes *Dune*. "Stop thinking about the things you can't control." He traces a soapy trail down my chest with his index finger. "And know this." His eyes lock onto mine. "No matter what happens," he says, his body solid, real, and pressed up against mine. "I'm here for you."

"Please, come in." Torres ushers me into his office.

"Raleigh, so good to see you." Sofia Perez stands to greet me with a hand shake. "Do take a seat."

My nerves ratchet into the stratosphere. If Perez has come down from her ivory tower for this meeting, it can't be good. Brennan is here—I hadn't been expecting that. He gives me a wink from across the room, looking relaxed and happy. Does that mean the inquiry has been closed and he still has a job? Or have we both been given the boot?

"You are a phenomenon, Raleigh," Perez says. "You have truly astounded us all."

"Is that a good thing?"

"It's an opportunity." Torres settles behind his desk and we all take our seats.

"The inquiry into Mr. Cozens and exactly what happened during your psychscape trial has been concluded," Perez says. "While there are some irregularities"—She gives Brennan a pointed look—"we've been authorized to proceed as usual." Hope fills my heart fit to bursting. Does this mean I got in?

"Regarding your results," Dr. Torres says, "our findings proved inconclusive." My heart plummets, shattering between my feet. "To be honest, your mental health history made this test a little tricky to conduct, and that's one of the reasons why the results might be more difficult to interpret."

"But my doctor signed off on my health certificate. I haven't needed meds in more than a year. Besides, I was never officially diagnosed—"

"Raleigh, we know," Perez says gently.

Everyone in this room knows. If a big ol' black hole could open up right underneath me that would be great, but no one's looking at me with pity or disdain.

"Are you saying I wouldn't have been medicated at all if I had just told my shrink the truth?" *Please, please, please don't let past mistakes destroy my future.*

"Hard to say." Torres taps his fingers on his desk. "But you certainly don't have borderline personality disorder."

Torres gives me a stern look that I find oddly comforting. "Now, onto business." He takes a breath. "Thanks to the additional analysis provided by Mr. Cozens here, we believe you would be a great asset to MarsLife and the work we do." Torres continues and my heart catapults into my throat. I'm going to be sick all over Perez's Jimmy Choos.

"You're accepting me as a MarsLife cadet?" I can barely get the words out.

"Actually, no." Perez folds her manicured fingers in her lap. "Instead of a place in our academy, we'd like to offer you a paid position in our simulations department."

"What?" I swallow down the disbelief, not sure I heard correctly.

"You'll still receive all the same basic training as a cadet," Torres says. "In addition to that we'd like you to work with our specialists on developing better 'scape technology as well as on producing new interactive simulations, the ones we've been using to help long-term astronauts adapt and adjust to their lives on Mars."

"Um, what does that mean?" I cast a glance at Brennan who's grinning like a dog with a juicy bone.

"It means you'll work with one of the teams I oversee," Torres says. "And closely with Cozens while developing these programs. Then, should you pass basic training and be considered fit for space travel, we'd like to send you both on a short-term trip to Mars to implement our new protocols for astronauts already stationed there. But…" Torres pauses and here comes the caveat. "All our cadets meet once a month with our in-house psychology team. It's part of the continuous screening required in the corps. I'm recommending weekly sessions for you. Does that sound reasonable?"

"Are you serious?" *Inhale.* This is really happening. *Exhale.* I can't believe it. *Inhale.* This is more than I ever dared to dream. *Exhale.* Dealing with weekly shrink sessions will be a piece of sheet cake if it means I get to go to Mars. "I'll do whatever it takes. Heck, I'll do daily sessions if you want."

"Then welcome to MarsLife, Mr. Williams." Sofia Perez beams.

"But— I mean, really? Are you sure?" I want to believe

this is happening, but I'm half expecting to wake up any second from this dream.

"We've all got our demons," Perez says. "Some bigger and meaner than others. We're not looking for someone without issues for the MarsLife Corps. We're looking for someone who isn't afraid of facing the demons they have to live with and that, Raleigh Alaska Williams, is you." She smiles, and I feel like I've stepped into a zero gravity zone, all light and floaty.

"You've already been emailed the complete contract and terms of employment. We'll give you the weekend to think it over and, if possible, we'd like an answer by Monday so that we can move forward with these projects," Torres says.

"This is— I'm, I mean— Thank you. Thank you so much." I pump Torres's hand then Perez's and catch Brennan smirking in the corner.

I stumble out of Torres's office and lean against the wall for a moment, trying to catch my breath. Brennan emerges a few minutes later, a stupid grin plastered on his face.

"I'm going to Mars." No matter how many times I say it, it still doesn't seem real. "I'm actually going to Mars."

"Me too." He takes my hand and tugs me down the corridor into the privacy of his own office.

"Did you know?" I pin him against the closed door.

"Found out an hour ago after a severe knuckle rapping for what they're calling a lax attitude toward protocols."

He kisses me, his hands creeping under my shirt.

"Holy shit, Bren. We're going to Mars." I know Crow was just a computer program, but I wish I could thank him for getting me to where I am. I reckon Crow was less AI and more spirit guide, helping me navigate the fractured landscape of my own mind just so I could stand right here holding Brennan, about to embark on the journey to a brand new everything.

"But first," Brennan says, extracting me from my thoughts.

"We're going to see the ocean and then we're going to swing by Dead Rock to pick up your brother."

"Thank you." It's hard to talk. "You have no idea how much this means to me."

"Actually, I do." He kisses me again, and I surrender to his touch, to the need burning up both of us.

I'm going to Mars. One day in the not too distant future, I'm going to kick my feet through rusted regolith and watch the sun set blue. I'm going to keep my promise to Weston and make all my dreams a reality.

Epilogue

Our booted feet scud through the iron-rich dust of Mars as the dying sun spills blue across the red rock skyline.

"Beautiful, isn't it?" Brennan stands beside me, his face obscured by the suit's visor, his gaze on the horizon.

"We're on Mars." It still doesn't seem real. The past eighteen months of preparation could never have prepared me for the actuality of standing on the red planet.

"Just like you always dreamed." Brennan scoops up a handful of dust and lets it fall through his gloved fingers.

"How did we get here?" Onboard the Entropy III, I know it and yet it's still so surreal.

"Blood, sweat, and smiles." He laughs, the sound reverberating in my earpiece. "Look." He points over my shoulder into the darkening west where the stars are glowing. "That's Earth." Our home world has been reduced to a polka dot of light in the sky.

"This is real, right? I mean, this isn't another simulation."

I scuff my boots through the dirt.

"This is as real as it gets, man." He punches me on the shoulder. I barely feel it through the insulating layers of my space suit.

"Wish West could've seen this." The urn holding my brother's ashes rests heavy in my hands.

"He'll do one better, you know," Brennan says. "He'll be a part of it. His atoms will go on to be new stars, but you have to let him go." His voice softens, and I clutch the urn to my chest. The Martian wind blasts sand against our legs, the same wind that'll tear apart all that remains of my brother. Brennan stands beside me, his shoulder pressed against mine. "It's time."

Slowly, my fingers open the lid and I take a deep breath. *Inhale*. I'm on Mars, and I came here to keep a promise. *Exhale*. I'm letting go of Weston.

I tip the urn and the wind steals away my brother's ashes in a gray and red vortex. The ashes spin and ribbon across the craters, dispersing into the universe. My brother is gone and with him so much of the guilt and self-loathing I've carried all these years.

"You okay?" Brennan takes my hand. Given our suits, it's more like an awkward squishing of enlarged fingers, but I'm grateful for the contact.

"I was just thinking that if West hadn't killed himself, I might've handled it."

"Handled what?"

"You know what."

"You know you can say it, right?" This guy knows me inside out; he knows all the darkness and still chooses to love me. If I can't say it to him, then I'll never be able to get rid of the thing that's festering inside of me. We're on Mars. I've made a new life for myself. There's no point holding on to the rotten carcass of the past. I couldn't do it while we were on Earth, but maybe here I can finally jettison the last of my baggage.

"Wayne…" The words stick in my throat like cactus, but I spit them out anyway. "He…he raped me." I thought the words would be razor blades, that saying it out loud would leave me cut up on the inside and rip the scabs off old wounds. Instead, I feel lighter than helium. "He thought he'd destroyed me, but now I'm a fucking astronaut."

"Yes, you are." I can hear the smile in Brennan's voice. "And I love you, Raleigh." He leans his padded shoulder against mine and together we watch the sun set on Mars.

Acknowledgments

This book took far too much chocolate, copious quantities of wine, and more than two years to write. This book never would've happened at all had it not been for some seriously awesome people who helped me on this journey by uncorking the wine and supplying the chocolate, among other things.

I owe a huge debt of thanks to the lovely people over at Scribophile who provided me with plenty of honest and humorous anecdotes about life in Texas, allowing me to better understand the brittle, bleak world where Raleigh lived. Next, the #wipmarathon gang – Ifeoma Dennis, Amy McNulty, Emma Adams, Yael Itamar, Krystal Jane, Cheyenne Campbell, and Jessica Gunn. Without the pressure of monthly check-ins and their enthusiasm for this novel, shared 200 words at a time, I might never have had the confidence to even finish this book. All amazing authors in their own right, this group of writers has helped me dig deeper and fight harder for all the words. I owe very special thanks to Jessica Gunn whose critique helped shape Scardust into the book it is today. Similarly, thank you Eliot Baker for reading and taking the time to comment—you were absolutely right and it couldn't have been fixed without your insights.

I owe huge and everlasting thanks to my friend Louise Gornall for being an endless source of support, love, and silly stickers on Facebook. Without her constant encouragement, I wouldn't have made it across the finish line. One day soon I'll thank her properly with a pot of tea and rainbow cupcakes.

I'd also like to thank the rest of the #WO2016 author gang for all their support!

More thanks are owed to the Helsinki Writers' Group, particularly Karoliina Vesa, who made an excellent critique partner and renewed my love for this story. Another Finnish friend in need of thanks is Sini Neuvonen. Thank you Sini for being my unofficial publicist in the north, for getting me involved in Nordic cons, for tirelessly plugging my books, and for always wanting to read more of my words. Kiitos paljon kaikesta!

Of course, I couldn't have done this without my editors Lydia Sharp and Stacy Abrams at Entangled. Thank you Lydia and Stacy for having faith in this book, for loving Raleigh and Crow as much as I did, and for believing that this book could be so much more than I ever imagined. Thank you to the entire Entangled team for helping me make my dream come true and seeing this book in the hands of readers!

As always, I owe my agent Jordy Albert, a ton of thanks. When I finished writing Scardust, I honestly didn't know if anyone would ever like it, let alone love it, but Jordy saw the potential in my word baby and helped my book find the perfect home. Thank you so much!

There are some people closer to home without whom this book would still be in the "unfinished and abandoned" file on my hard drive. My mom, for always being an eager reader and correcting my first draft grammar. My dog, Lego, who endured countless hours of plot discussion and never once disagreed with my choices! My partner in life and love, Mark, for helping me re-plot the umpteenth draft, for advising me on all things AI and computer code related, and for putting up with being ignored for several months while I rewrote this book, determined that this time I would get it right. I finally did!

And now my final thanks is owed to you, dear reader, for holding this book in your hands and giving Raleigh the chance to tell you his story.

About the Author

A genderqueer and tattooed storyteller from South Africa, Suzanne van Rooyen is the author of the YA novels *The Other Me* and *I Heart Robot*. She currently lives in Sweden and is busy making friends with the ghosts of her Viking ancestors. Although she has a Master's degree in music, Suzanne prefers conjuring strange worlds and creating quirky characters. When she grows up, she wants to be an elf—until then, Suzanne spends her time writing, wall climbing, buying far too many books, and entertaining her shiba inu, Lego.